Imaging Anatomy of the Human Spine

Imaging Anatomy of the Human Spine

A Comprehensive Atlas Including Adjacent Structures

Scott E. Forseen, MD
Assistant Professor, Neuroradiology Section
Department of Radiology and Imaging
Georgia Regents University
Augusta, Georgia

Neil M. Borden, MD
Neuroradiologist
Associate Professor of Radiology
The University of Vermont Medical Center
Burlington, Vermont

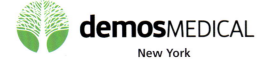

demosMEDICAL

New York

Visit our website at www.demosmedical.com

ISBN: 978-1-936287-82-6
e-book ISBN: 978-1-617051-32-6

Acquisitions Editor: Beth Barry
Compositor: diacriTech

Medicine is an ever-changing science. Research and clinical experience are continually expanding our knowledge, in particular our understanding of proper treatment and drug therapy. The authors, editors, and publisher have made every effort to ensure that all information in this book is in accordance with the state of knowledge at the time of production of the book. Nevertheless, the authors, editors, and publisher are not responsible for errors or omissions or for any consequences from application of the information in this book and make no warranty, expressed or implied, with respect to the contents of the publication. Every reader should examine carefully the package inserts accompanying each drug and should carefully check whether the dosage schedules mentioned therein or the contraindications stated by the manufacturer differ from the statements made in this book. Such examination is particularly important with drugs that are either rarely used or have been newly released on the market.

Library of Congress Cataloging-in-Publication Data
Forseen, Scott E., author.
  Imaging anatomy of the human spine : a comprehensive atlas including adjacent structures / Scott E. Forseen, Neil M. Borden.
     p. ; cm.
  Includes bibliographical references and index.
  ISBN 978-1-936287-82-6 — ISBN 978-1-61705-132-6 (e-book)
  I. Borden, Neil M., author. II. Title.
  [DNLM: 1. Spine—anatomy & histology—Atlases. 2. Multimodal Imaging—Atlases. 3. Spinal Cord—anatomy & histology—Atlases. 4. Spine—physiology—Atlases. WE 17]
  QP371
  612.8′3—dc23
                    2015036140

Special discounts on bulk quantities of Demos Medical Publishing books are available to corporations, professional associations, pharmaceutical companies, health care organizations, and other qualifying groups. For details, please contact:

Special Sales Department
Demos Medical Publishing, LLC
11 West 42nd Street, 15th Floor
New York, NY 10036
Phone: 800-532-8663 or 212-683-0072
Fax: 212-941-7842
E-mail: specialsales@demosmedical.com

Printed in the United States of America by Bang Printing.
15 16 17 18 / 5 4 3 2 1

Contents

Preface

To my mind, the spine is a constant source of wonderment. There is no other anatomic structure that can match the spine in terms of the combination of strength, structural stability, and the capability of multidirectional motion. On superficial inspection, the spine appears to be a simple structure with a repetitive design. However, a deeper look reveals an exceptionally complex structure with highly specialized anatomy at each level.

An overarching goal of this text is to introduce the reader to the subtleties of the spine that may not be commonly covered in radiological anatomy textbooks. Components of this work will resemble the traditional anatomic atlas. However, the reader will also notice several points of departure from the anatomic atlas model. Radiological anatomy is presented in multiple imaging modalities, including plain radiographs, fluoroscopy, myelography, computed tomography, and magnetic resonance imaging. The configuration and composition of the spine presents unique challenges to conventional imaging studies. Wherever possible, detailed anatomic concepts are presented in the imaging modality that is best suited to displaying that anatomy. Text is used sparingly to broaden the reader's understanding of the anatomic concepts and to provide a foundation upon which the anatomy displayed on the images can be understood. The result is something of a hybrid between an anatomic atlas and an anatomic textbook, designed to provide the best of both worlds to the reader.

The greatest point of departure of this work from standard radiological anatomy textbooks is the introduction of the reader to the world of spine intervention, a discipline that has its base in a firm understanding of spine imaging anatomy. Numerous images from spine intervention procedures are included to buttress the principles of spinal anatomy covered in the text and to illustrate how a detailed knowledge of spinal anatomy is exploited by the interventionalist.

Each chapter is organized into a brief introduction, a detailed gallery of images in a traditional atlas format, discussion of developmental anatomy, image gallery of developmental anatomy, a detailed description of adult anatomy with accompanying detailed figures, a gallery of anatomic variants and common congenital anomalies, and an extensive collection of suggested readings. The final chapter is a collection of computed tomographic and magnetic resonance images displaying the anatomy of the paraspinal musculature.

This work is written with the lifelong learner in mind, from the earliest exposure to this material in medical or graduate school to the resident, fellow, and practicing attending physician in the fields of diagnostic radiology, interventional radiology, neurology, neurosurgery, anesthesia, general surgery, orthopedics, and other closely related fields. Ultimately, it is my hope that readers gain an appreciation of the complex anatomy of the spine that carries them through their training into practice.

Scott E. Forseen

Acknowledgments

This work would not be possible without the seemingly endless patience of my wife of 20 years, Caralee. In the process of preparing this manuscript, she assumed nearly all of the primary responsibilities of our daily lives, allowing me to slip into a prolonged zombie-like state. My sons Mathias and Brendan have shown patience beyond their years in waiting for their father to return to the basketball court to play with them. Boys, it's me versus the two of you . . . your ball first.

William B. Bates III has been a tireless advocate for my wife and me since our earliest days at the Medical College of Georgia. Much of the venous imaging in this text comes directly from his early morning calls to let me know about the good cases he has encountered since our last conversation. It is my hope that the vascular imaging contained within meets his expectations for "pretty pictures."

Thanks is due to several people who assisted in this project, including Dr. Bruce Gilbert for his advice on many aspects of the manuscript, Dr. Brenten Heeke for generating 3D reformats of the sacrum, and Kyle Osteen for his willingness to share his talents in creating beautiful book quality MR images. Thanks is also due to Dr. Nathan Yanasak and Teresa Mills who set the standard for MR imaging quality at Georgia Regents University.

Last, I would like to thank Neil Borden for inviting me to co-author this book. I am honored that he would consider me to be a worthy contributor to this project. He sets the bar for excellence in the practice of neuroradiology and I strive to meet his expectations each time I log onto the workstation or step into the procedure room.

In the late stages of completing this manuscript, Dr. Bruce Dean of the Barrow Neurological Institute (BNI) passed on after a long battle with multiple myeloma. The outpouring of praise for this exceptional man by current and former BNI fellows after his passing had a profound impact on me. Dr. Dean motivated others not just to be better neuroradiologists, but to be better persons. We will miss you.

Imaging Anatomy of the Human Spine

The Craniocervical Junction

1

*T*he craniocervical junction is the anatomic region located at the transition from the skull to the cervical spine that houses the medulla, cervical spinal cord, multiple cranial nerves, blood vessels, and lymphatics. Included in the craniocervical junction are the occipital bone, atlas (C1), and axis (C2), six synovial joints, and multiple ligamentous structures. The paired atlanto-occipital (C0–C1) and atlantoaxial (C1–C2) joints allow for significant multidirectional mobility at the craniocervical junction that is distinct from the subaxial spine. In fact, most of the movement of the cervical segments takes place at the craniocervical junction.

EMBRYOLOGY OF THE CRANIOCERVICAL JUNCTION

In order to understand the common anatomic variations that occur at the craniocervical junction, a basic overview of embryology is needed. As the primitive streak is regressing, the paraxial mesoderm segments into somites. At the fourth week of gestation, there are four occipital and eight cervical somites. The somites will eventually differentiate into sclerotomes, myotomes, and dermatomes, which will eventually form the vertebrae, rib cartilage, muscles, tendons, ligaments, and skin of the back.

The craniocervical junction is ultimately derived from the four occipital sclerotomes and the first three cervical sclerotomes. There is general agreement that the transition from the skull to the cervical spine is located between the fourth and fifth sclerotomes. The first occipital somite and sclerotome form the basiocciput. The second and third occipital somites and sclerotomes form the jugular tubercles. The caudal aspect of the fourth somite and the rostral aspect of the fifth somite combine to form the proatlas sclerotome.

The proatlas sclerotome forms the occipital condyles, basion, opisthion, lateral rim of the foramen magnum, apical segment of the dens, and lateral masses of the atlas. Ligamentous structures derived from the proatlas sclerotome include the apical, alar, and cruciform ligaments. The proatlas and C1 sclerotomes both contribute to the posterior arch of the atlas.

The caudal aspect of the fifth somite and the rostral aspect of the sixth somite form the C1 sclerotome. The C1 sclerotome forms the basal segment of the dens, the anterior arch of the atlas, and contributes to the posterior arch of the atlas.

The C2 sclerotome is derived from the sixth and seventh somites. The centrum of the C2 sclerotome forms the body of the axis. The neural arch forms the posterior arch and facets of the axis. Thus, the axis is formed from three sclerotomes: the proatlas, C1, and C2.

The intervertebral border zones located between the apical and basal segments of the dens and between the basal segment and the body of the dens do not ultimately differentiate into nucleus pulposis and annulus fibrosis, as is the case in the subaxial cervical spine. This mesenchyme eventually forms the upper ("apicodental") and lower ("subdental") dental synchondroses. Remnants of the regressed subdental disc elements can occasionally be seen following fusion of the C2 ossification centers, referred to as the *ossiculum Albrecht* (**Figure 1.1**).

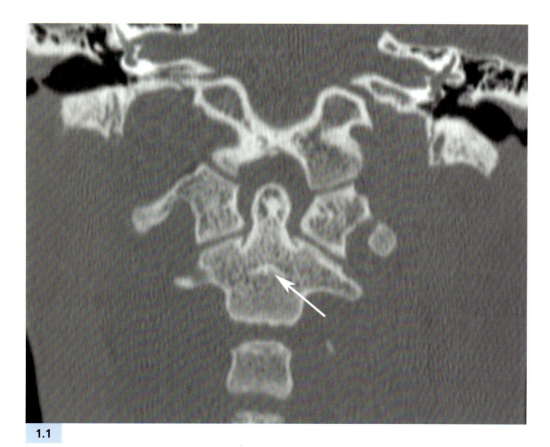

1.1

FIGURE 1.1 Coronal reformatted CT image demonstrates a remnant of the regressed subdental disc elements, called the ossiculum Albrecht.

DEVELOPMENTAL ANATOMY OF THE CRANIOCERVICAL JUNCTION

The atlas (C1) is typically derived from three primary ossification centers, one anterior and two posterior. The anterior ossification center forms the anterior arch. The posterior ossification centers form the lateral masses and neural arch. Neurocentral synchondroses are located between the anterior and posterior ossification centers on both sides of the midline. The intraneural synchondrosis is located between the two posterior ossification centers, generally at the midline. Ossification of the anterior arch and the neurocentral synchondroses is complete in most individuals by twelve years of age. The posterior arch and intraneural synchondrosis are generally ossified by 4 to 5 years of age. The atlas has no secondary ossification centers. The developmental anatomy of the atlas is depicted in **Figures 1.2a–f**.

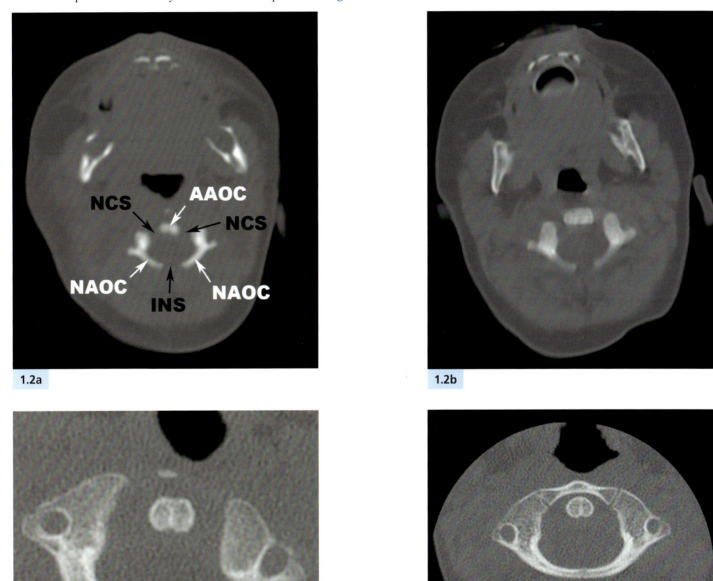

1.2a

1.2b

1.2c

1.2d

FIGURES 1.2a–f The primary ossification centers of the atlas (C1) at various ages: (a) newborn, (b) 6 months, (c) 2 years, (d) 3 years, (e) 10 years, and (f) 13 years. There is a wide range of normal ossification of the anterior and posterior arches. AAOC—anterior arch ossification center, INS—intraneural synchondrosis, NAOC—neural arch ossification center, NCS—neurocentral synchondrosis.

(continued)

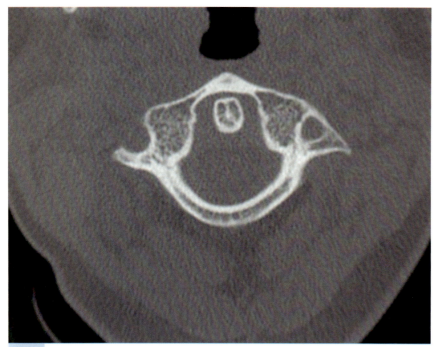

1.2e

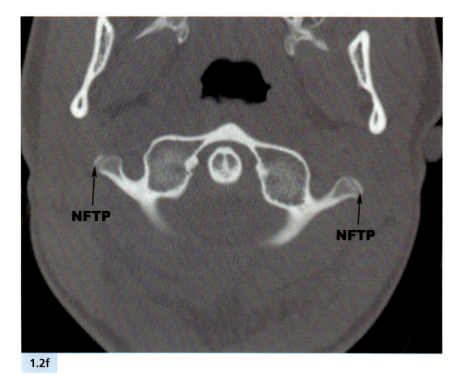

1.2f

FIGURES 1.2e,f   *(continued)* Occasionally, the posterior ossification centers do not completely ossify at the transverse processes which can simulate fractures. NFTP—nonfused transverse process.

The axis (C2) is typically made up of five primary ossification centers and four synchondroses. The centrum is separated from the laterally positioned neural arches by the neurocentral synchondroses. The subdental synchondrosis separates the centrum from the paired, mirror image ossification centers that form the base of the dens. The apicodental synchondrosis separates the apical and basal ossification centers. The neurocentral and subdental synchondroses are generally ossified after 9 years of age. The secondary ossification center at the dens apex, the *ossiculum terminale Bergmann*, begins to ossify between years 3 to 6 and fuses to the body of the dens by 12 years of age. Additional secondary ossification centers that arise and fuse in adolescence are found at the tips of the transverse processes, tips of the bifid spinous processes, and ring apophysis along the inferior margin of the centrum. The developmental anatomy of the axis is depicted in **Figures 1.3a–r**.

1 month

6 months

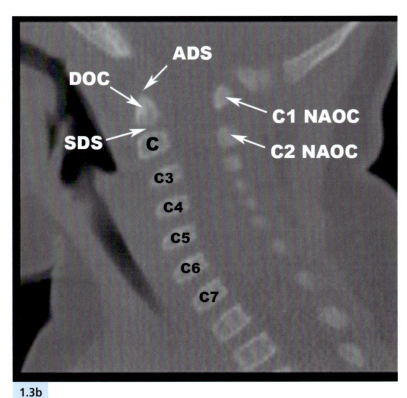

1.3a

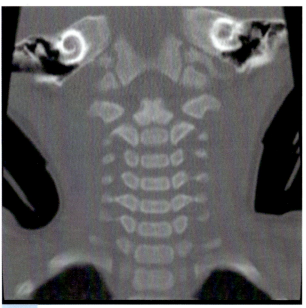

1.3c

1.3b

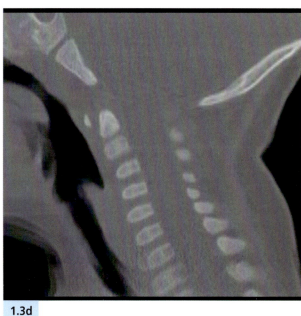

1.3d

FIGURES 1.3a–r   Typical appearance of the primary ossification centers of the atlas (C1) and axis (C2) at various ages: (a,b)—1 month, (c,d)—6 months, (e,f)—9 months, (g,h)—12 months, (i,j)—2 years, (k,l)—3 years, (m,n)—6 years, (o,p)—10 years, and (q,r)—17 years. ACS—acrocentral synchondrosis, ADS—apicodental synchondrosis, C—centrum, C1 NAOC—neural arch ossification center of C1, C2 NAOC—neural arch ossification center of C2, DOC—dens (basal) ossification centers, NCS—neurocentral synchondrosis, SDS—subdental synchondrosis.

(continued)

9 months

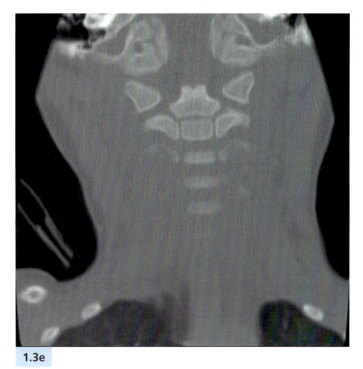

1.3e

12 months

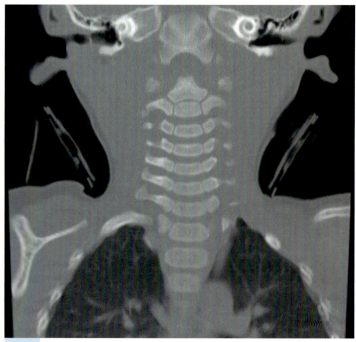

1.3g

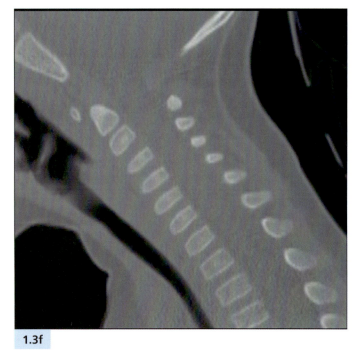

1.3f

FIGURES 1.3e–h

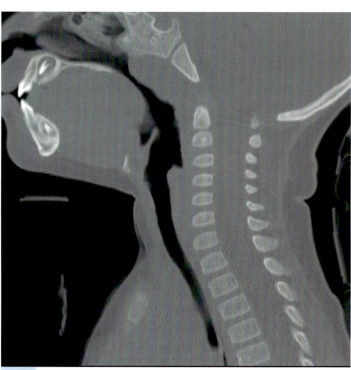

1.3h

(continued)

2 years

3 years

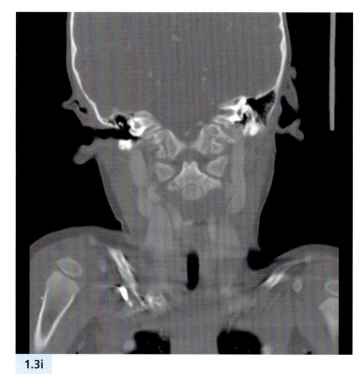

1.3i

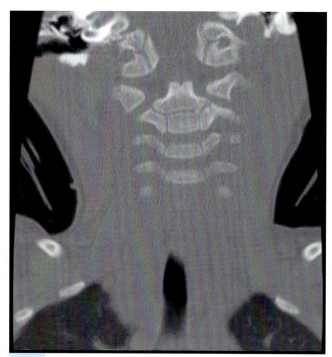

1.3k

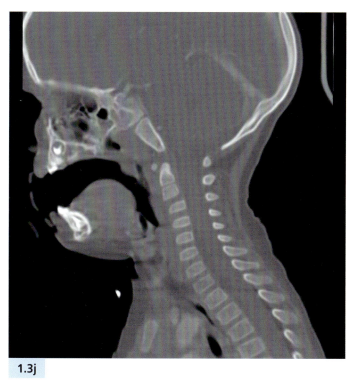

1.3j

FIGURES 1.3i–l

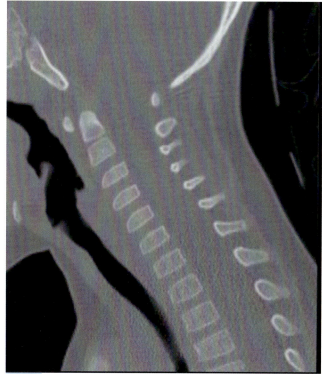

1.3l

(continued)

6 years

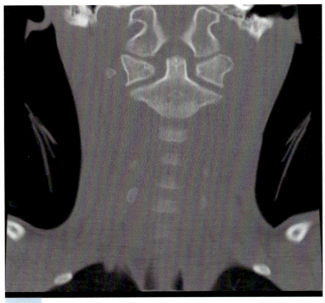

1.3m

10 years

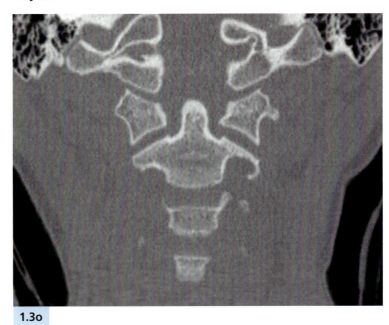

1.3o

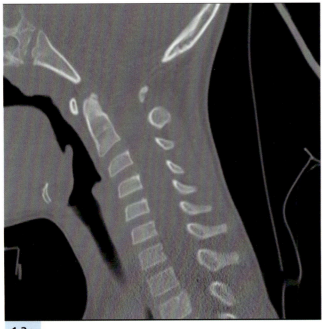

1.3n

1.3p

FIGURES 1.3m–p

(continued)

12 years

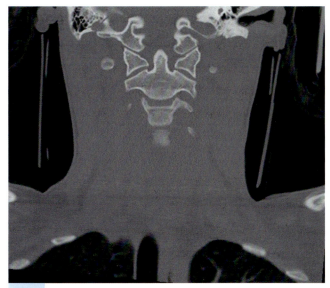

1.3q

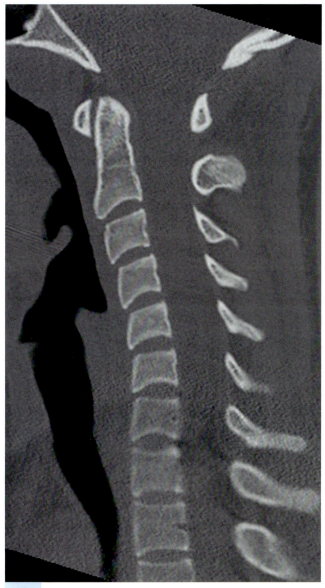

1.3r

FIGURES 1.3q–r

THE OCCIPUT

The occipital bone (**Figure 1.4**) forms the superior-most aspect of the craniocervical junction. The occipital condyles are bony protuberances arising from the exoccipital portion of the occipital bone, forming the lateral borders of the foramen magnum along with the basiocciput anteriorly and the supraocciput posteriorly.

The occipital condyles are most commonly oval or round in shape, as viewed in the sagittal plane (**Figure 1.5**). Occasionally, there is a small divot at the articular surface of the occipital condyle, referred to as the *synchondrosis intraoccipitalis anterior* (**Figure 1.6**). This represents the ossification border between the basioccipital and exoccipital portions of the chondrocranium and is considered a normal anatomic variant.

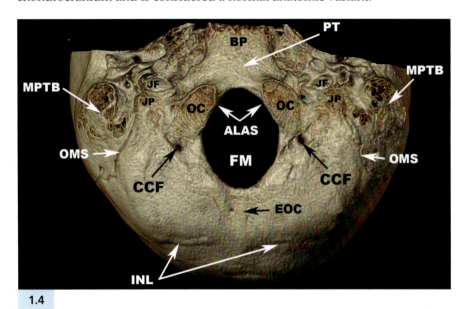

1.4

FIGURE 1.4   3D surface reconstructed CT image of the occipital bone. ALAS—alar ligament attachment sites, BP—basilar part of occipital bone, CCF—condylar canal/fossa, EOC—external occipital crest, FM—foramen magnum, INL—inferior nuchal line, JF—jugular foramen, JP—jugular process, MPTB—mastoid portion temporal bone, OC—occipital condyle, OMS—occipitomastoid suture, PT—pharyngeal tubercle.

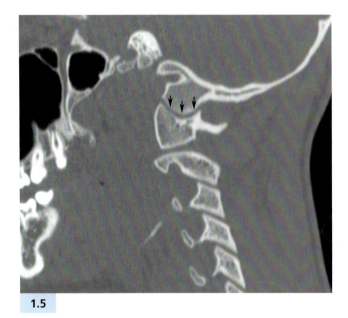

1.5

FIGURE 1.5   Sagittal CT image of the cervical spine demonstrating the typical convex inferior, rounded contour of the occipital condyles (arrows).

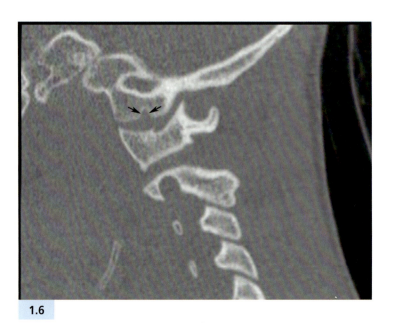

1.6

FIGURE 1.6   Sagittal CT image of the cervical spine demonstrating a small divot in the occipital condyle, the synchondrosis intraoccipitalis anterior (arrows).

THE ATLAS

The atlas (**Figures 1.7a–b**) is a bony ring that lacks a vertebral body and a spinous process. Superior and inferior articular processes arise from lateral masses on each side of the midline, forming the atlanto-occipital and atlantoaxial joints with the occipital condyles and superior articular processes of the axis, respectively. The lateral masses and foramina transversaria of the atlas are more laterally located than that of the rest of the cervical spine. There is a small anterior midline tubercle upon which the anterior longitudinal ligament attaches. There is a shallow groove on the dorsal margin of the anterior arch that forms an articular facet with the anterior surface of the dens. The medial tubercles arise from the lateral masses and serve as attachments for the transverse ligament. Along the superior surface of the neural arch, just posterior to the lateral masses on both sides of the midline, are shallow grooves for the vertebral arteries. The C1 nerves course with the vertebral arteries within these grooves. In approximately 15% of the population, a partial or complete bony arch forms that spans from the retroglenoid tubercle to the neural arch, most commonly referred to as the *ponticulus posticus* (**Figure 1.8**). The rectus capitus posterior minor muscles attach to the posterior tubercle.

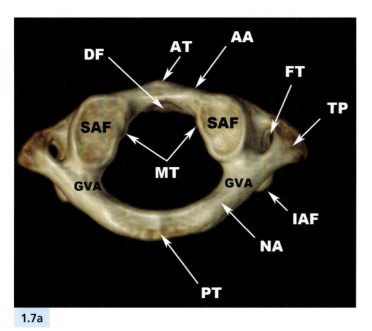

1.7a

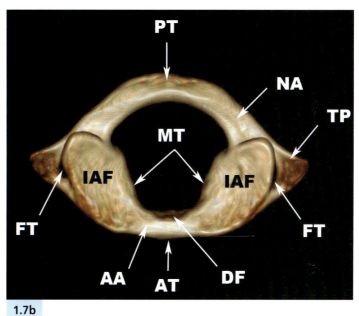

1.7b

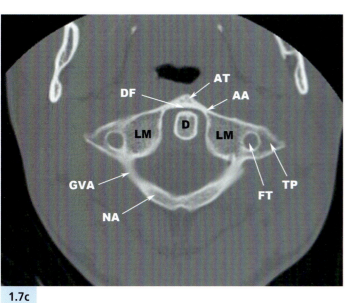

1.7c

FIGURES 1.7a–c Bony surface anatomy of the atlas (C1) depicted in (a) superior oblique 3D, (b) inferior 3D, and (c) axial reformatted CT images. AA—anterior arch, AT—anterior tubercle, D—dens, DF—dens facet, FT—foramen transversarium, GVA—groove for vertebral artery, IAF—inferior articular facet, LM—lateral mass, MT—medial tubercles (transverse ligament attachments), NA—neural arch, PT—posterior tubercle, SAF—superior articular facet, TP—transverse process.

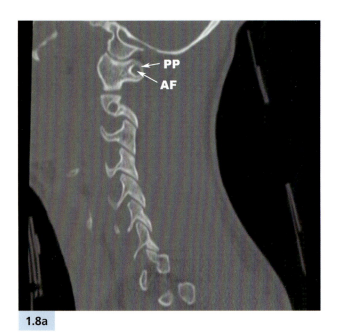

1.8a

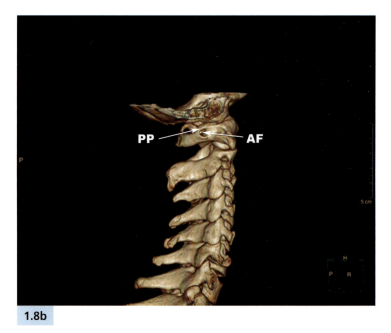

1.8b

FIGURES 1.8a,b Sagittal (a) and surface (b) reconstructed CT images demonstrating the arcuate foramen (AF) and ponticulus posticus (PP).

THE AXIS

The unique configuration of the axis (**Figures 1.9a–c**) is primarily due to the dens, an elongated bony process that extends superiorly from the C2 vertebral body and forms a pivot joint with the atlas. The lateral masses give rise to superior and inferior articular processes that articulate with the C1 inferior articular processes and C3 superior articular processes, respectively. There are shallow depressions along the dorsolateral surface of the dens at the alar ligament attachment sites. Inferior to the alar ligament attachments on the dorsal surface of the dens is a transversely oriented groove for the transverse ligament. The anterior surface of the dens is an articular facet with the anterior arch of the atlas. There is a small midline anterior tubercle that serves as the attachment for the anterior longitudinal ligament. The spinous process is generally bifid and is the attachment for the ligamentum nuchae and several muscles, including semispinalis cervicis, spinalis cervicus, inferior oblique, rectus capitis posterior major, interspinalis, and multifidus.

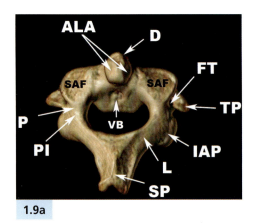

1.9a

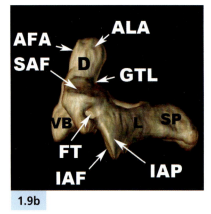

1.9b

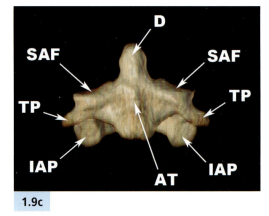

1.9c

FIGURES 1.9a–c Bony anatomy of the axis (C2) depicted in (a) superior oblique 3D (b) lateral, and (c) anterior 3D reformatted CT images. AFA—articular facet for the atlas, ALA—alar ligament attachments, AT—anterior tubercle for anterior longitudinal ligament attachment, D—dens, FT—foramina transversarium, GTL—groove for the transverse ligament, IAF—inferior articular facet, IAP—inferior articular process, L—lamina, P—pedicle, PI—pars interarticularis, SAF—superior articular facet, SP—spinous process, TP—transverse process, VB—vertebral body.

THE C0–C1 JOINT COMPLEX

The C0–C1 (occipitoatlantal) joints are formed by convex surfaces of the occipital condyles and the concave superior articular facets of the atlas (**Figures 1.10a–c**). They are oriented superolateral to inferomedial in the coronal plane and angled medially from posterior to anterior. Both C0–C1 joints are lined by synovium and surrounded by loose capsular ligaments. The mechanical properties of the C0–C1 joint are mostly determined by bony structures. The primary movements at the C0–C1 joint are flexion and extension. The orientation and shape of the C0–C1 joints restricts axial rotation and lateral bending.

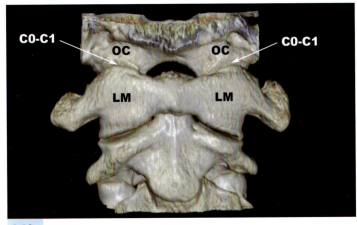

1.10a

FIGURES 1.10a–c   The anatomy of the occipitoatlantal (C0–C1) joint demonstrated with (a) surface reformatted anterior, (b) coronal reformatted, and (c) sagittal reformatted CT images. C0–C1—occipitoatlantal joints (C0–C1 joints), D—dens of axis, IAF—inferior articular facet, LM—lateral mass, OC—occipital condyle, SAF—superior articular facet.

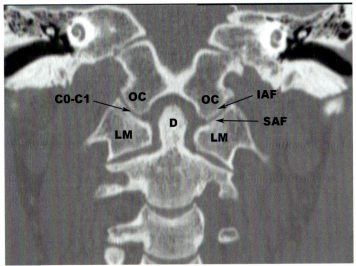

1.10b

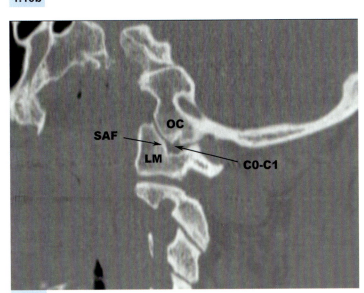

1.10c

THE C1–C2 JOINT COMPLEX

The C1–C2 (atlantoaxial) joint is a four part joint that includes a synovium lined articulation between the posterior surface of the C1 arch and anterior surface of the dens, a synovium lined articulation between the posterior surface of the dens and the anterior surface of the transverse ligament, and two synovium lined joints between the C1 and C2 lateral masses that are surrounded by loose capsular ligaments. The mechanical properties of the C1–C2 joint are predominantly determined by ligamentous structures. Axial rotation is the primary movement at C1–C2, with lesser degrees of flexion, extension, and lateral bending possible at this articulation. The anatomy of the C1–C2 joints is demonstrated in **Figures 1.11a–d**.

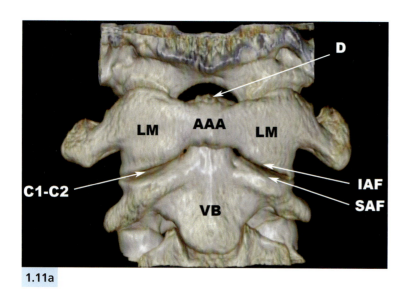

1.11a

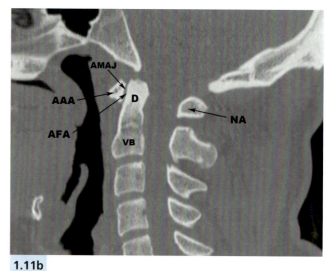

1.11b

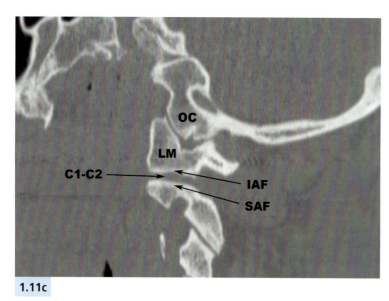

1.11c

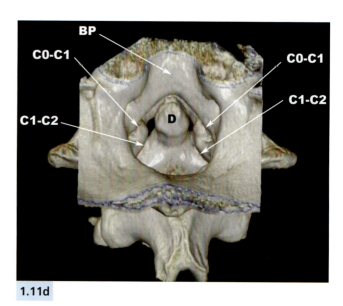

1.11d

FIGURES 1.11a–d The anatomy of the atlantoaxial (C1–C2) joints demonstrated with (a) surface rendered anterior, (b) sagittal reformatted, (c) sagittal reformatted, and (d) surface rendered superior oblique CT images. C0–C1—occipitoatlantal joint (C0–C1), C1–C2—atlantoaxial joint (C1–C2), AAA—anterior arch of C1, AFA—articular facet for the atlas, AMAJ—anterior median atlantoaxial joint, BP—basilar part of the occipital bone, D—dens, IAF—inferior articular facet of C1, LM—lateral mass of C1, NA—neural arch of C1, OC—occipital condyle, SAF—superior articular facet of C2, VB—vertebral body of C2.

LIGAMENTOUS ANATOMY OF THE CRANIOCERVICAL JUNCTION

The *anterior longitudinal ligament* attaches to the anterior tubercles of C1 and C2. The *anterior occipitoatlantal membrane* is the craniad extension of the anterior longitudinal ligament that attaches to the anterosuperior margin of the C1 arch and to the clivus (**Figure 1.12**). The weak *apical ligament* attaches to the apex of the dens and to the clivus. The *cruciform ligament* has three components: the transverse, ascending, and descending bands. The transverse band or *transverse ligament* attaches to the medial tubercles of the C1 lateral masses and courses dorsal to the dens and posterior median atlantoaxial joint capsule, providing the primary stabilization of the atlantoaxial joint (**Figures 1.13a–c**). This ligament is one of the most important ligaments of the body. The ascending and descending bands of the cruciform ligament attach to the dorsal clivus and posterior body of C2, respectively. Immediately posterior to the cruciform ligament is the *tectorial membrane*, which arises as the craniad continuation of the posterior longitudinal ligament that attaches to the dorsal surface of the clivus (Figure 1.12). The transition from the posterior longitudinal ligament to the tectorial membrane occurs imperceptibly at the level of the C2 vertebral body.

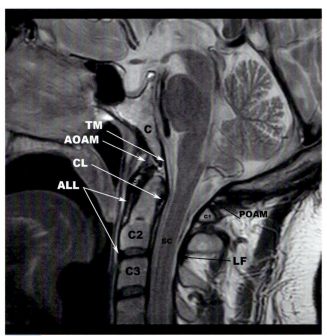

1.12

FIGURE 1.12   The ligamentous anatomy of the craniocervical junction demonstrated on a mid-sagittal T2 fast spin echo (FSE) image. ALL—anterior longitudinal ligament, AOAM—anterior occipitoatlantal membrane, C—clivus, CL—cruciform ligament (transverse band or transverse ligament), LF—ligamentum flavum, POAM—posterior occipitoatlantal membrane, SC—spinal cord, TM—tectorial membrane.

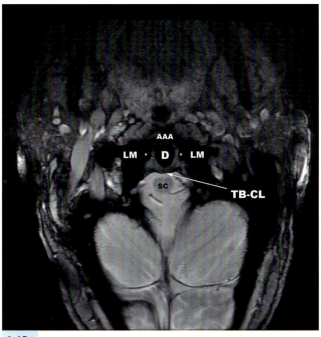

1.13a

FIGURES 1.13a–c   (a) Axial gradient-recalled echo (GRE) image at the C1–C2 level that demonstrates the transverse band of the cruciform ligament and its attachments to the medial tubercles of C1. AAA—anterior arch of atlas (C1), D—dens, LM—lateral mass, SC—spinal cord, TB-CL—transverse band of cruciform ligament, asterisks (*)—medial tubercles of C1.

(continued)

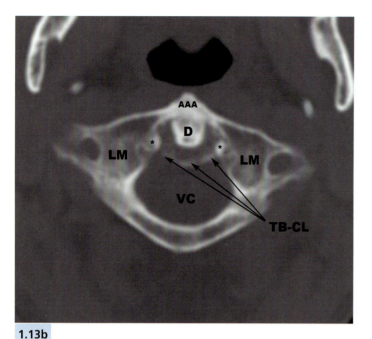

1.13b

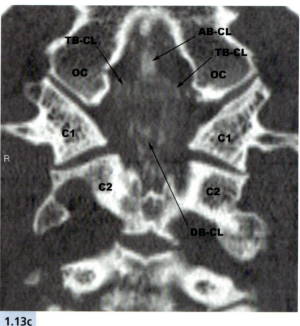

1.13c

FIGURES 1.13b,c (*continued*) (b) Axial CT showing a heavily calcified transverse band of the cruciform ligament. (c) Curved reformatted CT image demonstrating heavy calcification of the ascending, descending, and transverse bands of the cruciform ligament. AAA—anterior arch of atlas, AB-CL—ascending band of cruciform ligament, D—dens, DB-CL—descending band of cruciform ligament, LM—lateral mass, OC—occipital condyle, TB-CL—transverse band of cruciform ligament, VC—vertebral canal, (*)—medial tubercles of C1.

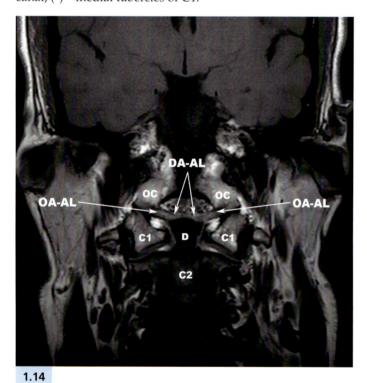

1.14

FIGURE 1.14 Coronal T1-weighted turbo spin echo (TSE) image demonstrating the odontoid and occipital attachments of the alar ligaments. C1—atlas vertebra, C2—axis vertebra, D—dens, DA-AL—dens attachment of the alar ligaments, OA-AL—occipital attachments of the alar ligaments, OC—occipital condyles.

The *alar ligaments* are strong ligaments that attach along the superolateral margins of the dens and project to the medial margins of the occipital condyles, where they attach to small tubercles (**Figure 1.14**). The left alar ligament limits axial rotation to the right and vice versa. The *ligament of Barkow* attaches to the anteromedial margins of the occipital condyles anterior to the odontoid process and alar ligaments. The exact function of the Barkow ligament is unknown, but it is thought to assist in containing the dens.

The *posterior occipitoatlantal membrane* (POAM) is a broad ligamentous sheet that attaches along the posterior margin of the foramen magnum and the superior margin of the C1 neural arch (Figure 1.12). Laterally, the POAM blends with the C0–C1 articular capsules. There are small rents in the lateral aspects of the POAM that transmit the V3h segments of the vertebral arteries. The ponticulus posticus (defined previously) forms along the superior margin of this ligamentous foramen. The *posterior atlantoaxial membrane* is also a ligamentous sheet that attaches to the inferior margin of the C1 neural arch and the superior margin of the C2 neural arch.

Additional ligaments at the craniocervical junction include the transverse occipital, lateral atlanto-occipital, and the accessory atlantoaxial ligaments. These are small ligaments that are generally not well visualized on conventional imaging examinations. The ligamentum nuchae is discussed in detail in Chapter 2.

ARTERIAL ANATOMY OF THE CRANIOCERVICAL JUNCTION

The primary blood supply to the craniocervical junction is derived from the vertebral arteries and branches of the internal carotid and external carotid arteries. The distal segments of the vertebral arteries (distal V2, V3, and V4) supply the structures of the craniocervical junction. The V3 segments extend from the C2 foramina transversaria to the dural opening at the level of the foramen magnum. The V4 segments begin at the dural opening and extend to the vertebrobasilar junction. This numbering convention is more commonly used in the spine literature and will be used in this text. This anatomy is displayed in **Figures 1.15a–h**.

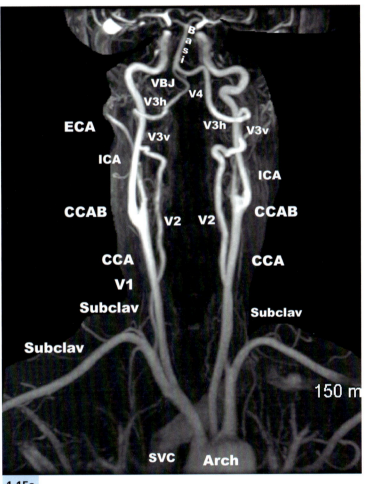

1.15a

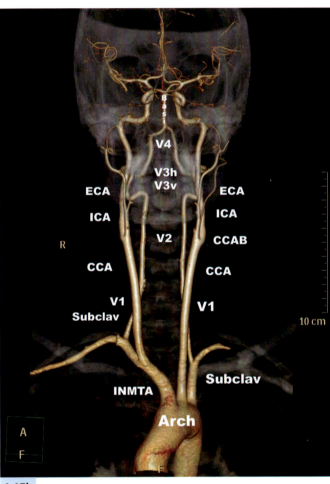

1.15b

FIGURES 1.15a–h Multimodality images demonstrating the arterial supply of the craniocervical junction: (a) coronal post contrast MR angiogram, (b,c) anterior surface rendered CT angiograms, (d) lateral surface rendered CT angiogram, (e) posterior surface rendered image CT angiogram, (f) axial CT angiographic image at the C1–C2 level displaying the horizontal segments of the V3 segments (V3h), (g) axial CT angiographic image at C2 displaying the vertical portion of the V2 segment on the left and the transition from V2 to V3v on the right, and (h) conventional angiogram of the right vertebral artery.

KEY					
Arch	aortic arch	**Subclav**	subclavian artery	**V3h**	horizontal portion V3 segment of vertebral artery
Basi	basilar artery	**SVC**	superior vena cava		
CCA	common carotid artery (R = right, L = left)	**VBJ**	vertebrobasilar junction	**V3v**	vertical portion V3 segment of vertebral artery
		V1	initial extraforaminal segment of vertebral artery		
CCAB	common carotid artery bifurcation			**V4**	intradural segment of vertebral artery
ECA	external carotid artery	**V2**	intraforaminal segment of vertebral artery		
ICA	internal carotid artery				
INMTA	innominate artery				

(continued)

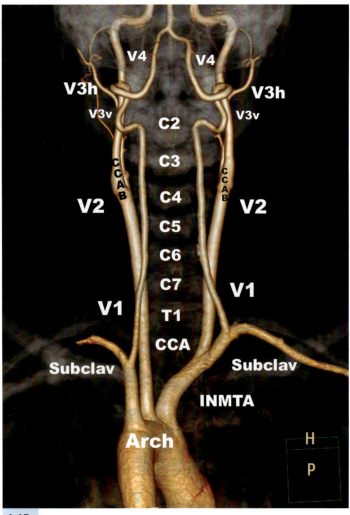

1.15c

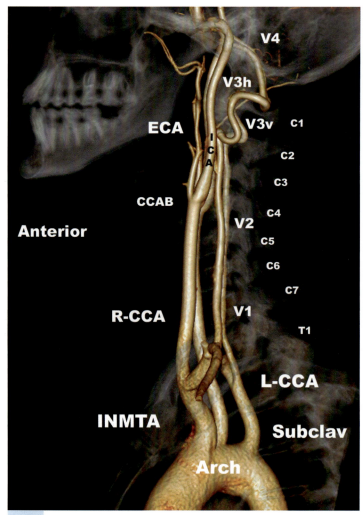

1.15d

FIGURES 1.15c–e

KEY	
Arch	aortic arch
CCA	common carotid artery (R = right, L = left)
CCAB	common carotid artery bifurcation
D	dens
ECA	external carotid artery
INMTA	innominate artery
MB	muscular branch
OCCA	occipital artery
Subclav	subclavian artery
V1	initial extraforaminal segment of vertebral artery
V2	intraforaminal segment of vertebral artery
V3h	horizontal portion V3 segment of vertebral artery
V3v	vertical portion V3 segment of vertebral artery
V4	intradural segment of vertebral artery

1.15e

(continued)

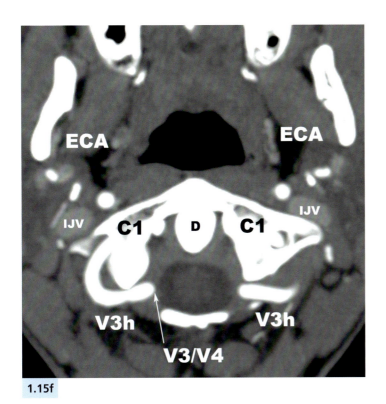

1.15f

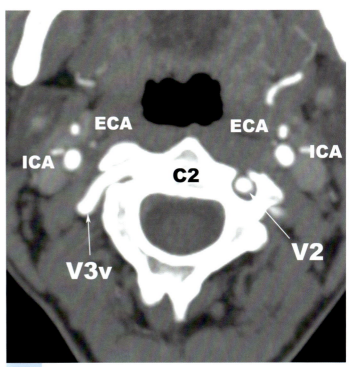

1.15g

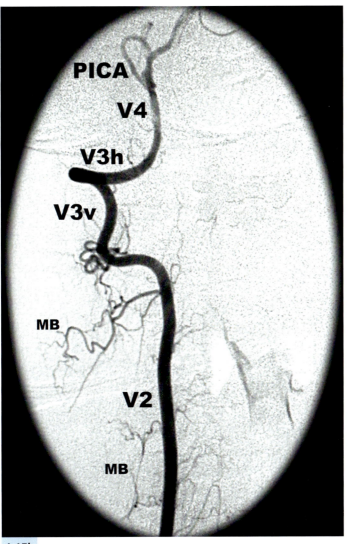

1.15h

FIGURES 1.15f–h

KEY	
D	dens
ECA	external carotid artery
ICA	internal carotid artery
IJV	internal jugular vein
MB	muscular branch
PICA	posterior inferior cerebellar artery
V2	intraforaminal segment of vertebral artery
V3h	horizontal portion V3 segment of vertebral artery
V3v	vertical portion V3 segment of vertebral artery
V3/V4	junction of V3 and V4 segments of vertebral artery
V4	intradural segment of vertebral artery

The vertical portions of the V3 segment (V3v) loop posterolaterally and slightly superiorly as they exit the C2 foramina transversaria, then course superiorly, anteriorly and slightly laterally prior to entering the C1 foramina transversaria. The horizontal portions (V3h) loop posteromedially and slightly inferiorly after they exit the C1 foramina transversaria, positioned within the grooves on the C1 neural arch and eventually turning anteriorly superiorly and medially to pierce the posterior occipitoatlantal membrane and dura mater at the level of the foramen magnum (Figure 1.15d,e).

There are two sets of segmental branches arising from the vertebral arteries, cervical and cranial. The *cervical branches* include muscular, osteoarticular, meningeal, and spinal branches. Branches of V2 at C1–C2 most commonly are muscular, supplying the semispinalis capitis, semispinalis cervicis, rectus capitis, and obliquus capitis musculature. The suboccipital muscles are also supplied by deep descending branches of the occipital arteries. The V3 segments typically do not give off radicular, medullary, or radiculomedullary branches. The *artery of Salmon* is a muscular branch of V3 that arises just proximal to the dural opening that anastomoses with branches of the ascending cervical (thyrocervical trunk) and occipital (external carotid) arteries. The posterior meningeal artery supplies the dura of the posterior fossa and typically arises from V3. A small caliber branch to the C0–C1 joints generally arises from V3. Osseous branches arise at each level and tend to arise ventrally. Intersegmental anastomoses between C1 and C2 are variably present.

The *cranial branches* include the posterior inferior cerebellar artery, posterior meningeal, anterior and posterior spinal arteries. The *posterior inferior cerebellar artery* is the largest branch of the vertebral arteries and typically arises from the V4 segment (**Figure 1.16**), less commonly

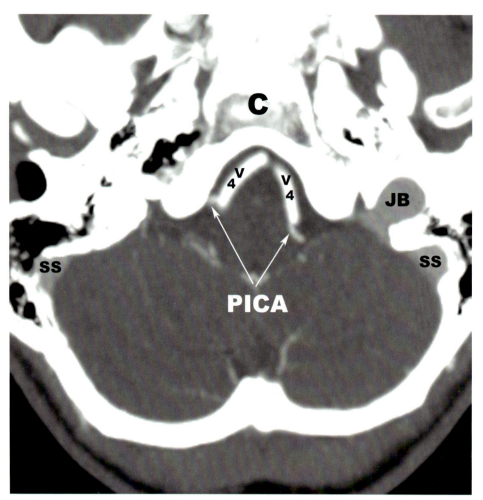

FIGURE 1.16 Axial CT angiographic image demonstrating the typical origin of the posterior inferior cerebellar arteries (PICA) from the V4 segments. C—clivus, JB—jugular bulb, SS—sigmoid sinus.

from the distal V3 segment (**Figures 1.17a,b**). Its branches supply the inferior medulla, inferior vermis, and posteroinferior cerebellar hemispheres. The *anterior spinal artery* (ASA) typically (45%–80%) forms from small branches arising from the medial aspects of the V4 segments that fuse at the midline. However, a wide range of variant origins of the ASA, including a number of unilateral origins, have been reported. Accessory ASAs are commonly encountered (40%). The posterior spinal arteries arise just outside of the dural openings along the posteromedial surface of the V3 segments of the vertebral arteries, the proximal V4 segments, or rarely from the posterior inferior cerebellar arteries. Thus, the vertebral arteries, posterior spinal arteries, and dorsal rami of C1 (suboccipital nerves) pass though the dural openings together. The posterior spinal arteries give off ascending and descending branches. The descending branches course inferiorly between the denticulate ligaments and the dorsal roots to supply the dorsal spinal cord. The ascending branch enters the foramen magnum.

The odontoid process of C2 is supplied by branches of the vertebral and carotid arteries. The anterior and posterior ascending arteries branch from the distal V2 segments and course superiorly along the ventral and dorsal surfaces of C2 meeting superiorly to form an apical arcade. Branches of the ascending pharyngeal arteries give off perforators that supply the superior portion of the odontoid.

The dura of the craniocervical junction is supplied by the anterior and posterior meningeal branches of the vertebral arteries, the ascending pharyngeal and occipital branches of the external carotid arteries, and the dorsal meningeal branches of the meningohypophyseal trunks of the internal carotid arteries.

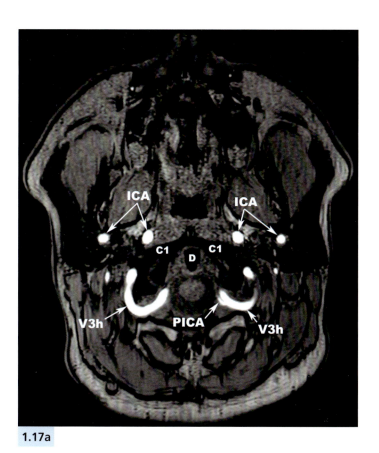 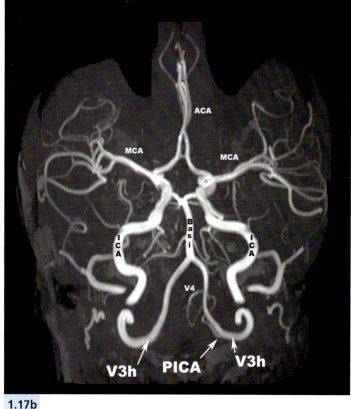

1.17a   1.17b

FIGURES 1.17a,b   Origin of the left posterior inferior cerebellar artery (PICA) from the horizontal portion of the V3 segment of the left vertebral artery (V3h): (a) 3D time-of-flight MR angiography and (b) maximum intensity projection (MIP) image. ACA—anterior cerebral artery, Basi—basilar artery, C1—atlas, D—dens, ICA—internal carotid artery, MCA—middle cerebral artery, V4—intradural segment of the vertebral artery.

VENOUS ANATOMY OF THE CRANIOCERVICAL JUNCTION

The *suboccipital cavernous sinus* (SCS) anchors the venous drainage of the craniocervical junction. The SCS is a venous network that surrounds the V3h segment of the vertebral artery (**Figure 1.18**) and has numerous interconnections, including the vertebral artery venous plexus, marginal sinus, suboccipital venous plexus, internal and external vertebral venous plexuses, and the anterior, lateral, and posterior condylar veins.

The *vertebral artery venous plexus* (VAVP) encompasses the V3v segment (**Figure 1.19**). It continues inferiorly as the vertebral veins and communicates with the internal and external

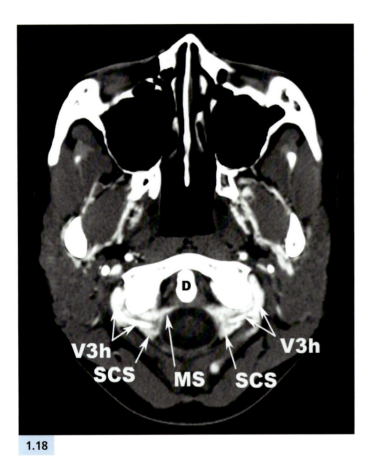

1.18

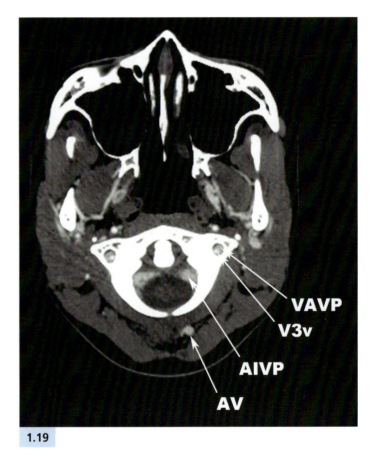

1.19

FIGURE 1.18 Axial CT angiographic image demonstrating the horizontal portions of the V3 segments of the vertebral arteries (V3h) coursing through dense venous plexuses, the suboccipital cavernous sinuses. D—dens, MS—marginal sinus, SCS—suboccipital cavernous sinus.

FIGURE 1.19 Axial CT angiographic image demonstrating the vertebral artery venous plexuses coursing with the vertical portions of the vertebral arteries (V3v) through the C1 foramina transversaria. Also visualized is the anastomotic vein, which is a communication between the vertebral artery venous plexus and the suboccipital venous plexus. AIVP—anterior internal vertebral venous plexus, AV—anastomosing vein, VAVP—vertebral artery venous plexus.

vertebral venous plexuses (**Figure 1.20**). The *marginal sinus* is contained within the dura at the level of C0–C1 and connects the occipital sinus and basilar venous plexus to the vertebral venous plexuses (Figure 1.18). The *suboccipital venous plexus* is located within the suboccipital triangle and communicates with the VAVP via an anastomotic vein (**Figure 1.21**) that traverses the posterior occipitoatlantal membrane with the vertebral artery, C1 dorsal ramus, and posterior spinal arteries. The vertebral venous plexuses are densely interconnected networks of epidural and paravertebral veins that connect to one another through the intervertebral veins, across the midline, and to the vertebral venous plexuses of adjacent segments. The vertebral venous plexuses are discussed in detail in Chapter 2.

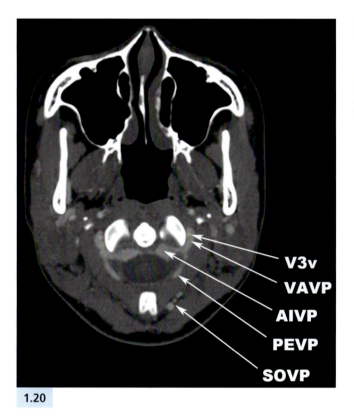

1.20

FIGURE 1.20   Axial CT angiographic image displaying interconnections between the vertebral artery venous plexus (VAVP), the anterior internal vertebral venous plexus (AIVP), and the posterior external vertebral venous plexus (PEVP). The suboccipital venous plexus (SOVP) is partially visible. V3v—vertical portion V3 segment of vertebral artery.

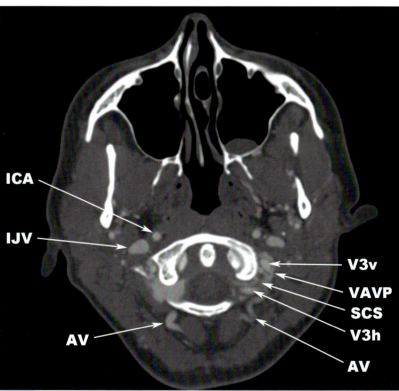

1.21

FIGURE 1.21   Axial CT angiographic image at the C0–C1 level showing large caliber anastomotic veins (AV), which connect the suboccipital cavernous sinuses (SCS) to the suboccipital venous plexus (not shown). The communications between the vertebral artery venous plexus (VAVP), suboccipital cavernous sinus (SCS), and anastomotic veins are also visualized. ICA—internal carotid artery, IJV—internal jugular vein, V3h—horizontal portion V3 segment of vertebral artery, V3v—vertical portion V3 segment of vertebral artery.

The *anterior condylar vein* arises from the anterior condylar confluence, projects through the hypoglossal canal, and extends along the internal margin of the occipital bone to the marginal sinus (**Figures 1.22a–c**). The *lateral condylar vein* also arises from the anterior condylar

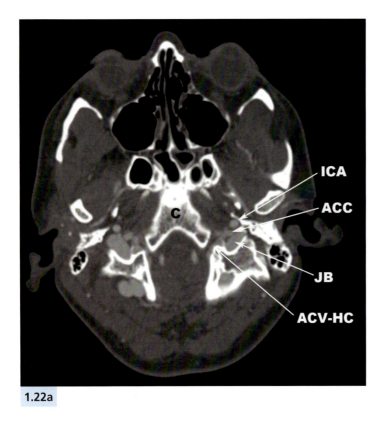

1.22a

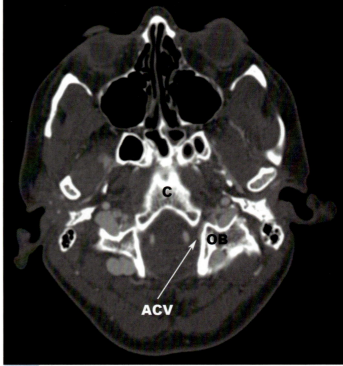

1.22b

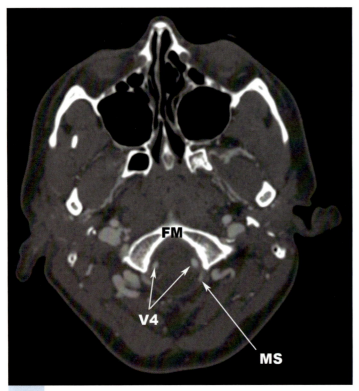

1.22c

FIGURES 1.22a–c   Axial CT angiographic images demonstrate: (a) the anterior condylar vein (ACV) arising from the anterior condylar confluence (ACC) and projecting through the hypoglossal canal (ACV-HC). (b) The ACV courses along the inner margin of the occipital bone (OB) and (c) drains into the marginal sinus (MS). C—clivus, FM—foramen magnum, ICA—internal carotid artery, JB—jugular bulb, V4—intradural segments of the vertebral arteries.

confluence and courses posteroinferolaterally to the SCS (**Figures 1.23a–c**). The *posterior condylar vein* originates from the sigmoid sinus, jugular bulb, or anterior condylar confluence and projects through the condylar canal to the SCS. The posterior condylar canal can be complete or incomplete (**Figures 1.24a–c**).

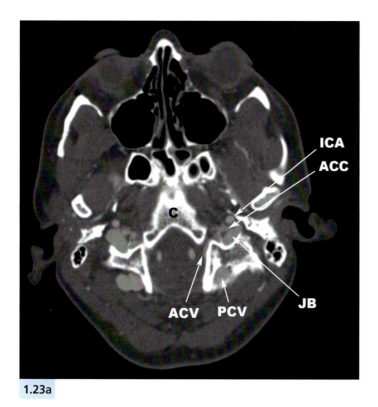

1.23a

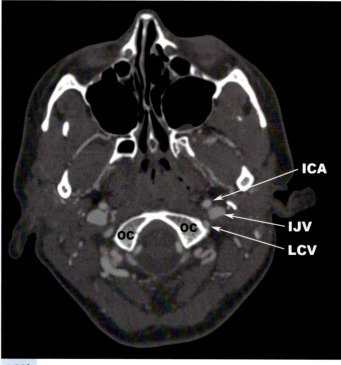

1.23b

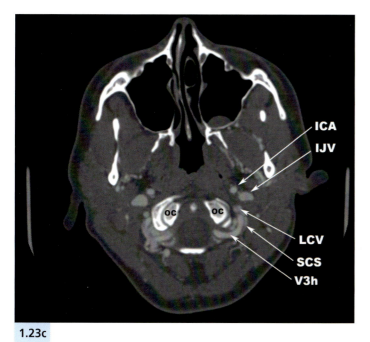

1.23c

FIGURES 1.23a–c   Axial CT angiographic images display the lateral condylar vein (LCV): (a) arising from the anterior condylar confluence (ACC), (b) coursing posteriorly and inferiorly along the lateral margin of the occipital condyle (OC), and (c) draining into the suboccipital cavernous sinus (SCS). ACV—anterior condylar vein, C—clivus, ICA—internal carotid artery, IJV—internal jugular vein, JB—jugular bulb, PCV—posterior condylar vein (in condylar canal), SCS—suboccipital cavernous sinus, V3h—horizontal portion V3 segment of vertebral artery.

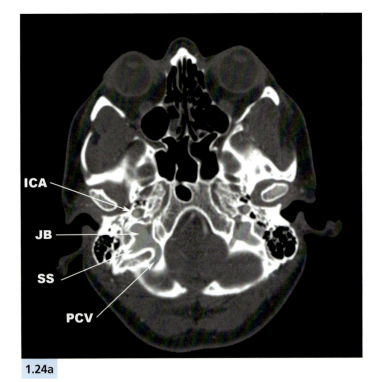

1.24a

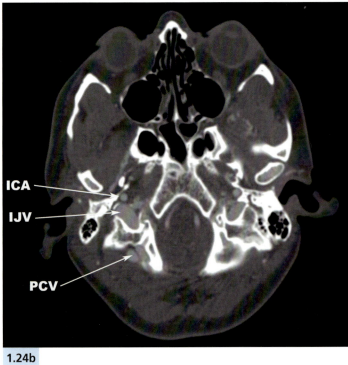

1.24b

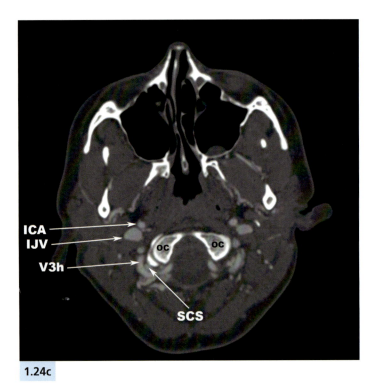

1.24c

FIGURES 1.24a–c Axial CT angiographic images show the course of the posterior condylar vein (PCV). (a) The PCV enters the condylar canal after arising from the sigmoid sinus (SS), (b) exits the condylar canal through the condylar fossa, and (c) drains into the suboccipital cavernous sinus (SCS). ICA—internal carotid artery, IJV—internal jugular vein, JB—jugular bulb, OC—occipital condyle, V3h—horizontal portion V3 segment of vertebral artery.

MENINGES AND SPACES OF THE CRANIOCERVICAL JUNCTION

The characteristics of the meninges and spaces of the craniocervical junction are similar to the rest of the spine. The features of the spinal meninges and spaces that are unique to the craniocervical junction will be discussed here. A detailed description of the spinal meninges is found in Chapter 2.

The denticulate ligaments are triangular, longitudinally-oriented extensions of the pia mater that extend from the lateral margins of the spinal cord to the lateral margins of the thecal sac between the ventral and dorsal nerve roots caudal to C1. The first denticulate ligaments arise along the lateral margins of the cervicomedullary junction and attach to the outer layer of the dura of the marginal sinus at the level of the foramen magnum. One-fifth of the time, the first denticulate ligaments attach to the proximal V4 segment. The first denticulate ligaments are broader medially and thicker laterally. They travel immediately superior to the vertebral arteries as they course through the posterior atlanto-occipital membrane and dural openings. The vertebral arteries are normally positioned along the anterior border of the denticulate ligaments. The spinal accessory nerves, C1 nerve roots, and posterior spinal arteries are positioned along the posterior border. The hypoglossal nerves are located just superior to the lateral attachments of the intracranial denticulate ligaments to the outer layer of the marginal sinuses.

The spinal cord occupies approximately one-half of the subarachnoid space at C1, versus three-quarters of the spinal canal in the subaxial cervical spine. Viewed on sagittal images, the subarachnoid space is greater in diameter, tapering superiorly to inferiorly and forming a funnel shape (**Figures 1.25a,b**).

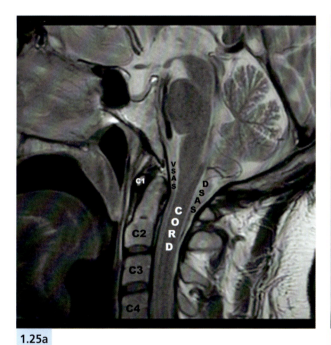
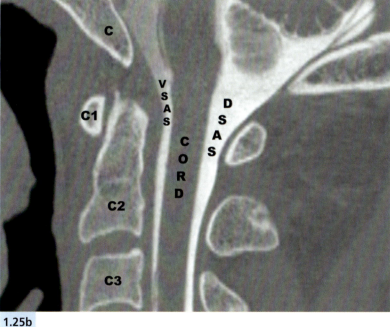

1.25a
1.25b

FIGURES 1.25a,b   The unique, tapering configuration of the subarachnoid spaces at the craniocervical junction demonstrated on (a) sagittal TSE and (b) sagittal CT myelography images. C—clivus, CORD—spinal cord, DSAS—dorsal subarachnoid space, VSAS—ventral subarachnoid space.

An anatomic space unique to the craniocervical junction is the supraodontoid space or *apical cave*. The primary contents of the apical cave are fat, the apical ligament, a tortuous venous plexus around the apical ligament, apical arcade, anterior and posterior ascending arteries. The floor of the apical cave is the superior margin of the alar ligaments and their covering fascia. The dens apex and anterior atlantodental joint capsule form the contour of the floor. The sites of attachment of the alar ligaments on the occipital condyles are the lateral margins of the floor. The roof is comprised of the anterior inferior foramen magnum, the medial aspects of the occipital condyles, and the intercondylar occipital bone. The anterior wall is formed by the anterior occipitoatlantal membrane and the posterior wall by the tectorial membrane (**Figure 1.26a,b**).

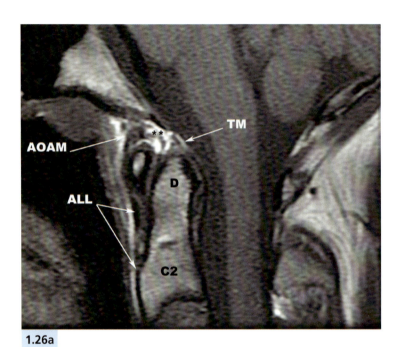
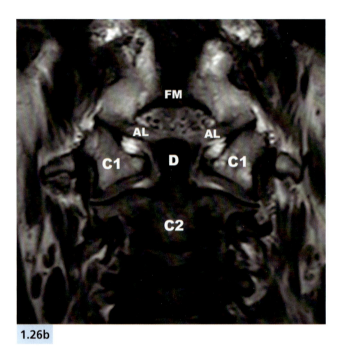

1.26a 1.26b

FIGURES 1.26a,b The boundaries of the apical cave demonstrated on sagittal and coronal T1-weighted TSE images. (a) The anterior wall is formed by the anterior occipitoatlantal membrane (AOAM) and the tectorial membrane (TM) forms the posterior wall. (b) The floor of the apical cave is the superior margin of the alar ligaments (AL) and the roof is the anterior inferior foramen magnum (FM). The primary content is fat, visualized as hyperintense signal (asterisks). ALL—anterior longitudinal ligament, D—dens.

NEURAL ANATOMY OF THE CRANIOCERVICAL JUNCTION

The transition from the medulla oblongata to the cervical spinal cord, the cervicomedullary junction (CMJ), is defined anatomically as the point of decussation of the corticospinal tracts. With MR or CT myelography, the CMJ position can be estimated by the position of regional structures. The CMJ is typically positioned 3.4 mm (± 0.9 mm) caudal to the inferior margin of the olivary bodies and 6.4 mm (± 1.3 mm) caudal to the obex. The CMJ can be estimated to reside near the superior margin of the C1 nerve roots, which can be visualized with high resolution MR and CT myelography (**Figure 1.27**).

The spinal cord at C1–C2 is more rounded in configuration than the more ovoid subaxial cervical spinal cord (**Figures 1.28a,b**). There are eight cervical cord segments, versus seven cervical vertebral segments, with the C1 segment located at the C0–C1 level. The average anterior to posterior (AP) measurements of the spinal cord at C2 and C4 are similar, but the average transverse measurements and cord area are greater at C4–C6. The surface anatomy, white matter, and gray matter anatomy are described in detail in Chapter 2.

The C1 spinal nerves arise from the C1 segment of the spinal cord, which is positioned just cranial to the atlas. The anatomy of the C1 spinal nerves is highly variable. Dorsal roots are absent around 50% of the time (**Figure 1.29**), dorsal root ganglia are variably present, and the spinal accessory nerves join with the dorsal rootlets in around 50% of patients.

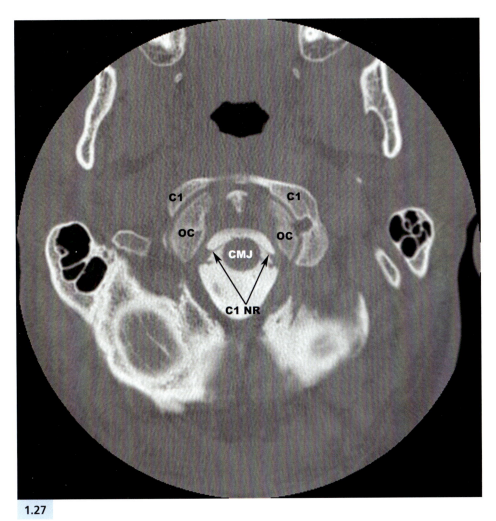

1.27

FIGURE 1.27   Axial CT myelogram demonstrating the approximate location of the cervicomedullary junction (CMJ) as estimated by the superior margins of the C1 nerve roots (C1 NR). C1—atlas, OC—occipital condyles.

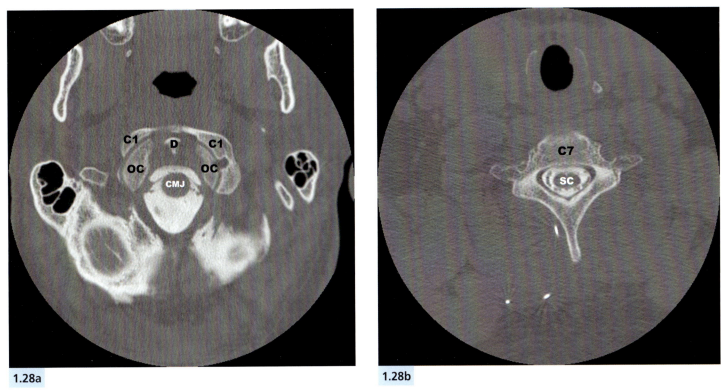

1.28a

1.28b

FIGURES 1.28a,b   Axial CT myelogram displaying the rounded shape of the (a) cervicomedullary junction (CMJ) and (b) ovoid shape of the spinal cord (SC) at C7. C1—atlas, D—dens, OC—occipital condyle.

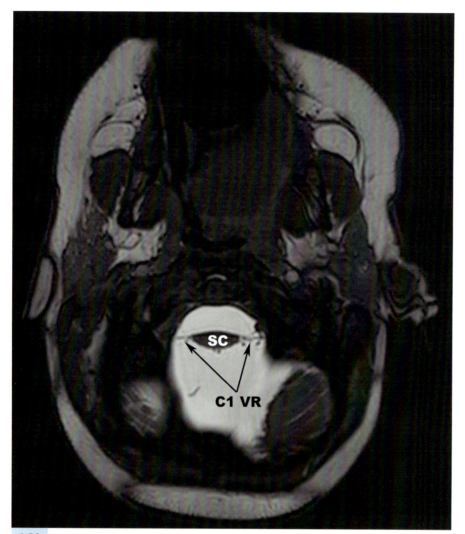

FIGURE 1.29 Axial balanced fast field echo (b-FFE) MR image demonstrating the ventral roots of C1 (C1 VR) arising from the spinal cord (SC). The C1 dorsal nerve roots are absent or very small in caliber.

1.29

The C1 ventral roots frequently share a communicating branch with the ipsilateral spinal accessory nerve, called the *nerve of McKenzie*. The C1 spinal nerves course anterior to the V3h segments of the vertebral arteries within the grooves for the vertebral arteries at the superior margins of the neural arches of the atlas. The C1 nerves accompany the vertebral arteries as they pierce the dura and the posterior occipitoatlantal membrane. The C1 spinal nerves then travel laterally and posteriorly along the posterior margin of the C1 superior articular facets, giving off ventral and dorsal rami. The C1 ventral rami wrap around the lateral margins of the C1 superior articular facets and medial to the C1 foramina transversaria. The C1 dorsal rami or *suboccipital nerves* innervate the musculature of the suboccipital triangle. The muscles innervated by the C1 ventral and dorsal rami are summarized in **Table 1.1**.

The C2 spinal nerve roots arise at the C1–C2 level (**Figure 1.30**). The C2 dorsal root ganglia and spinal nerves are located adjacent (lateral) to the lateral C1–C2 joint capsules, inferior to the C1 neural arch, superior to the C2 laminae, and lateral to the posterior atlantoaxial membrane. They provide extensive innervation of the C1–C2 lateral joint capsules and the C2–C3 zygapophyseal joint capsules. The C2 dorsal root ganglia and mixed spinal nerves are invested by a robust venous plexus that connects the posterior internal vertebral venous plexus and the vertebral veins (**Figures 1.31a,b**). The largest of the branches of the dorsal ramus is the *greater occipital nerve* that supplies the skin of the occipital scalp. The ventral rami are closely associated with the lateral C1–C2 joint capsules and ultimately join the cervical plexuses. This unique anatomic arrangement can explain some cases of cervicogenic headache.

The *spinal roots of the accessory nerves* coalesce from multiple rootlets that arise from the posterolateral sulcus of the spinal cord from C1–C5. They ascend between the denticulate ligaments anteriorly and the dorsal roots posteriorly (**Figures 1.32a–d**). There are variable connections of the spinal roots with the C1 dorsal root ganglia, if present. The spinal roots then enter the foramen magnum positioned just posterior to the vertebral arteries and travel superolaterally to exit the skull again through the pars vascularis of the jugular foramina. What has been previously characterized as the *cranial roots of the spinal accessory nerves* are best considered components of the vagus nerves.

The C1–C3 sinuvertebral nerves variably arise from the ventral ramus, dorsal root ganglia, mixed spinal nerve, vertebral artery sympathetic plexus, and gray rami communicans and reenter the intervertebral foramina to provide pain sensation to the dura, ligaments, and other components of the craniocervical junction. The C1 sinuvertebral nerves innervate the C0–C1 joint capsules, posterior arch of C1, and the dura mater. The C2 sinuvertebral nerves innervate the lateral C1–C2 joints, C2 pedicles, C1 neural arch, anterior internal vertebral venous plexus, tectorial membrane, transverse ligament, alar ligaments, hypoglossal foramina, and

TABLE 1.1   C1 Spinal Nerve Innervation

VENTRAL RAMUS

cervical plexus

rectus capitis anterior muscle

rectus capitis lateralis muscle

longus capitis muscle

sternothyroid muscle

sternohyoid muscle

omohyoid muscle

thyrohyoid muscle

geniohyoid muscle

Dorsal Ramus (Suboccipital Nerve)

rectus capitis posterior major muscle

obliquus capitis superior muscle

obliquus capitis inferior muscle

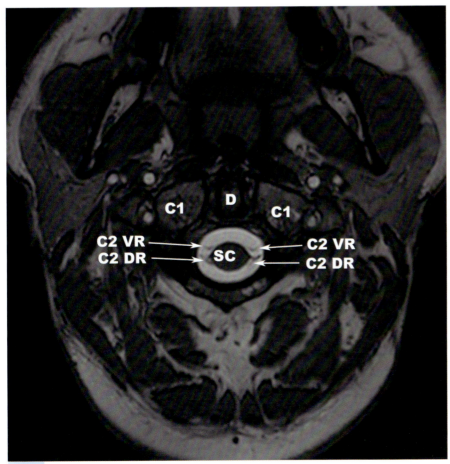

FIGURE 1.30   Axial b-FFE MR image demonstrating the C2 ventral (C2 VR) and dorsal (C2 DR) nerve roots arising from the spinal cord (SC) at the C1–C2 level. D—dens.

1.30

dura mater. The C3 sinuvertebral nerves innervate the median C1–C2 joints, C2 vertebral body and pedicles, tectorial membrane, alar ligaments, ascending band of the cruciform ligament, anterior internal vertebral venous plexus, posterior cranial fossa, and dura mater. The sinuvertebral nerves are not typically visible on conventional imaging examinations, but are mentioned here as potential cervicogenic pain generators.

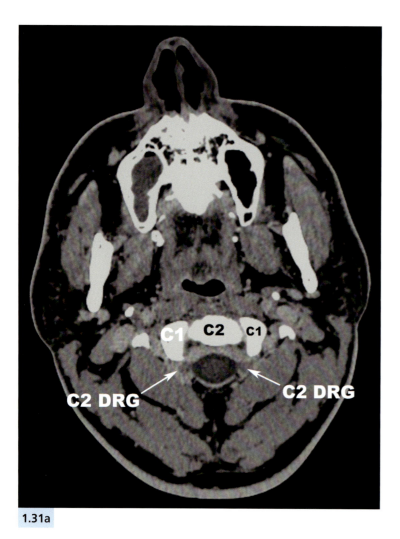

1.31a

FIGURES 1.31a,b The C2 dorsal root ganglia (C2 DRG) are demonstrated on (a) axial CT angiographic images as ovoid hypodensities against a backdrop of an extensive enhancing venous plexus. (b) Sagittal CT angiographic image demonstrates the position of the C2 DRG immediately posterior to the C1–C2 lateral joint capsules. V3h—horizontal portion V3 segment of vertebral artery.

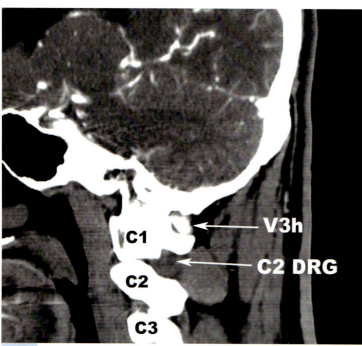

1.31b

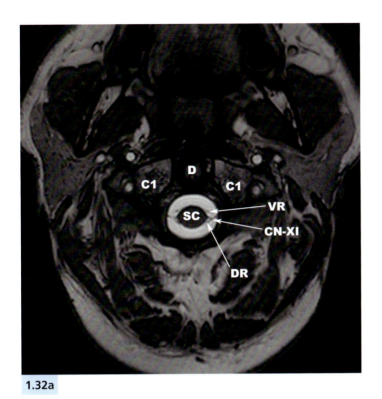

1.32a

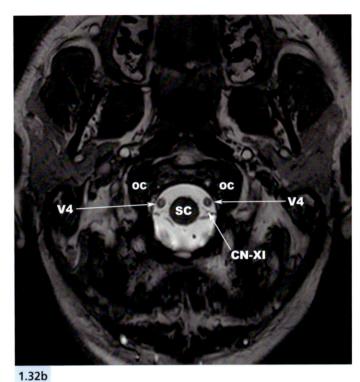

1.32b

1.32c

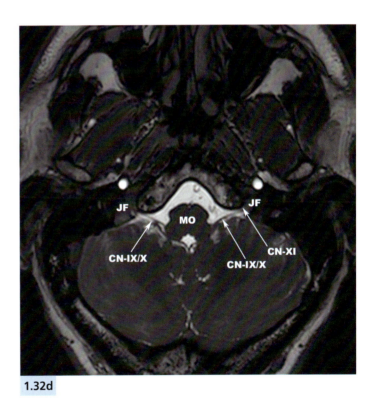

1.32d

FIGURES 1.32a–d   The course of the left spinal accessory nerve (CN-XI) is displayed on selected axial b-FFE images. (a) CN-XI forms from a coalescence of rootlets arising from C1 to C5 that course vertically between the dorsal roots and the denticulate ligament. (b) CN-XI is positioned posterior to the V4 segment of the left vertebral artery at the C0–C1 level. (c) CN-XI travels superolaterally between the occipital bone and cerebellum and (d) exits through the jugular foramen with the glossopharyngeal and vagus nerve complex (CN-IX/X). Basi—basilar artery, CN-XII—hypoglossal nerve, D—dens, DR—dorsal roots, HC—hypoglossal canal, JF—jugular foramen, MO—medulla oblongata, OC—occipital condyle, SC—spinal cord, V4—intradural segment of the vertebral artery, VR—ventral roots.

CRANIOMETRY AND MEASUREMENTS OF THE CRANIOCERVICAL JUNCTION

The complex interrelationships of the craniocervical junction structures can be assessed clinically with the use of several measurements, collectively referred to as *craniometry*. Most of these techniques were developed for use with lateral projection plain film radiographs. Several of these techniques have been modified for use with multidetector computed tomography (MDCT) or MR. As can be seen in **Table 1.2**, the plain radiography measurements do not necessarily translate to cross sectional imaging.

The *Welcher basal angle* is an indicator of skull base flattening. It is measured as the angle between lines drawn from the nasion to the tuberculum sella and from the basion to the tuberculum sella (**Figure 1.33**). A simplified version of the Welcher basal angle for use with MR has been developed by Koenigsberg et al. (2005). In this technique, the angle formed between a line drawn along the plane of the anterior cranial fossa and a line drawn through the dorsum sella along the plane of the clivus is measured (Figure 1.33).

The *Wackenheim clivus baseline* is drawn along the dorsal margin of the clivus (**Figure 1.34**). It is a measure of the position of the dens, which should not project above this line. When the dens projects through the foramen magnum above the Wackenheim line, either basilar invagination (congenital) or cranial settling (acquired) is diagnosed. The *clivus canal angle* is formed between a line drawn along the posterior vertebral body line and the Wackenheim clivus baseline (Figure 1.34). This angle is measured in flexion and extension. Spinal cord compression is more likely when the angle measures less than 150°.

TABLE 1.2 Craniocervical Junction Measurement Techniques

MEASUREMENT	NORMAL
Welcher basal angle	125°–143° (plain films) 104°–124° in children (MR); 105°–127° in adults (MR)
Welcher basal angle (modified)	113°–115° in children (MR); 116°–118° in adults
Clivus canal angle	150° in flexion to 180° in extension
Wackenhelm clivus baseline	Dens should be completely below this line
McCrae's line	Dens should be completely below this line (plain films, MDCT, MR)
Chamberlain's line	< 5–6 mm of dens above this line (plain films) < 6.2 mm of dens above this line (MDCT) < 5–6 mm of dens above this line (MR)*
McGregor's line	< 4.5 mm of dens above this line (plain films) < 6.5 mm of dens above this line (MDCT) < 5.1 mm of dens above this line (MR)*
Redlund-Johnell criterion	> 34 mm for men; > 29 mm for women (plain films) > 31.6 mm for men; > 27.4 mm for women (MDCT)
Ranawat criterion	> 15 mm for men; > 13 mm for women (plain films) > 23.7 mm for men; > 24.2 for women (modified for MDCT)
Basion to dens interval	< 12 mm for children (plain films) < 10.5 mm for children (MDCT); < 8.5 mm for adults (MDCT)
Basion-axial interval	< 12 mm (unreliable and not recommended)
Powers ratio	< 1.0 (plain films, MDCT, MR)
Atlantooccipital interval	< 5 mm for children (plain films) < 2.5 mm for children (MDCT); 0.5–1.4 mm for adults (MDCT)
Condylar sum	< 4.2 mm for adults (MDCT)
Anterior atlantal dental interval	< 4.5–5 mm for children (plain films); < 3 mm for adults (plain films) < 2.6 mm for children (MDCT); < 2 mm for adults (MDCT)
Posterior atlantal dental interval	>14 mm for adults (plain films)
C1–C2 spinolaminar line	< 7.8 mm for adults (MDCT)
Atlantoaxial interval	< 3.9 mm for children (MDCT); < 3.4 mm for adults (MDCT)

*potential for false positives
MDCT, multidetector computed tomography.

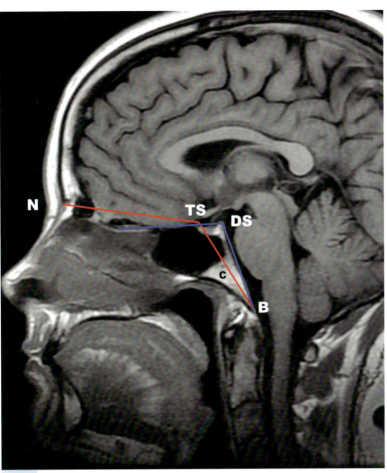

FIGURE 1.33 The Welcher basal angle (red) designed for use with plain films and a modified version of the Welcher basal angle (blue) designed for use in MR are demonstrated on a mid-sagittal T1-weighted TSE MR image. B—basion, C—clivus, DS—dorsum sella, N—nasion, TS—tuberculum sella.

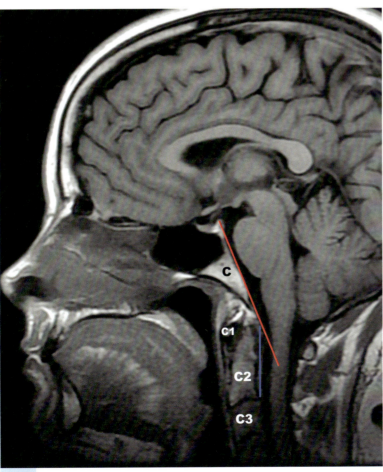

FIGURE 1.34 Mid-sagittal T1-weighted TSE image demonstrating the Wackenheim clivus baseline (red line) and the clivus canal angle (intersection of red and blue lines). C—clivus.

Other measures of basilar invagination or cranial settling include McCrae's line, Chamberlain's line, McGregor's line, and Clark's station. McCrae's line is drawn from the basion to the opisthion (**Figure 1.35**). Chamberlain's line is drawn from the hard palate to the opisthion (Figure 1.35). McGregor's line is used when the opisthion cannot be seen. It is drawn from the hard palate to the most inferior point of the occipital curve (Figure 1.35). Clark's station refers to the position of the anterior arch of the atlas relative to the dens (**Figure 1.36**). In this system, the dens is divided into thirds; upper (station I), middle (station II), and inferior (station III). The anterior arch of the atlas should be located in the rostral one third of the dens (station I).

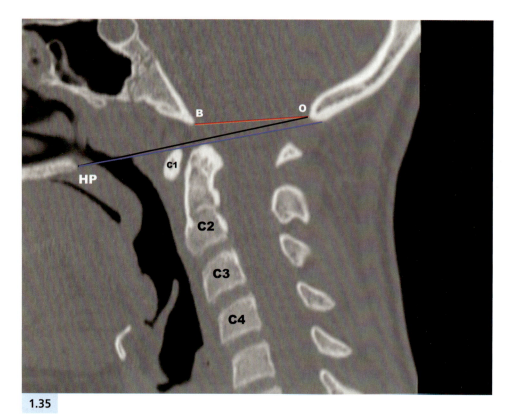

FIGURE 1.35 Mid-sagittal cervical spine CT image demonstrates McCrae's line (red), Chamberlain's line (black), and McGregor's line (blue). B—basion, HP—hard palate, O—opisthion.

1.35

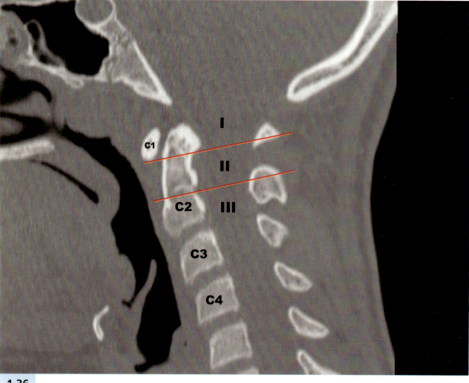

FIGURE 1.36 Clark's stations demonstrated on a mid-sagittal cervical spine CT. If the anterior arch of C1 is level with station II or III, basilar invagination is diagnosed.

1.36

When the dens cannot be visualized, different measurement techniques are available to evaluate for basilar invagination or cranial settling, including the Redlund-Johnell and Ranawat criterion. The *Redlund-Johnell criterion* is the distance from the McGregor line to the inferior margin of the C2 vertebral body (**Figure 1.37**). The *Ranawat criterion* is the distance from the transverse axis of C1 to the center of the C2 pedicle (**Figure 1.38**).

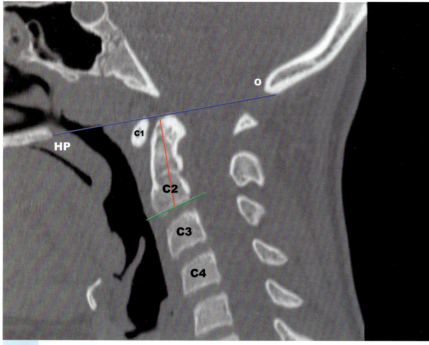

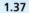
1.37

FIGURE 1.37   The Redlund-Johnell criterion is the distance between the McGregor line and the midpoint of a line drawn along the inferior endplate of C2 (red line) as demonstrated on a mid-sagittal CT of the cervical spine. HP—hard palate, O—opisthion.

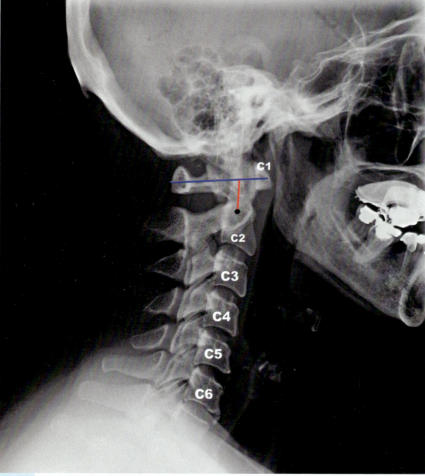
1.38

FIGURE 1.38   The Ranawat criterion is the distance (red line) from the transverse axis of C1 (blue line) to the center of the C2 pedicle (black dot) and is demonstrated on a lateral radiograph of the cervical spine.

Techniques designed to predict occipitoatlantal (C0–C1) dissociation include the basion-dens interval, basion-axial interval, Powers ratio, and the condylar sum. The *basion-dens interval* is the distance from the tip of the dens to the basion (**Figure 1.39**). The *basion-axial interval* is the distance from the basion to the posterior axial line, a line drawn along the posterior margin of C2 and extended superiorly (Figure 1.39). The *Powers ratio* is the distance from the basion to the internal margin of the C1 neural arch divided by the distance from the opisthion to the internal margin of the C1 anterior arch (**Figure 1.40**). The *condylar sum* is the addition of the

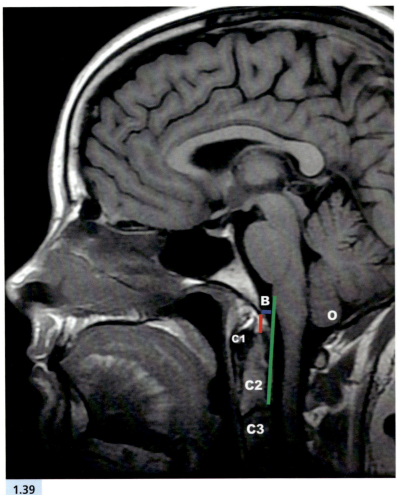

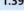

FIGURE 1.39   Mid-sagittal T1-weighted TSE MR image demonstrates the basion to dens interval (red line) and the basion-axial interval (blue line), which is the distance from the basion to the posterior axial line (green line). B—basion, O—opisthion.

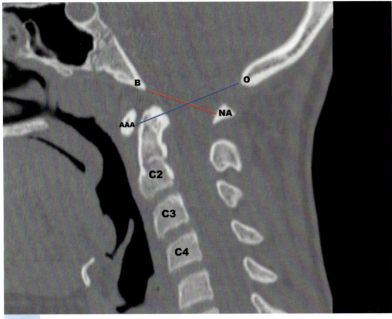

FIGURE 1.40   The Powers ratio is the distance between the basion and the internal margin of the C1 neural arch divided by the distance between the opisthion and the internal margin of the C1 anterior arch. AAA—anterior arch of atlas, B—basion, NA—neural arch of C1, O—opisthion.

distances from the points of greatest separation of the occipital condyles and the C1 superior articular processes, measured perpendicular to the articular surfaces (**Figure 1.41**).

The integrity of the atlantoaxial (C1–C2) joints is assessed with a variety of techniques that include the anterior atlantodental interval, posterior atlantodental interval, C1–C2 spinolaminar line, and atlantoaxial interval. The *anterior atlantodental interval* (AADI) is measured from the inner margin of the C1 anterior arch to the anterior margin of the dens (**Figure 1.42**). The measured AADI is greater in children due to relative ligamentous laxity in childhood. The *posterior atlantodental interval* (PADI) is measured from the posterior margin

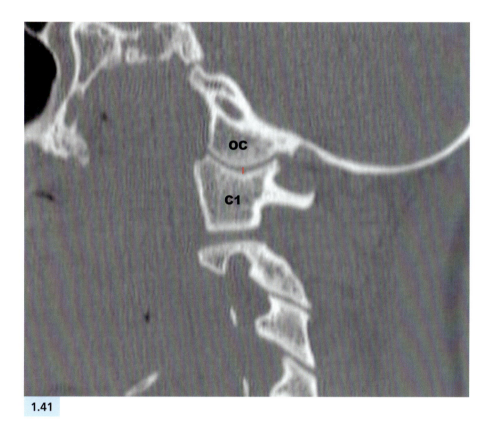

1.41

FIGURE 1.41   Sagittal cervical spine CT image demonstrating the measurement of the C0–C1 joint space (red line). The C0–C1 joint space measurements from each side are added together to give the condylar sum. OC—occipital condyle.

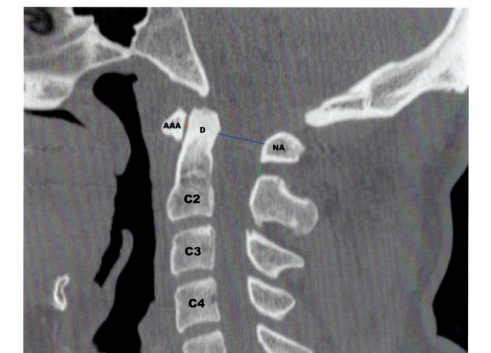

1.42

FIGURE 1.42   Mid-sagittal cervical spine CT demonstrating the anterior atlantodental interval (red line), which is drawn between the internal margin of the C1 anterior arch (AAA) to the anterior margin of the dens (D). The posterior atlantodental interval (blue line) is drawn from the posterior margin of the dens to the internal margin of the C1 neural arch (NA). The green line shows the C1–C2 spinolaminar line.

of the dens to the anterior margin of the C1 lamina (Figure 1.42). The PADI provides an indication of the residual spinal canal diameter in the setting of atlantoaxial instability. The *C1–C2 spinolaminar line* is the distance between the inferior margin of the C1 neural arch to the superior margin of the C2 neural arch, measured at the midline (Figure 1.42). The *atlantoaxial interval* is measured from the inferior surface of the C1 inferior articular process to the C2 superior articular process at three points (medial, intermediate, lateral; **Figure 1.43**).

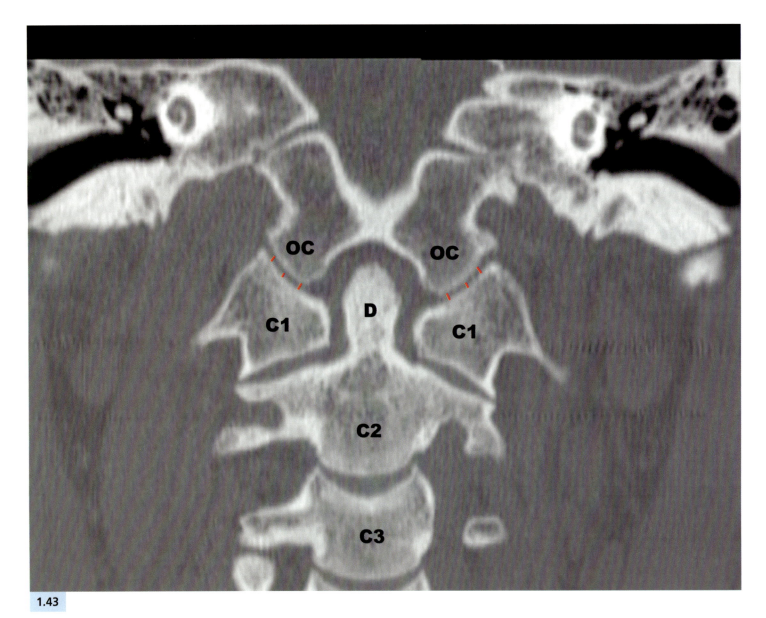

1.43

FIGURE 1.43   The atlantoaxial interval is measured from the inferior surface of the C1 inferior articular process to the C2 superior articular process at three points: medial, lateral, and intermediate (red lines). D—dens, OC—occipital condyle.

GALLERY OF COMMON ANATOMIC VARIANTS

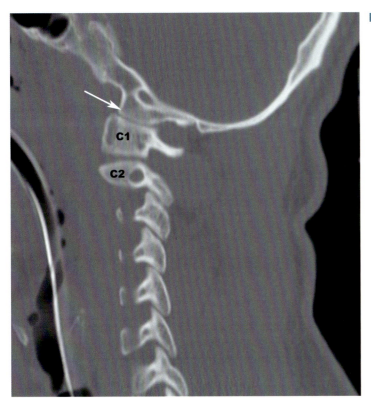

IMAGE 1   Flat occipital condyles (arrow).

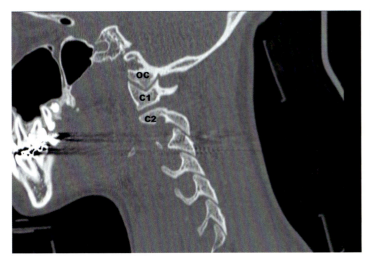

IMAGE 2   Triangular occipital condyles. OC—occipital condyle.

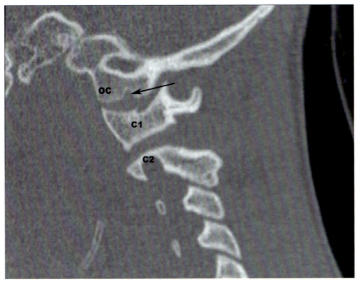

IMAGE 3   Synchondrosis intraoccipitalis anterior (arrow). OC—occipital condyle.

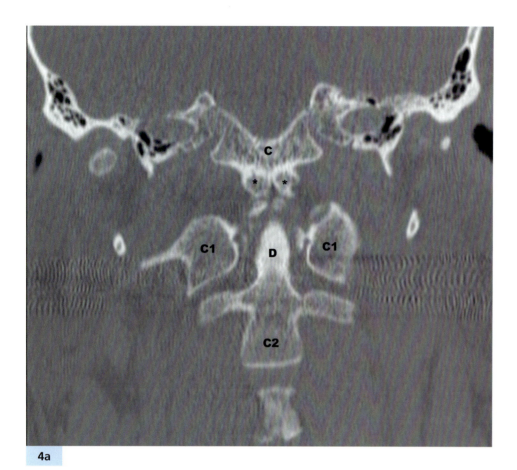

4a

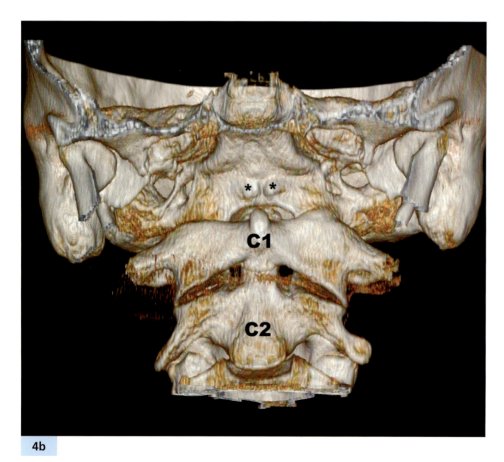

4b

IMAGES 4a,b   Processus basilaris (asterisks). C—clivus, D—dens.

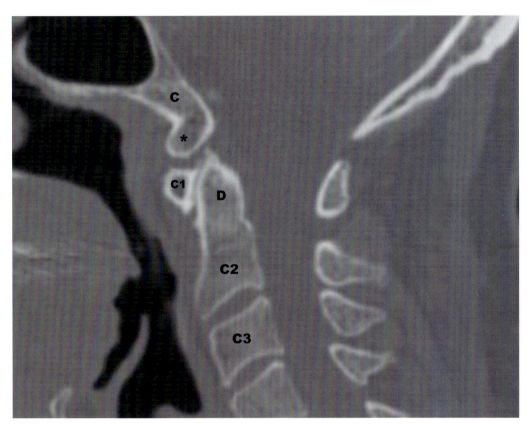

IMAGE 5   Prebasioccipital arch (asterisk). C—clivus, D—dens.

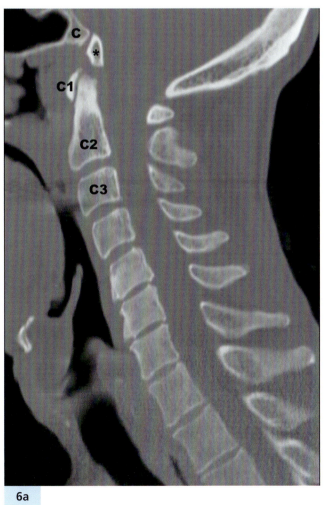

6a

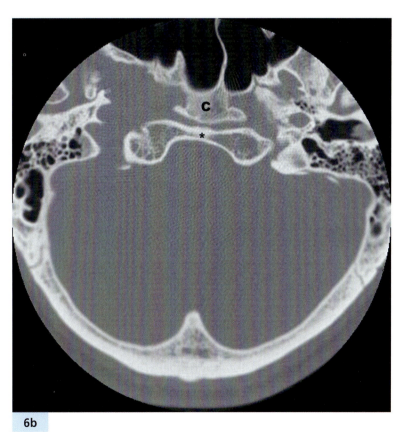

6b

IMAGES 6a,b   Occipital vertebra (asterisk). C—clivus.

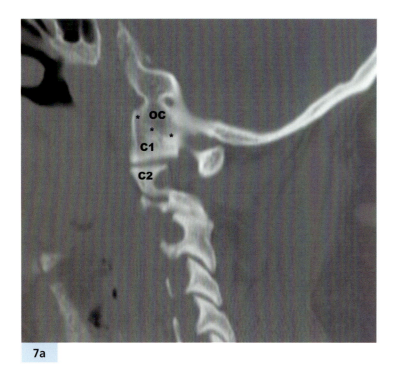

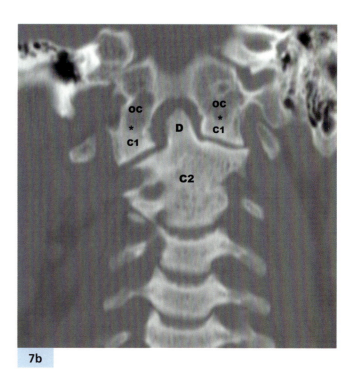

IMAGES 7a,b   Occipitalized atlas (asterisks mark the site of fusion). D—dens, OC—occipital condyle.

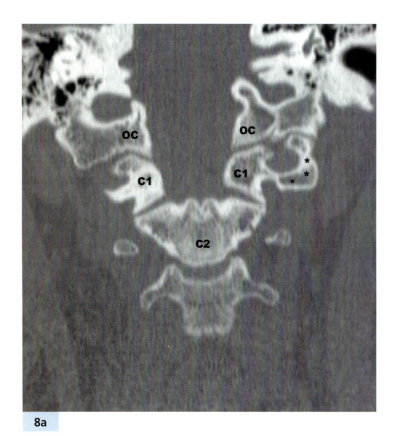

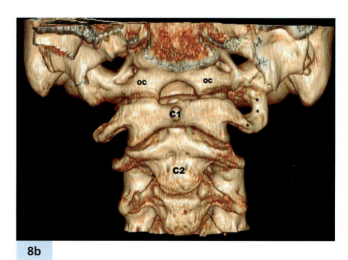

IMAGES 8a,b   Paracondylar process (asterisks). OC—occipital condyle.

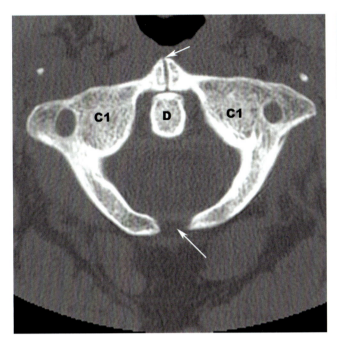

IMAGE 9   Split atlas (white arrows). D—dens.

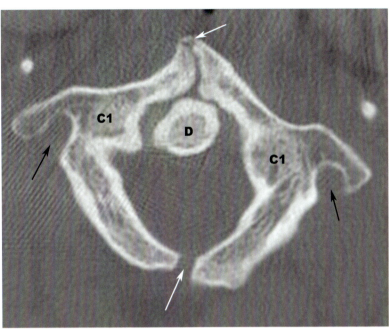

IMAGE 10   Split atlas (white arrows) and nonfusion of the C1 foramina transversaria (black arrows). D—dens.

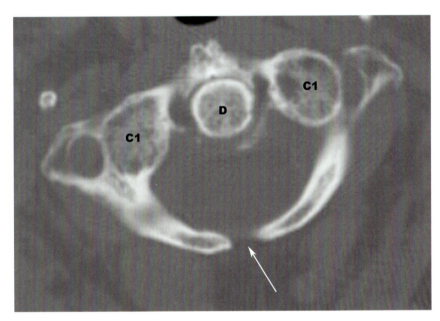

IMAGE 11   Nonfused C1 neural arch centrally (white arrow). D—dens.

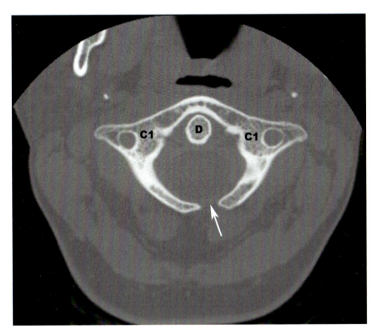

IMAGE 12   Nonfused C1 neural arch on the left (white arrow). D—dens.

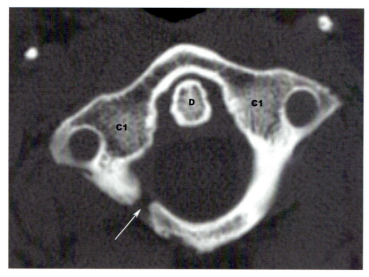

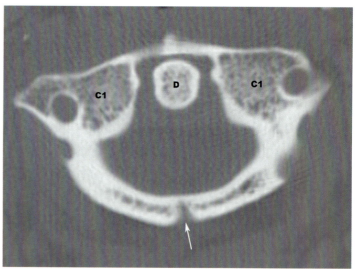

IMAGE 13   Nonfused C1 neural arch on the right (white arrow). D—dens.

IMAGE 14   Partially nonfused neural arch centrally (white arrow). D—dens.

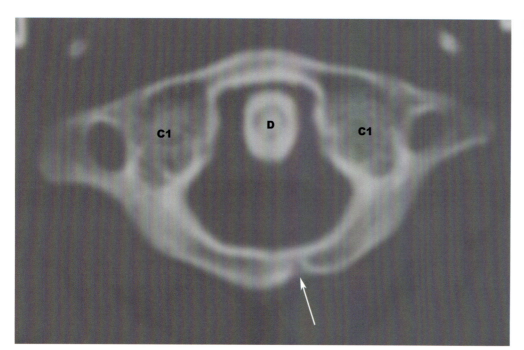

IMAGE 15   Partially nonfused neural arch on the left (white arrow). D—dens.

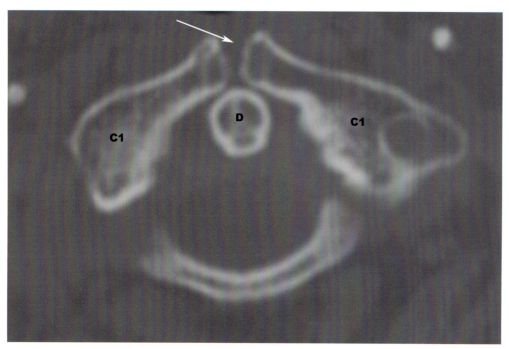

IMAGE 16   Nonfused anterior arch (white arrow). D—dens.

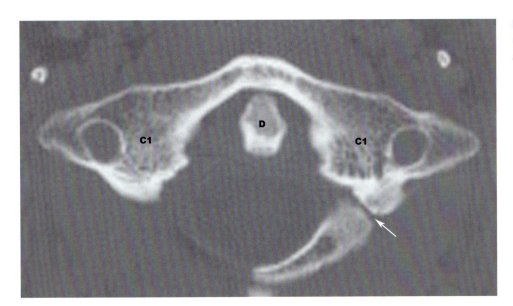

IMAGE 17 Nonfused left neural arch (white arrow) and absent right neural arch. D—dens.

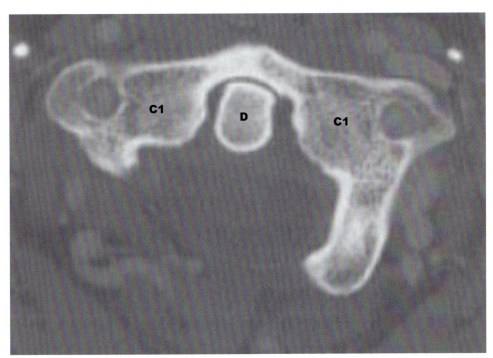

IMAGE 18 Absent right neural arch. D—dens.

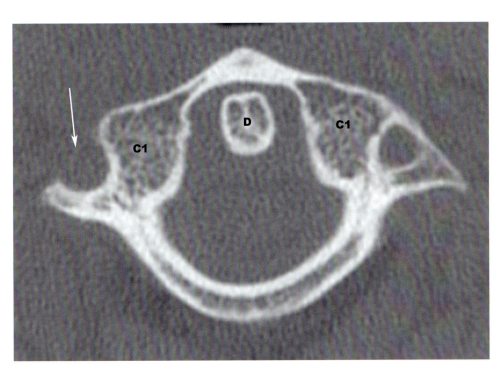

IMAGE 19 Nonfused right C1 transverse foramen (white arrow). D—dens.

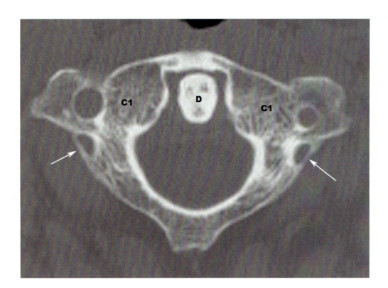

IMAGE 20   Variant arcuate foramina (white arrows). D—dens.

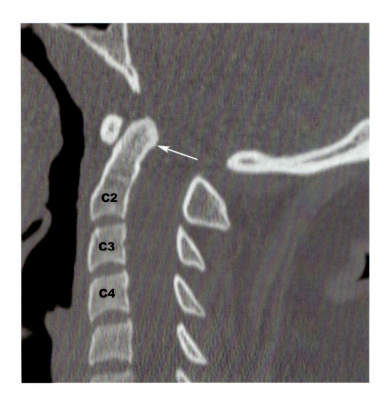

IMAGE 21   Retroverted dens (white arrow).

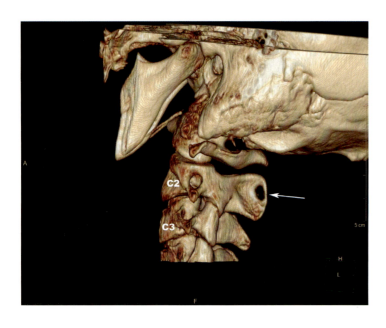

IMAGE 22   Variant C2 spinous process (white arrow).

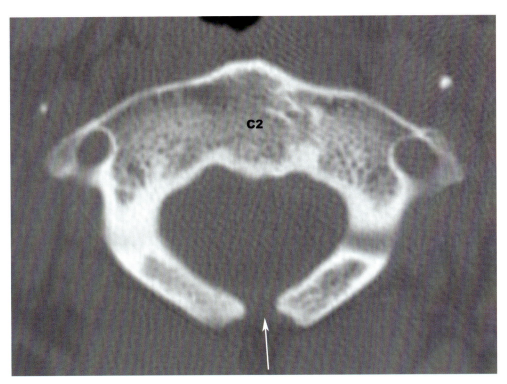

IMAGE 23   Nonfused C2 neural arch (white arrow).

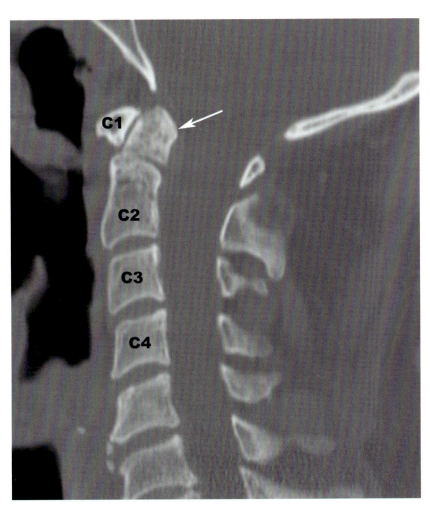

IMAGE 24   Os odontoideum (white arrow).

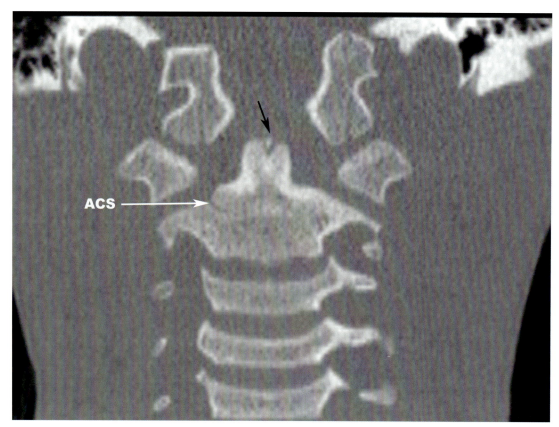

IMAGE 25   Asymmetric fusion of the right acrocentral synchondrosis (ACS). Normal ossiculum terminale (black arrow).

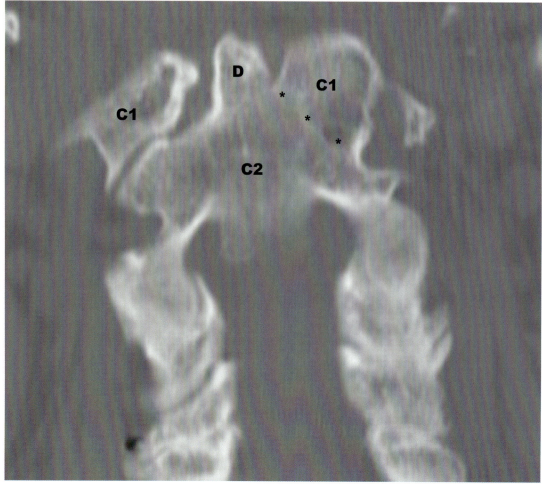

IMAGE 26   Fused left C1-C2 lateral masses (asterisks). D—dens.

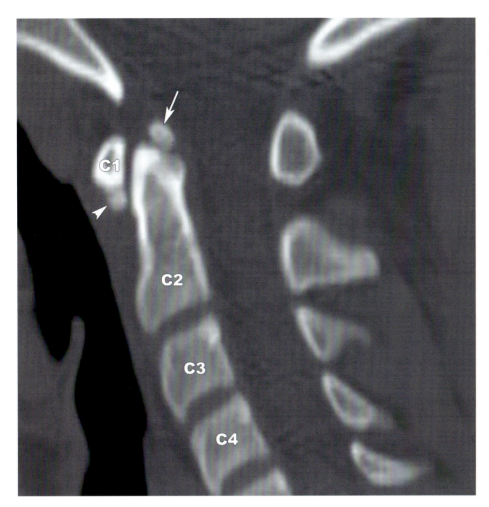

IMAGE 27   Ossiculum terminale of Bergmann (arrow) and a small ossicle located at the inferior margin of the C1 anterior arch (arrowhead).

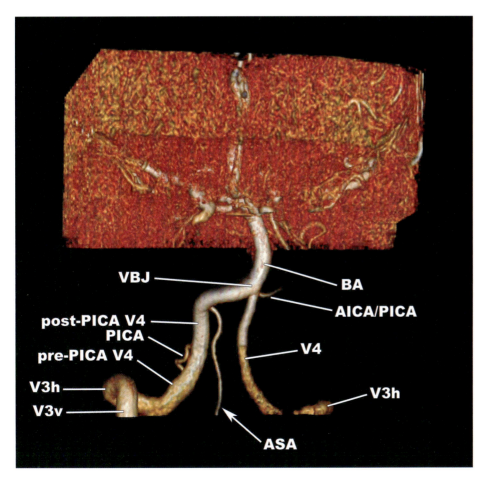

IMAGE 28   Large caliber anterior spinal artery (ASA) arising from the post-PICA V4 segment of the right vertebral artery. AICA/ PICA—common trunk of the anterior inferior cerebellar and posterior inferior cerebellar arteries, BA—basilar artery, PICA—posterior inferior cerebellar artery, VBJ—vertebrobasilar artery, V3h—horizontal portion V3 segment of vertebral artery, V3v—vertical portion V3 segment of vertebral artery, V4—intradural segment of the vertebral artery.

SUGGESTED READINGS

Arnautovic KI, Al-Mefty O, Pait TG, et al. The suboccipital cavernous sinus. *J Neurosurg.* 1997;86:252–262.

Ballesteros L, Forero P, Quintero I. Morphological expression of the anterior spinal artery and the intracranial segment of the vertebral artery: a direct anatomic study. *Rom J Morphol Embryol.* 2013;54(3):513–518.

Benke M, Yu WD, Peden SC, et al. Occipitocervical junction: imaging, pathology, instrumentation. *Am J Orthop.* 2011;40(10):E205-E215.

Bertozzi JC, Rojas CA, Martinez CR. Evaluation of the pediatric craniocervical junction on MDCT. *Am J Roentgenol.* 2009;192:26–31.

Cacciola F, Phalke U, Goel A. Vertebral artery in relationship to C1-C2 vertebrae: an anatomical study. *Neurol India.* 2004;52(2):178–184.

Campos D, Goerck ML, Ellwanger JH, et al. Anatomy of the first spinal nerve—a review. *J Morphol Sci.* 2012;29(2):65–68.

Caruso RD, Rosenbaum AE, Chang JK, et al. Craniocervical junction venous anatomy on enhanced MR images: the suboccipital cavernous sinus. *Am J Neuroradiol.* 1999;20:1127–1131.

Chamberlain WE. Basilar impression (platybasia). A bizarre developmental anomaly of the occipital bone and upper cervical spine with striking and misleading neurologic manifestations. *Yale J Biol Med.* 1939;11(5):487–496.

Chang W, Alexander MT, Mirvis SE. Diagnostic determinants of craniocervical distraction injury in adults. *Am J Roentgenol.* 2009;192:52–58.

Cronin CG, Lohan DG, Ni Mhuircheartigh J, et al. MRI evaluation and measurement of the normal odontoid peg position. *Clin Radiol.* 2007;62:897–903.

Duan S, Lv S, Ye F, et al. Imaging anatomy and variation of vertebral artery and bone structure at craniocervical junction. *Eur Spine J.* 2009;18:1102–1108.

Dickman CA, Lekovic GP: Biomechanical considerations for stabilization of the craniovertebral junction. *Clin Neurosurg.* 2005;53:205–213.

Dvorak J, Panjabi M. Functional anatomy of the alar ligaments. *Spine.* 1987;12(2):183–189.

Er U, Fraser K, Lanzino G. The anterior spinal artery origin: a microanatomical study. *Spinal Cord.* 2008;46(1):45–49.

Gire JD, Roberto RF, Bobinski M, et al. The utility and accuracy of computed tomography in the diagnosis of occipitocervical dissociation. *The Spine Journal.* 2013;13:510–519.

Gray H. Osteology. In: Howden R, Jex-Blake AJ, Fedden WF, eds. *Anatomy, Descriptive and Applied.* 18th ed. New York, NY: Lea & Febiger; 1913:210.

Haffajee MR. A contribution by the ascending pharyngeal artery to the arterial supply of the odontoid process of the axis vertebra. *Clin Anat.* 1997;10(1):14–18.

Haffajee MR, Thompson C, Govender S. The supraodontoid space or "apical cave" at the craniocervical junction: a microdissection study. *Clin Anat.* 2008;21:405–415.

Harris JH Jr, Carson GC, Wagner LK. Radiologic diagnosis of traumatic occipitovertebral dissociation: 1. Normal occipitovertebral relationships on lateral radiographs of supine subjects. *Am J Roentgenol.* 1994;162:881–886.

Harris JH Jr, Carson GC, Wagner LK. Radiologic diagnosis of traumatic occipitovertebral dissociation: 2. Comparison of three methods of detecting occipitovertebral relationships on lateral radiographs of supine subjects. *Am J Roentgenol.* 1994;162:887–892.

Hovorka MS, Uray NJ. Microscopic clusters of sensory neurons in C1 spinal nerve roots and in the C1 level of the spinal accessory nerve in adult humans. *Anat Record.* 2013;296:1588–1593.

Is M, Sevinc O, Safak AA, et al. Assessment of the atlanto-occipital junction in the MRI of subjects with cervical disc herniation. *Neurosciences.* 2007;12(4):289–292.

Junewick JJ, Chin MS, Meesa IR, et al. Ossification patterns of the atlas vertebra. *AJR.* 2011;197:1229–1234.

Kaufman RA, Carroll CD, Buncher CR. Atlantooccipital junction: standards for measurement in normal children. *Am J Neuroradiol.* 1987;8:995–999.

Karwacki GM & Schneider JF. Normal ossification patterns of atlas and axis: a CT study. *Am J Neuroradiol.* 2012;33(10):1882–1887.

Koenigsberg RA, Vakil N, Hong TA, et al. Evaluation of platybasia with MR imaging. *Am J Neuroradiol.* 2005;26:89–92.

Kwong Y, Rao N, Latief K. Craniometric measurements in the assessment of craniovertebral settling: are they still relevant in the age of cross-sectional imaging? *Am J Roentgenol.* 2011;196:W421-W425

McGregor M. The significance of certain measurements of the skull in the diagnosis of basilar impression. *Br J Radiol.* 1948;21:171–181.

McRae DL. Bony abnormalities in the region of the foramen magnum: correlation of the anatomic and neurologic findings. *Acta Radiol.* 1953;40(2–3):335–354.

Middlebrooks EH, Tagmurlu K, Bennett JA, et al. Normal relationship of the cervicomedullary junction with the obex and olivary bodies: a comparison of cadaveric dissection and in vivo diffusion tensor imaging. *Surg Radiol Anat.* doi:10.1007/s00276-014-1387-2

Moon WJ, Roh HG, Chung EC. Detailed MR imaging anatomy of the cisternal segments of the glossopharyngeal, vagus, and spinal accessory nerves in the posterior fossa: the use of 3D balanced fast-field echo MR imaging. *Am J Neuroradiol*. 2009;30:1116–1120.

Paluzzi A, Belli A, Lafuente J, et al. Role of the C2 articular branches in occipital headache: an anatomical study. *Clin Anat*. 2006;19:497–502.

Panjabi M, Dvorak J, Crisco J III, et al. Flexion, extension, and lateral bending of the upper cervical spine in response to alar ligament transections. *J Spinal Disord*. 1991;4:157–167.

Panjabi M, Dvorak J, Yamamoto I, et al. Three dimensional movements of the upper cervical spine. *Spine*. 1988;13:726–730.

Poppel MH, Jacobson HG, Duff BK, et al. Basilar impression and platybasia in Paget's disease. *Radiology*. 1953;61:639–644.

Powers B, Miller MD, Kramer RS, et al. Traumatic anterior atlanto-occipital dislocation. *Neurosurgery*. 1979;4:12–17.

Ranawat CS, O'Leary P, Pellicci P, et al. Cervical spine fusion in rheumatoid arthritis. *J Bone Joint Surg Am*. 1979;61(7):1003–1010.

Redlund-Johnell, Pettersson H. Radiographic measurements of the craniovertebral region. Designed for evaluation of abnormalities in rheumatoid arthritis. *Acta Radiol Diagn (Stockh)*. 1094;25(1):23–28.

Rennie C, Haffajee MR, Ebrahim MAA. Sinuvertebral nerves at the craniovertebral junction: a microdissection study. *Clin Anat*. 2013;26:357–366.

Rojas CA, Bertozzi JC, Martinez CR, et al. Reassessment of the craniocervical junction: normal values on CT. *Am J Neuroradiol*. 2007;28:1819–1823.

Rojas CA, Hayes A, Bertozzi JC, et al. Evaluation of the C1-C2 articulation on MDCT in healthy children and young adults. *Am J Roentgenol*. 2009;193:1388–1392.

Ruiz DSM, Gailloud P, Rufenacht DA, et al. The craniocervical venous system in relation to cerebral venous drainage. *Am J Neuroradiol*. 2002;23:1500–1508.

Ryan S, Blyth P, Duggan N, et al. Is the cranial accessory nerve really a portion of the accessory nerve? Anatomy of the cranial nerves in the jugular foramen. *Anat Sci Int*. 2007;82(1):1–7.

Schilling J, Schilling A, Suazo GI. Ponticulus posticus on the posterior arch of atlas, prevalence analysis in asymptomatic patients. *Int J Morphol*. 2010;28(1):317–322.

Sherman JL, Nassaux PY, Citrin CM. Measurements of the normal cervical spinal cord on MR imaging. *Am J Neuroradiol*. 1990;11(2):369–372.

Smoker WR. Craniovertebral junction: normal anatomy, craniometry, and congenital anomalies. *Radiographics*. 1994;14(2):255–277.

Smoker WR. Imaging of the craniovertebral junction. *Magn Reson Imaging Clin North Am*. 2000;8(3):635–650.

Stanoue S, Kiyosue H, Sagara Y, et al. Venous structures at the craniocervical junction: anatomical variations evaluated by multidetector row CT. *Br J Radiol*. 2010;83:831–840.

Steinmetz MP, Mroz TE, Benzel EC. Craniovertebral junction: biomechanical considerations. *Neurosurgery*.2010; 66:A7–A12.

Stubs DM. The arcuate foramen: variability in distribution related to race and sex. *Spine*. 1992;17(12):1502–1504.

Takahashi S, Sakuma I, Omachi K, et al. Craniocervical junction venous anatomy around the suboccipital cavernous sinus: evaluation by MR imaging. *Eur Radiol*. 2005;15:1694–1700.

Tassanawipas A, Mokkhavesa S, Chatchavong S, et al. Magnetic resonance imaging study of the craniocervical junction. *J Orthop Surg*. 2005;13(3):228–231.

Tubbs RS, Grabb P, Spooner A, et al. The apical ligament: anatomy and functional significance. *J Neurosurg Spine*. 2000;92(2 suppl):197–200.

Tubbs RS, Ammar K, Liechty P, et al. The marginal sinus. *J Neurosurg*. 2006;104:429–431.

Tubbs RS, Hansasuta A, Loukas M, et al. The basilar venous plexus. *Clin Anat*. 2007;29(7):755–759.

Tubbs RS, Loukas M, Slappey JB, et al. Clinical anatomy of the C1 dorsal root, ganglion, and ramus: a review and anatomical study. *Clin Anat*. 2007;20:624–627.

Tubbs RS, Shah NA, Sullivan BP, et al. Surgical anatomy and quantitation of the branches of the V2 and V3 segments of the vertebral artery. *J Neurosurg Spine*. 2009;11:84–87.

Tubbs RS, Dixon J, Loukas M, et al. Ligament of Barkow of the craniocervical junction: its anatomy and potential clinical and functional significance. *J Neurosurg Spine*. 2010;12:619–622.

Tubbs RS, Hallock JD, Radcliff V, et al. Ligaments of the craniocervical junction: a review. *J Neurosurg Spine*. 2011;14:697–709.

Tubbs RS, Benninger B, Loukas M, et al. The nerve of McKenzie: anatomic study with application to intradural rhizotomy for spasmodic torticollis. *Br J Neurosurg*. 2014;28(5):650–652.

Wackenheim A. *Roentgen Diagnosis of the Cranio-vertebral Region*. New York, NY: Springer-Verlag; 1974.

The Subaxial Cervical Spine

2

*T*he subaxial cervical spine is the anatomic region that includes the C3–C7 vertebrae, the cervical spinal cord, C3–C8 spinal nerves, the spinal accessory nerve, blood vessels, multiple synovial joints, ligaments, and lymphatics. As opposed to the specialized structure and function of the C1 and C2 segments, the subaxial cervical segmental morphology is more uniform. As such, the subaxial cervical segments are commonly referred to as the *typical cervical segments*.

DEVELOPMENTAL ANATOMY OF THE SUBAXIAL CERVICAL SPINE

The subaxial segments are formed from three primary ossification centers: a centrum, right, and left neural arches. The neurocentral synchondroses are located between the centrum and each neural arch. The intraneural synchondrosis is located between the dorsal tips of the neural arches (**Figure 2.1**).

The subaxial segments develop over the first 4 months of fetal life, starting with C7 early in fetal life and progressing rostrally to C3. At birth, the subaxial segments are characterized by shallow divots along the anterolateral margins of the neural arches at the sites of the developing foramina transversaria. The centra have a characteristic configuration in the sagittal plane, with slight downward sloping of the superior endplates, flat inferior endplates, and rounded anterior superior corners.

The neural arches fuse posteriorly around 2 years of age and fuse to the centra around 3 to 4 years of age. The ventral bars of the transverse processes ossify between 3 and 4 years of age, forming complete foramina transversaria. The subaxial segments typically have six secondary ossification centers that fuse in adolescence, including the tips of the transverse processes, tips of the bifid spinous processes, and ring apophyses along the superior and inferior endplates. A single secondary ossification center arises at the tip of the monofid C7 spinous process. The developmental sequence of the subaxial cervical vertebrae is displayed in **Figures 2.2a–t**.

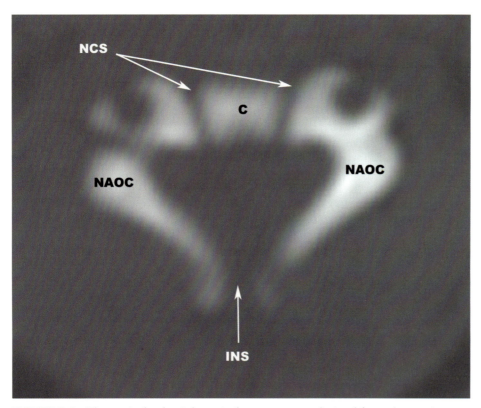

FIGURE 2.1   The typical subaxial cervical segments are derived from three primary ossification centers, a centrum (C) and two neural arch ossification centers (NAOC). The neurocentral synchondroses (NCS) are located between the centrum and the neural arch ossification centers. The intraneural synchondrosis (INS) is located between the neural arch ossification centers posteriorly.

Newborn

3 months

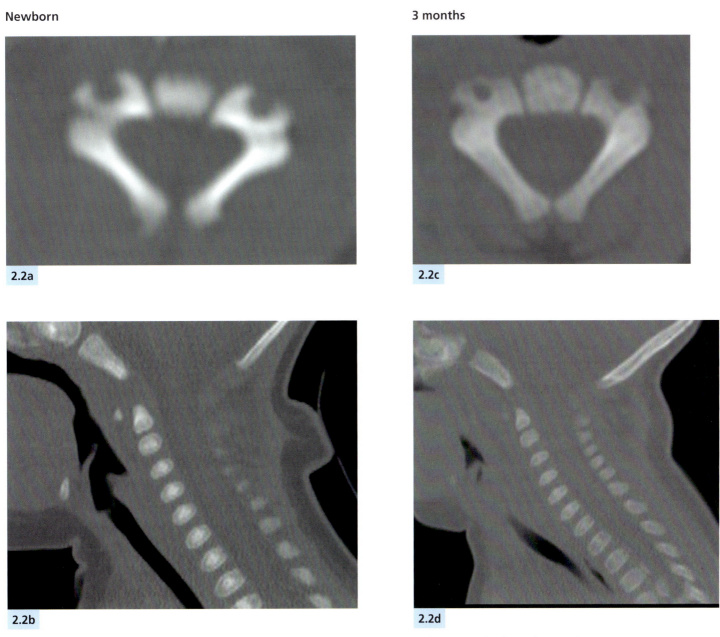

FIGURES 2.2a–t
2.2a
2.2b
2.2c
2.2d

FIGURES 2.2a–t   The typical appearance of the primary ossification centers of the typical subaxial cervical segments at various ages: (a,b)—newborn, (c,d)—3 months, (e,f)—6 months, (g,h)—12 months, (i,j)—2 years, (k,l)—3 years, (m,n)—4 years, (o,p)—5 years, 10 years (q,r), and 18 years (s,t).

(continued)

6 months

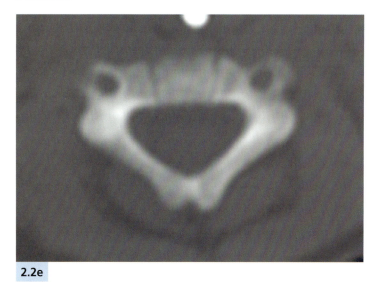

2.2e

12 months

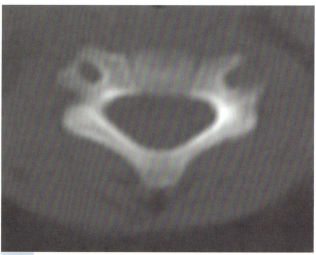

2.2g

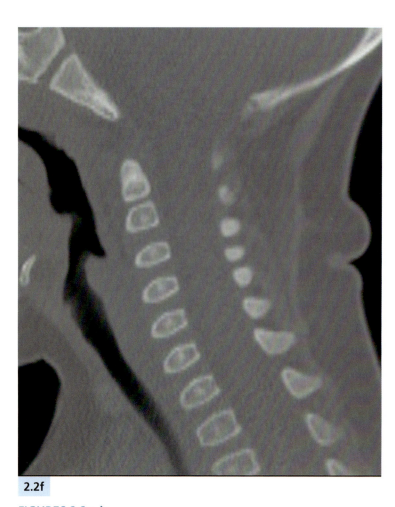

2.2f

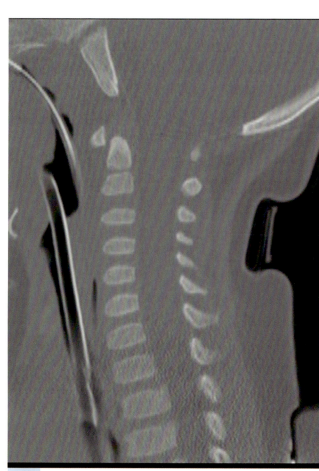

2.2h

FIGURES 2.2e–h

(continued)

2 years

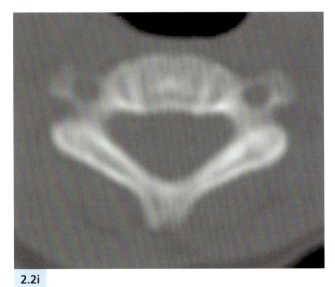

2.2i

3 years

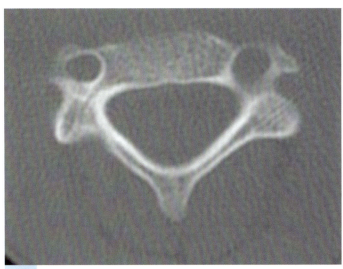

2.2k

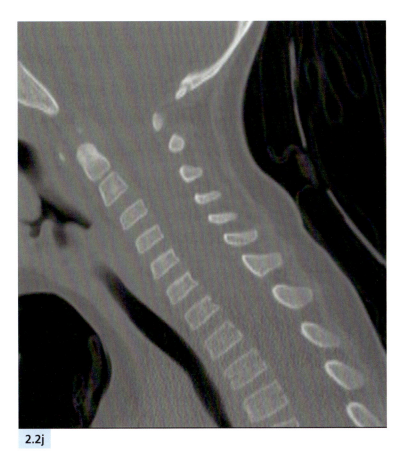

2.2j

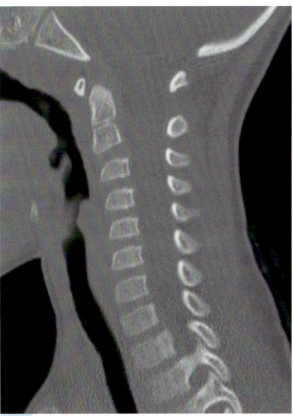

2.2l

FIGURES 2.2i–l

(continued)

4 years

5 years

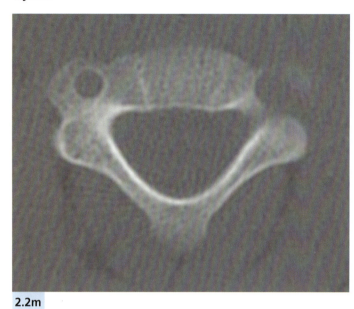

2.2m

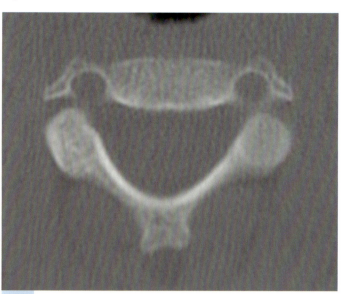

2.2o

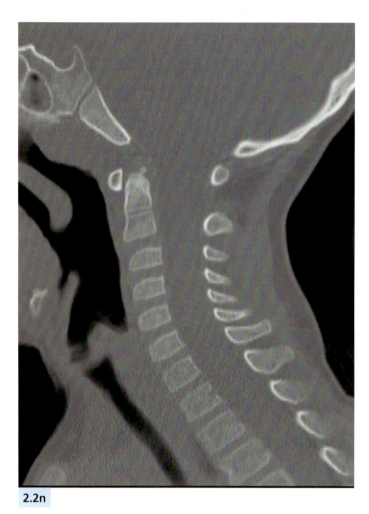

2.2n

2.2p

FIGURES 2.2m–p

(continued)

10 years

18 years

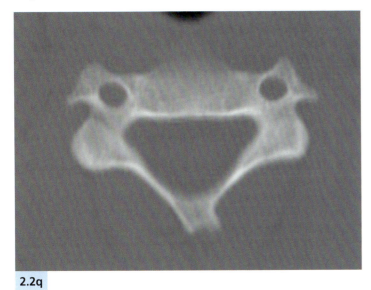

2.2q

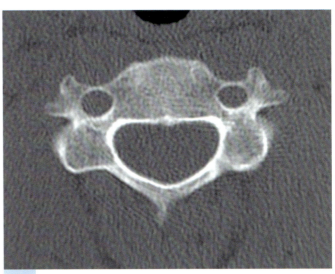

2.2s

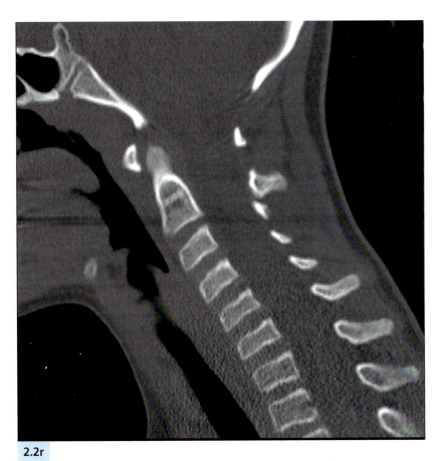

2.2r

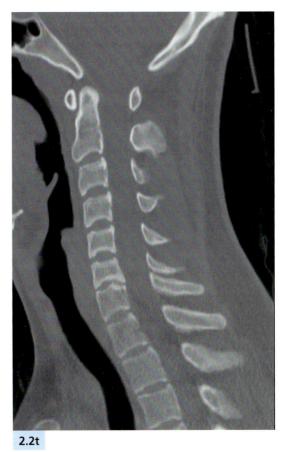

2.2t

FIGURES 2.2q–t

MULTIMODALITY ATLAS IMAGES OF THE SUBAXIAL CERVICAL SPINE

The primary modalities used to image the subaxial cervical spine are plain films, computed tomography (CT), and magnetic resonance imaging (MRI). The basic anatomy of the subaxial cervical segments is presented in **Figures 2.3a–r** in order to provide a foundation prior to the more detailed anatomic descriptions to follow.

■ PLAIN FILMS (FIGURES 2.3a–2.3e)

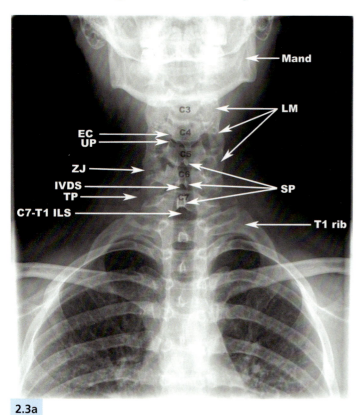

2.3a

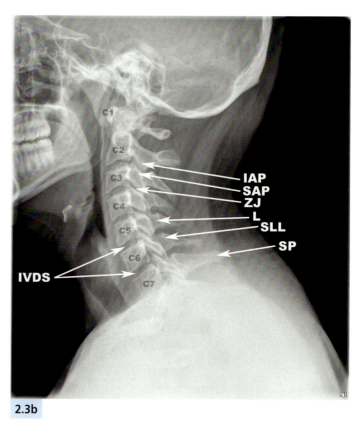

2.3b

FIGURES 2.3a–r Multimodal image gallery demonstrating the anatomy of the subaxial cervical spine on plain films (a–e), CT (f–l), and MR (m–r).

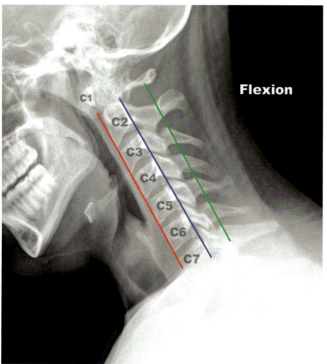

2.3c

KEY			
EC	echancrure	SLL	spinolaminar line
IAP	inferior articular process	SP	spinous process
		TP	transverse process
ILS	interlaminar space	UP	uncinate process
IVDS	intervertebral disc space	ZJ	zygapophyseal joint
L	lamina	**red line**	anterior spinal line
LM	lateral mass	**blue line**	posterior spinal line
Mand	mandible	**green line**	spinolaminar line
SAP	superior articular process		

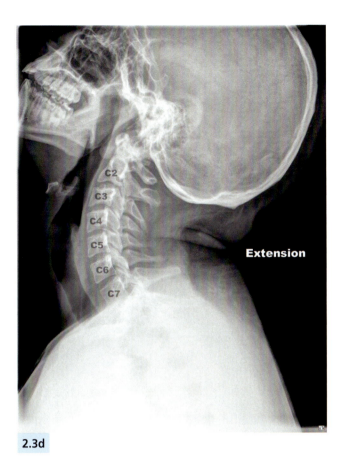

2.3d

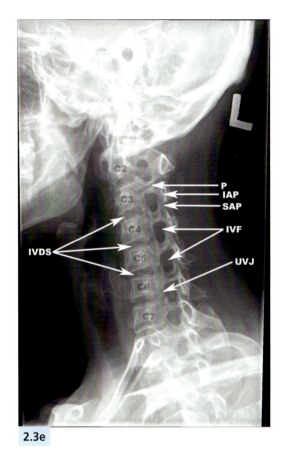

2.3e

FIGURES 2.3d,e

KEY					
IAP	inferior articular process	**IVF**	intervertebral foramen	**SAP**	superior articular process
IVDS	intervertebral disc space	**P**	pedicle	**UVJ**	uncovertebral joint

(continued)

■ CT (FIGURES 2.3f–2.3l)

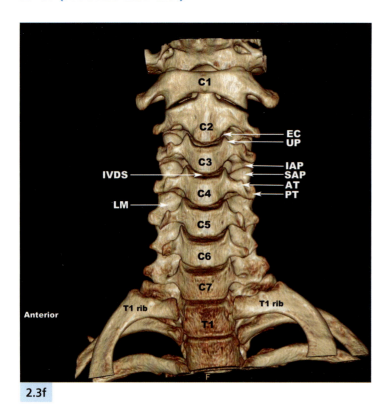

2.3f

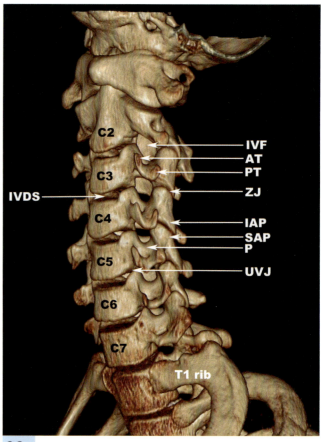

2.3g

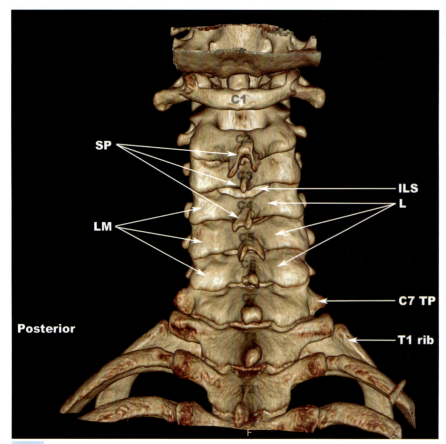

2.3h

FIGURES 2.3f–h

KEY

AT	anterior tubercle
EC	echancrure
IAP	inferior articular process
ILS	interlaminar space
IVDS	intervertebral disc space
IVF	intervertebral foramen
L	lamina
LM	lateral mass
P	pedicle
PT	posterior tubercle
SAP	superior articular process
SP	spinous process
TP	transverse process
UP	uncinate process
UVJ	uncovertebral joint
ZJ	zygapophyseal joint

(continued)

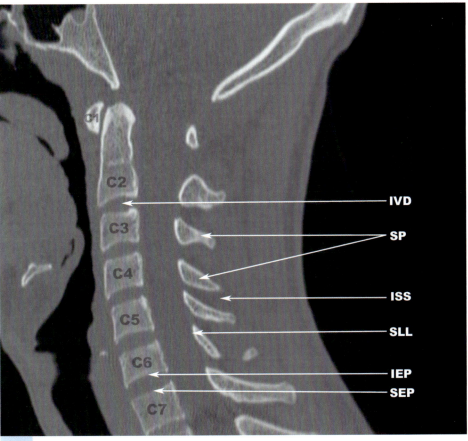

2.3i

FIGURES 2.3i,j

KEY			
IAP	inferior articular process	**SAP**	superior articular process
IEP	inferior endplate	**SEP**	superior endplate
ISS	interspinous space	**SLL**	spinolaminar line
IVD	intervertebral disc	**SP**	spinous process
IVF	intervertebral foramen	**ZJ**	zygapophyseal joint
P	pedicle		

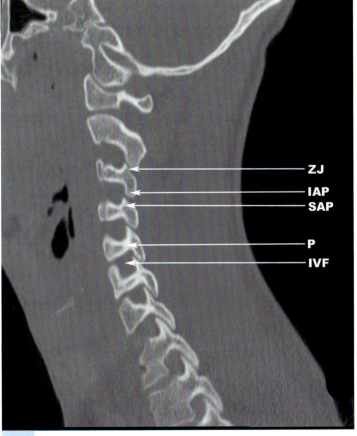

2.3j

(continued)

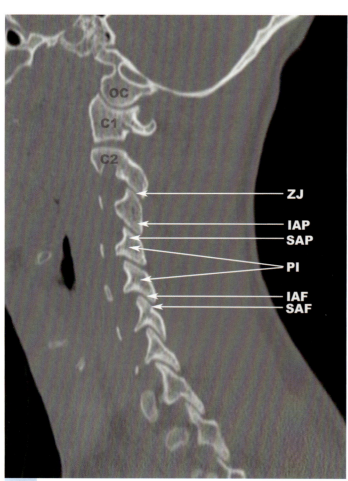

2.3k

FIGURES 2.3k,l

KEY

AT	anterior tubercle
C	centrum
CP	costal process
CTB	costotransverse bar
FT	foramina transversarium
IAF	inferior articular facet
IAP	inferior articular process
L	lamina
LM	lateral mass
OC	occipital condyle
P	pedicle
PI	pars interarticularis
PT	posterior tubercle
SAF	superior articular facet
SAP	superior articular process
SP	spinous process
ZJ	zygapophyseal joint

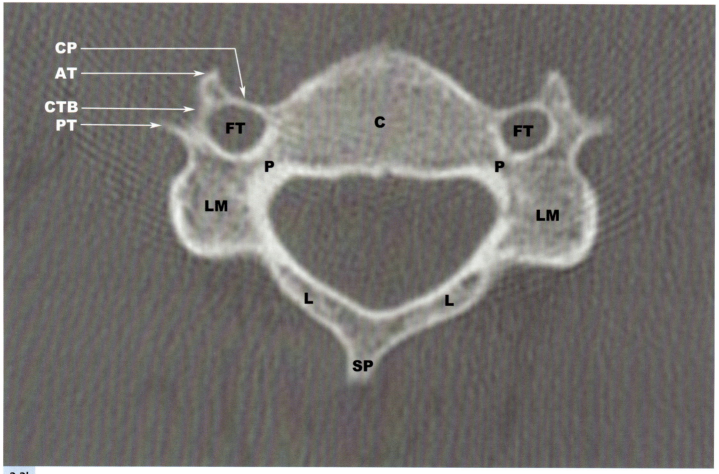

2.3l

(continued)

■ MR (FIGURES 2.3m–2.3r)

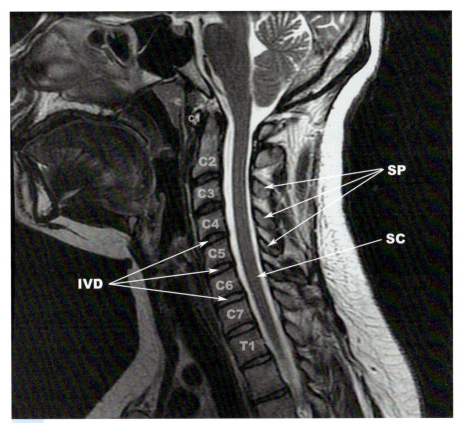

2.3m

FIGURES 2.3m,n

KEY	
IVD	intervertebral disc
SC	spinal cord
SP	spinous process

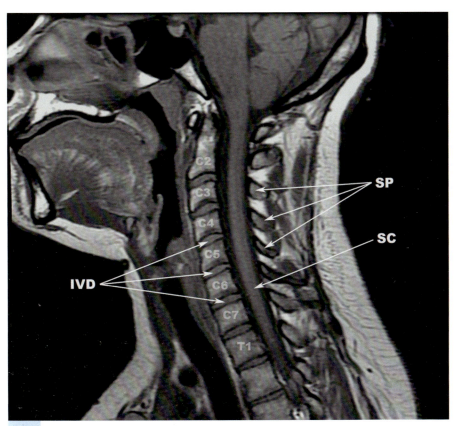

2.3n

(continued)

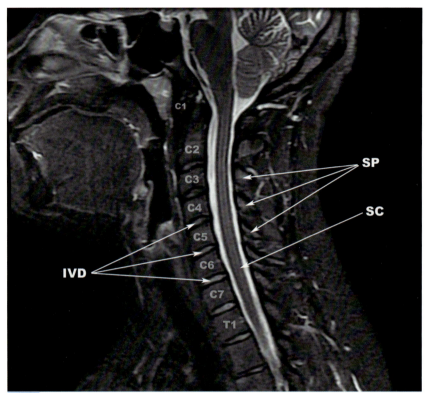

2.3o

FIGURES 2.3o,p

KEY	
CTB	costotransverse bar
DRG	dorsal root ganglion
IAP	inferior articular process
IVD	intervertebral disc
OC	occipital condyle
SAP	superior articular process
SC	spinal cord
SN	spinal nerve
SP	spinous process
V2	intraforaminal segment of vertebral artery
V3h	horizontal portion V3 segment of vertebral artery
ZJ	zygapophyseal joint

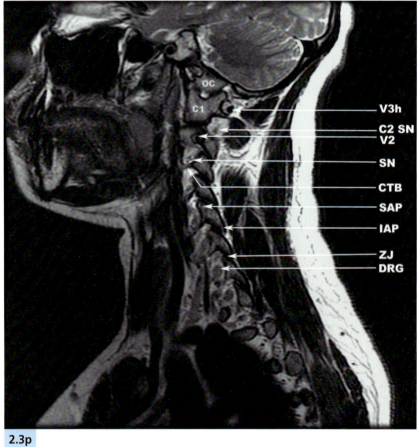

2.3p

(continued)

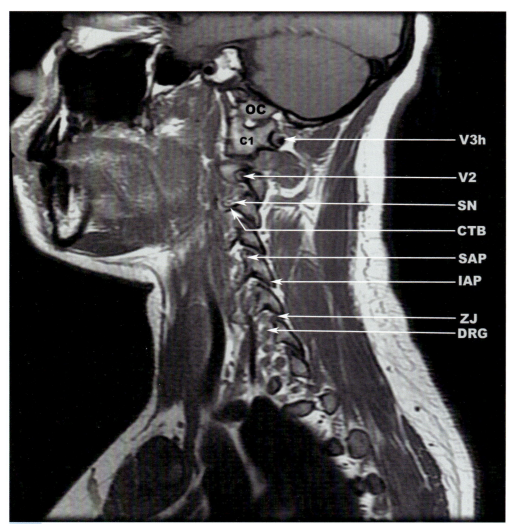

2.3q

FIGURES 2.3q,r

KEY

C	centrum
CTB	costotransverse bar
DRG	dorsal root ganglion
IAP	inferior articular process
L	lamina
LM	lateral mass
OC	occipital condyle
P	pedicle
SAP	superior articular process
SC	spinal cord
SN	spinal nerve
V2	intraforaminal segment of vertebral artery
V3h	horizontal portion V3 segment of vertebral artery
ZJ	zygapophyseal joint

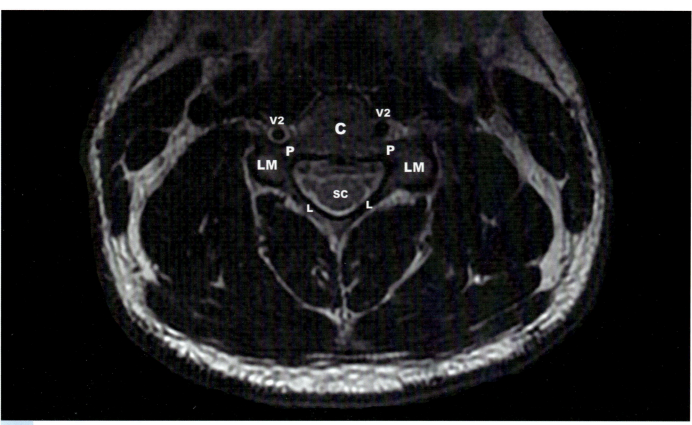

2.3r

OSTEOLOGY OF THE C3–C7 SEGMENTS

The long axis of the C3–C7 vertebral bodies is transverse. There is relatively little difference between the anterior and posterior heights of the C3–C7 vertebral bodies. The cervical lordosis is primarily derived from the configuration of the intervertebral discs in the subaxial cervical segments. The anterior to posterior length and transverse width of the vertebral bodies increases from C3 to C7. The anterior to posterior length of the inferior endplates is consistently larger than that of the adjacent superior endplate of the next caudal vertebral body. Projecting superiorly from the posterolateral margins of the C3–C7 superior endplates are the uncinate processes. The uncinate processes articulate with shallow depressions in the posterolateral margins of the adjacent inferior endplates, forming the uncovertebral or Luschka joints (**Figures 2.4a–d**).

The transverse processes arise from the lateral aspects of the vertebral bodies on both sides of the midline. The transverse processes are composed of ventral and dorsal bony bars that terminate laterally in the anterior and posterior tubercles, respectively. The anterior bar is the homologue of the thoracic rib and is called the *costal process or costal element*. The anterior tubercles progressively increase in size from C3 to C6. The anterior tubercles at C6 are variable in shape and size and are referred to as the *carotid tubercles of Chassaignac* (**Figures 2.5a–c**), against which the carotid arteries can be compressed. The Chassaignac tubercles are also a target for the stellate ganglion blockade. The anterior and posterior tubercles are joined laterally by a short bony bridge referred to as the *costotransverse bar* or *costotransverse lamella*. The foramina transversaria are formed by the pedicles medially, anteriorly by the ventral bar and anterior tubercle, laterally by the costotransverse lamella, and posteriorly by the transverse process. Rarely, the transverse foramina are duplicated or triplicated. The foramina transversaria arise more anteriorly from the vertebral bodies from C3 to C6 and return to a more posterior position at C7. The distance between the foramina transversaria increases progressively from C3 to C7. The C7 foramina transversaria tend to be smaller in caliber due to the fact that they typically do not transmit the vertebral arteries.

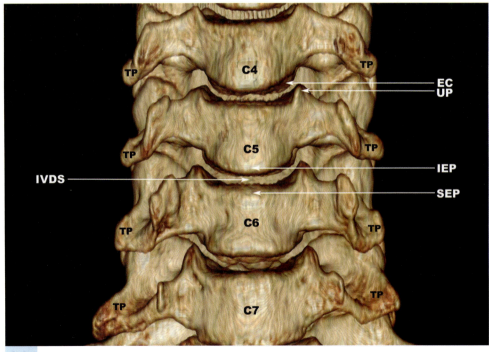

2.4a

FIGURES 2.4a–d (a) coronal surface rendered CT, (b) curved reformatted CT, (c) axial CT, and (d) axial T2 turbo spin echo (TSE) images demonstrating the anatomy of the uncovertebral joints. EC—echancrure, IEP—inferior endplate, IVDS—intervertebral disc space, SEP—superior endplate, TP—transverse process, UP—uncinate process.

(continued)

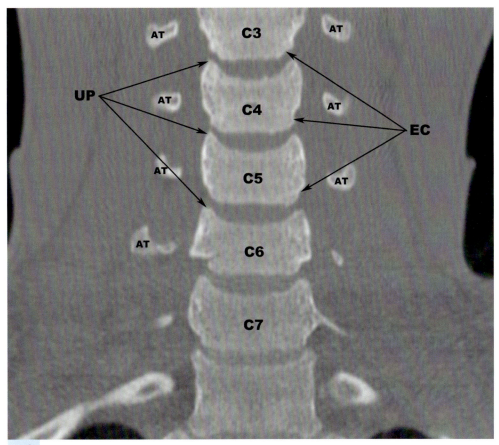

2.4b

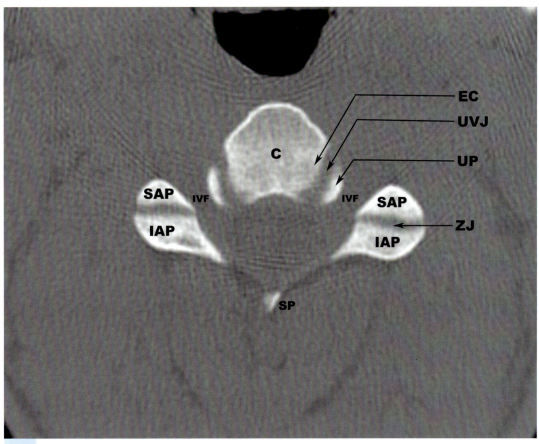

2.4c

FIGURES 2.4b,c   (*continued*) AT—anterior tubercle, C—centrum, EC—echancrure, IAP—inferior articular process, IVF—intervertebral foramen, SAP—superior articular process, SP—spinous process, UP—uncinate process, UVJ—uncoverteberal joint, ZJ—zygapophyseal joint.

(*continued*)

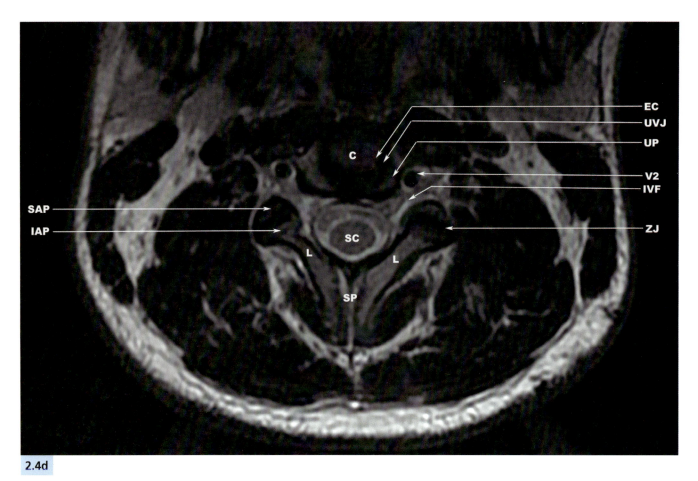

2.4d

FIGURE 2.4d   (*continued*) C—centrum, EC—echancrure, IAP—inferior articular process, IVF—intervertebral foramen, L—lamina, SAP—superior articular process, SC—spinal cord, SP—spinous process, UP—uncinate process, UVJ—uncoverteberal joint, V2—intraforaminal segment vertebral artery, ZJ—zygapophyseal joint.

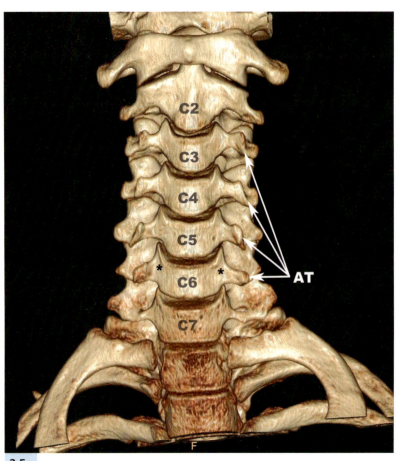

2.5a

FIGURES 2.5a–c   The anterior tubercles of C6 (carotid tubercles of Chassaignac) are displayed in (a) an anterior projection surface rendered 3D CT image, (b) AP radiograph of the cervical spine, and (c) axial CT image. The asterisks (*) mark the sites of fluoroscopically guided stellate ganglion block at the junction of the anterior tubercle and vertebral body within the vertebral gutter (VG), just inferior to the uncinate process of C6. AP—articular pillar, AT—anterior tubercle, C—centrum, CP—costal process, CTB—costotransverse bar, FT—foramina transversaria, L—lamina, P—pedicle, PT—posterior tubercle.

(*continued*)

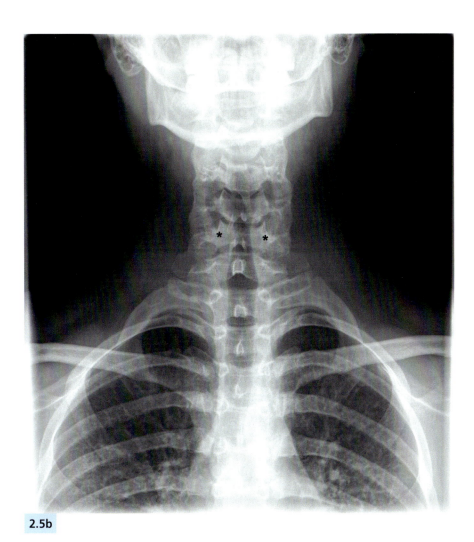

2.5b

FIGURES 2.5b,c   The anterior tubercles of C6 (carotid tubercles of Chassaignac) are displayed in (a) an anterior projection surface rendered 3D CT image, (b) AP radiograph of the cervical spine, and (c) axial CT image. The asterisks (*) mark the sites of fluoroscopically guided stellate ganglion block at the junction of the anterior tubercle and vertebral body within the vertebral gutter (VG), just inferior to the uncinate process of C6. AP—articular pillar, AT—anterior tubercle, C—centrum, CP—costal process, CTB—costotransverse bar, FT—foramina transversaria, L—lamina, P—pedicle, PT—posterior tubercle.

2.5c

The pedicles arise just inferior to the uncinate processes along the posterolateral aspects of the vertebral bodies. At the junction of the pedicles and lamina are the articular pillars, including the superior articular processes, inferior articular processes, and the pars interarticularis. The lamina meet at the midline posterior to the spinal canal to form the spinous process. The C3–C6 spinous processes are bifid. The C7 spinous process is elongated and monofid, similar to the thoracic spinous processes (**Figure 2.6**).

The subaxial cervical spinal canal is formed by the posterior margin of the vertebral body, medial margins of the pedicles, anterior margins of the lamina, and anterior margin of the spinous process (**Figure 2.7**). The cervical spinal canal is triangular or trefoil in shape. The *effective* spinal canal dimensions are reduced in the subaxial segments due to the cervical enlargement at C3–T1 (Figure 2.35). The lateral borders of the spinal canal are funnel-shaped with apex oriented laterally toward the neural foramina, forming the cervical equivalent of the lateral recess that is found in the lumbar segments (**Figure 2.8**).

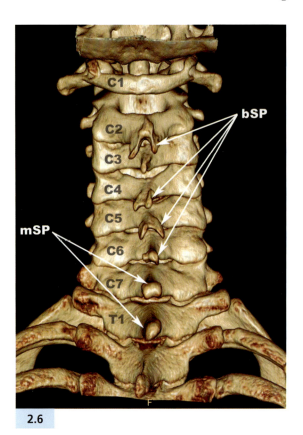

FIGURE 2.6 Surface rendered reformatted image of the cervical spine from a posterior projection shows characteristically bifid upper spinous processes (bSP) and a monofid (mSP), thoracic-type spinous process at C7. Variation of the subaxial cervical spinous processes is common, as seen in this case with a monofid C3 spinous process.

2.6

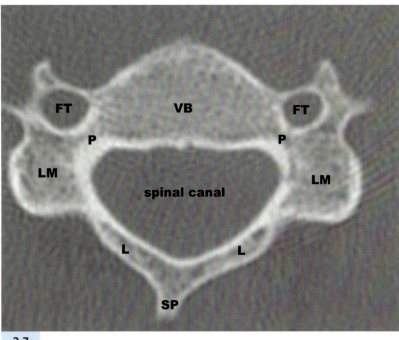

FIGURE 2.7 The subaxial cervical spinal canal is bounded anteriorly by the posterior margin of the vertebral body (VB), anterolaterally by the medial margins of the pedicles (P), posterolaterally by the lamina (L), and posteriorly by the spinous process (SP). FT—foramina transversaria, LM—lateral mass.

2.7

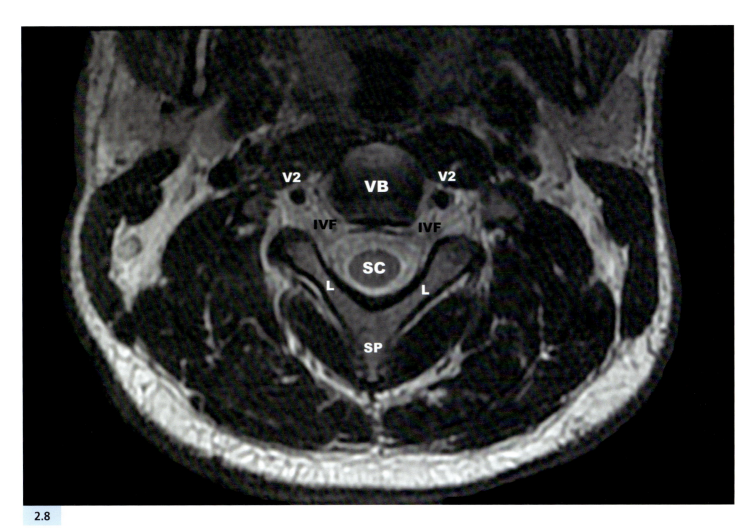

2.8

FIGURE 2.8   Axial T2-weighted TSE image displaying the funnel-shaped anterolateral aspects of the spinal canal that point to the intervertebral foramina (IVF). L—lamina, SC—spinal cord, SP—spinous process, V2—intraforaminal segment of the vertebral artery, VB—vertebral body.

The borders of the neural foramina are formed by the uncovertebral joints medially and the zygapophyseal joints laterally (Figure 2.4d). The floors of the neural foramina are formed by the superior margins of the pedicles medially and the dorsal bony bars and costotransverse lamella laterally. The superior surface of the costotransverse lamella is concave and forms a shallow groove in which the anterior ramus of the exiting spinal nerve resides at each level (**Figures 2.9a,b**).

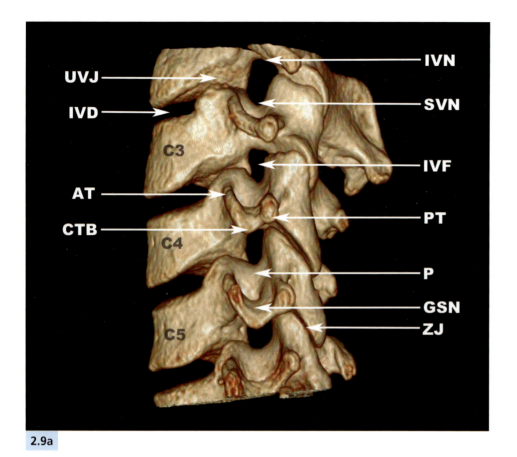

2.9a

FIGURES 2.9a,b (a) Lateral oblique surface rendered CT image demonstrating the anatomy of the subaxial cervical intervertebral foramina. The superior margin of the intervertebral foramen (IVF) is formed by the inferior vertebral notch (IVN) and the inferior margin is formed by the superior vertebral notch (SVN) of the pedicle (P). The anterior margin is the uncovertebral joint (UVJ) and the posterior margin is the zygapophyseal joint (ZJ). The exiting spinal nerve is bounded anteriorly by the anterior tubercle (AT), posteriorly by the posterior tubercle (PT), and inferiorly by a groove for the spinal nerve (GSN) in the costotransverse bar (CTB). (b) Sagittal T2-weighted TSE image displays the subaxial cervical spinal nerves (SN) surrounded by fat and positioned within shallow grooves of the costotransverse bars (CTB) as they exit the intervertebral foramina. AP—articular pillar, DRG—dorsal root ganglia, IVD—intervertebral disc, OC—occipital condyle.

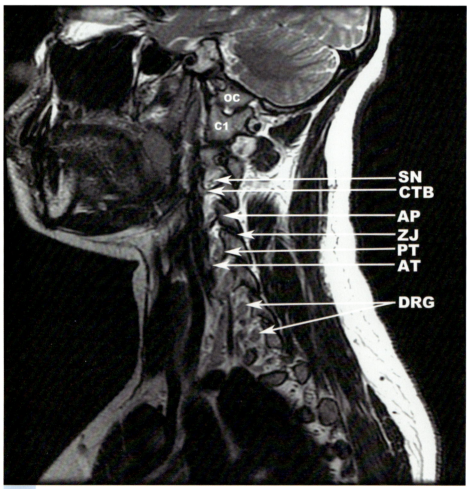

2.9b

THE INTERVERTEBRAL DISCS OF THE SUBAXIAL CERVICAL SPINE

Intervertebral disc morphology is the primary determinant of the cervical lordosis. The ventral height of the subaxial cervical intervertebral discs is greater than the dorsal height (Figure 2.3m). The structure of the annulus fibrosis in the subaxial cervical segments differs from that in the thoracic and lumbar segments. The anterior annulus is thick and progressively thins posterolaterally to the margin of the uncinate processes. There is no significant substance to the annulus fibrosis in the region of the uncovertebral joints. The posterior annulus consists of a single band of vertically oriented fibers. In the transverse plane, this results in a crescentic configuration.

The composition of the cervical intervertebral discs differs from that of the thoracic and lumbar discs. At birth, the nucleus pulposis comprises approximately one quarter of the entire disc. Early in life, the cervical intervertebral disc has greater collagen composition and relatively lower proteoglycan content. By the end of the third decade, the nucleus pulposis is nearly indistinguishable from the annulus fibrosis. A well-defined nucleus pulposis is generally only observed in children and young adults. This corresponds to more homogeneous low T2 signal within the cervical intervertebral discs (**Figures 2.10 a–d**).

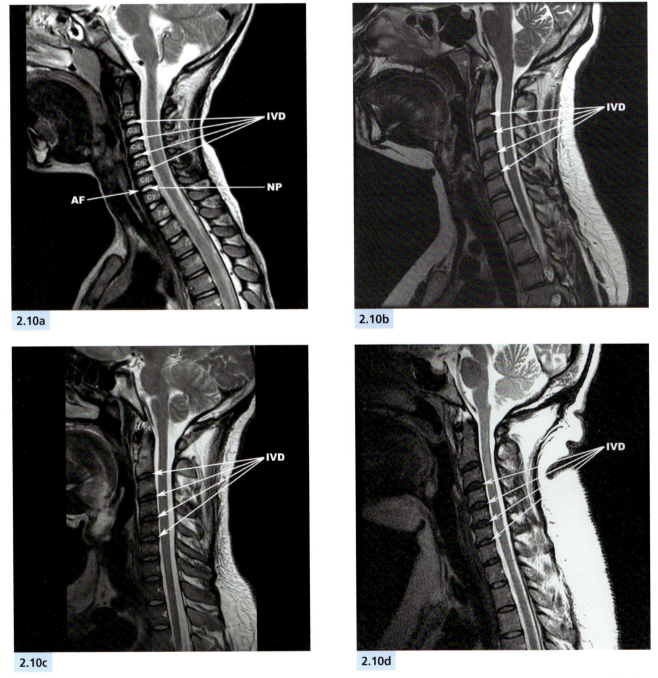

2.10a

2.10b

2.10c

2.10d

FIGURES 2.10a–d   Sagittal T2-weighted TSE images of the cervical spine demonstrating the typical appearance of the intervertebral discs (IVD) at various ages: (a) 5 years, (b) 20 years, (c) 30 years, and (d) 40 years. AF—annulus fibrosis, NP—nucleus pulposis.

THE ZYGAPOPHYSEAL (FACET) JOINTS

The superior and inferior articular processes arise from the pedicle lamina junction. The superior articular facets arise on the dorsal surface of the superior articular process and face superiorly. The inferior articular facets arise on the ventral surface of the inferior articular process and face inferiorly (**Figure 2.11**). The facet surfaces are lined by a thin layer of smooth articular cartilage, are surrounded by a fibrous capsule, and are lubricated by synovial fluid. The cervical zygapophyseal joint capsules are lax and elongated compared with the thoracic and lumbar segments.

The zygapophyseal joints are variable in their orientation within the subaxial cervical spine. The C3 superior articular facets are oriented posteromedially. Approximately 75% of the time, the C4 superior articular facets are oriented posteromedially. The C7 superior articular facets are oriented posterolaterally. The transition from posteromedial to posterolateral facet orientation most commonly occurs at C6 and is gradual. The angle of inclination of the zygapophyseal joints, as measured in the sagittal plane, increases progressively from C3 to T1.

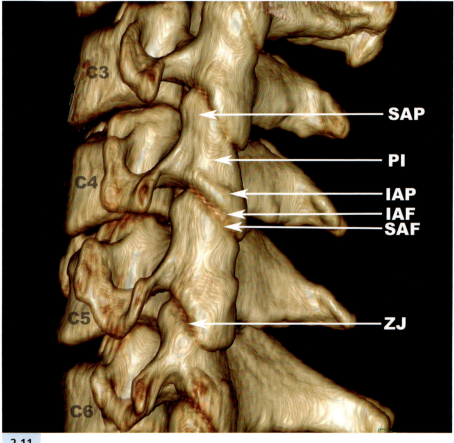

2.11

FIGURE 2.11 Lateral projection surface rendered CT image demonstrating the zygapophyseal joints (ZJ) of the subaxial cervical spine. Superior (SAP) and inferior articular processes (IAP) arise from the lateral masses that have relatively flat articular facets (SAF, IAF) that appose to form the ZJ. The bone located between the superior and inferior articular processes is the pars interarticularis (PI).

THE UNCOVERTEBRAL (LUSCHKA) JOINTS

The uncovertebral joints are formed by the uncinate processes and the *echancrures*. The uncinate processes arise from the posterolateral margins of the C3–C7 superior endplates. The echancrures are shallow depressions located along the posterolateral margins of the inferior endplates that appose the uncinate processes. The uncovertebral joints form the anterior wall of the neural foramina from C3 to C7 and are in close proximity to the medial wall of the transverse foramina (Figures 2.4a–d).

Distinct capsules surround the uncovertebral joints and synoviocytes have been demonstrated in the lateral capsular tissue. The uncinate processes progressively shift from a more anterior position at C3 to a more posterior position at C7. The C7 uncinate processes are occasionally absent and distinct uncinate processes are rarely observed at T1 and T2. Rudimentary uncinate processes are visible in full-term neonates and continue to enlarge until 9 to 14 years of age.

LIGAMENTOUS ANATOMY OF THE SUBAXIAL CERVICAL SPINE

The major ligaments of the subaxial cervical spine include the anterior longitudinal ligament, posterior longitudinal ligament, ligamenta flava ("yellow ligaments"), interspinous ligaments, ligamentum nuchae, and supraspinous ligament. The bulk of the supraspinous ligament is found in the thoracic and lumbar spine and will be discussed in depth within those chapters. The intertransverse ligaments are not well-developed in the subaxial cervical segments and not well demonstrated on neuroimaging studies.

The *anterior longitudinal ligament* (ALL) is a multilayered structure that extends inferiorly from a cord-like attachment to the anterior tubercle of the atlas and gradually increases in width from C3 to C7 (**Figures 2.12a,b** and **2.13a,b**). The anterior to posterior thickness of the ALL is greatest at the vertebral body levels and thinnest at the intervertebral disc levels. The ALL is firmly adherent to the anterior superior and inferior endplates, infrequently adherent to the intervertebral discs (20%), and variably adherent to the central portion of the vertebral bodies (40%) of the subaxial cervical segments. The deepest layer of the ALL projects laterally to the anterior margin of the uncovertebral joints. It plays a major role in spine stability, resists hyperextension, and supports the intervertebral discs.

The *posterior longitudinal ligament* (PLL) arises inconspicuously from the inferior margin of the tectorial membrane at the C2 body level and extends to the sacrum. Like the ALL, the PLL contains multiple layers that are variable in length and configuration. The transverse dimension and anterior to posterior thickness of the PLL are greatest in the cervical spine. The PLL attaches to the dorsal annulus and posterior margins of the vertebral bodies, with loose attachments in the central regions of the vertebral bodies. The deepest layer of the PLL extends laterally to the margin of the uncovertebral joint. The functions of the PLL include support of the intervertebral discs, resisting hyperflexion, and enhancing zygapophyseal joint stability. The PLL is displayed in Figures 2.12a,b and **2.14a,b**.

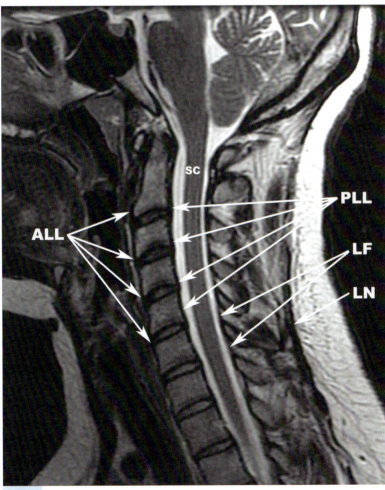

2.12a

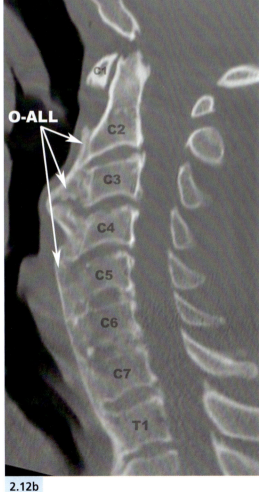

2.12b

FIGURES 2.12a,b   (a) Sagittal T2-weighted TSE image showing the normal anterior longitudinal ligament (ALL), posterior longitudinal ligament (PLL), ligamenta flava (LF), and ligamentum nuchae (LN). (b) ossification of the anterior longitudinal ligament (O-ALL), also known as diffuse idiopathic skeletal hyperostosis. SC—spinal cord.

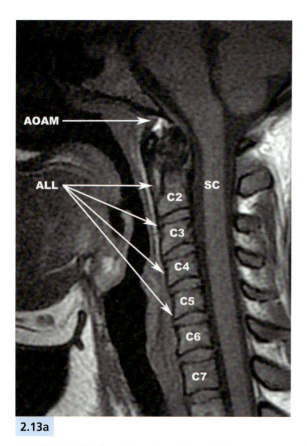

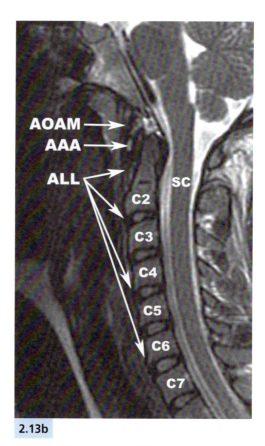

2.13a

2.13b

FIGURES 2.13a,b   The subaxial cervical component of the anterior longitudinal ligament (ALL) is demonstrated with
(a) T1-weighted TSE and (b) T2-weighted TSE images. AAA—anterior arch of atlas, AOAM—anterior occipitoatlantal membrane,
SC—spinal cord.

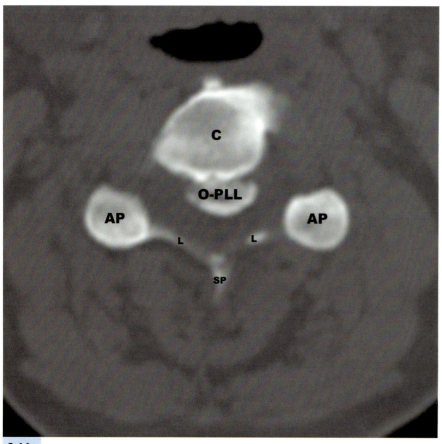

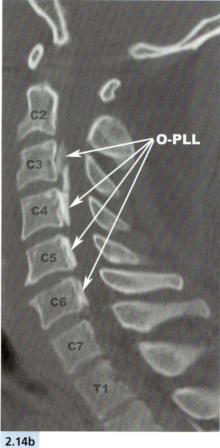

2.14a

2.14b

FIGURES 2.14a,b   (a) axial and (b) sagittal CT images showing mixed type ossification of the posterior longitudinal ligament
(O-PLL) that is continuous at C3–C4 and segmental at C5 and C6. AP—articular pillar, C—centrum, L—lamina, SP—spinous
process.

The *ligamenta flava* are found from C1–C2 to L5–S1. The ligamenta flava increase in size proportional to the increase in the interlaminar distances from C2–C3 to C7–T1. The ligamenta flava are thinnest in anterior to posterior dimension in the cervical segments, becoming more prominent in the thoracic and lumbar segments. The ligamenta flava are paired ligaments that are positioned on either side of the midline, extending from the anterior inferior margin of the lamina above to the posterior superior margin of the lamina below. The lateral aspects of the ligamenta flava cover and support the medial portions of the zygapophyseal joints (Figures 2.12a and **2.15a–d**). The ligamenta flava contain approximately 80% elastin, which may prevent spinal canal encroachment resulting from ligamentous buckling during extension.

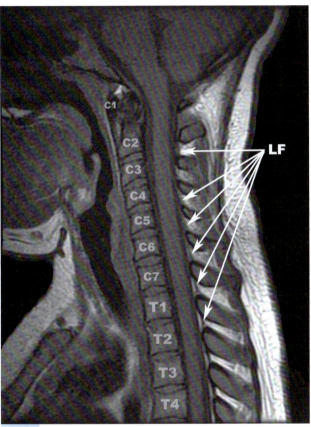

2.15a

FIGURES 2.15a–d   (a) Sagittal T1-weighted TSE image demonstrating the increase in size of the ligamenta flava (LF) from craniad to caudad. (b) Axial T2-weighted TSE image showing the LF as hypointense bands along the inner margins of the lamina. A small gap between the LF is present at the midline between the left ligamentum flavum (LF - left) and right ligamentum flavum (LF - right), a finding commonly observed on MR. C—centrum, DRG—dorsal root ganglion, ICA—internal carotid artery, IJV—internal jugular vein, SC—spinal cord, SP—spinous process, T—trachea, ZJ—zygapophyseal joint.

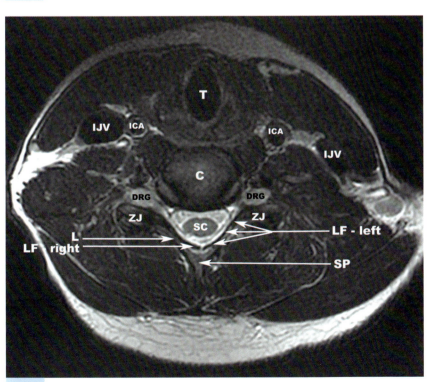

2.15b

(*continued*)

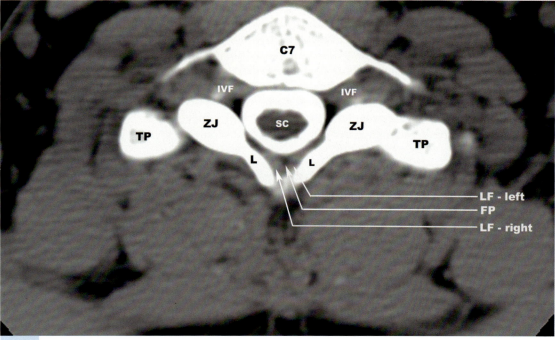

2.15c

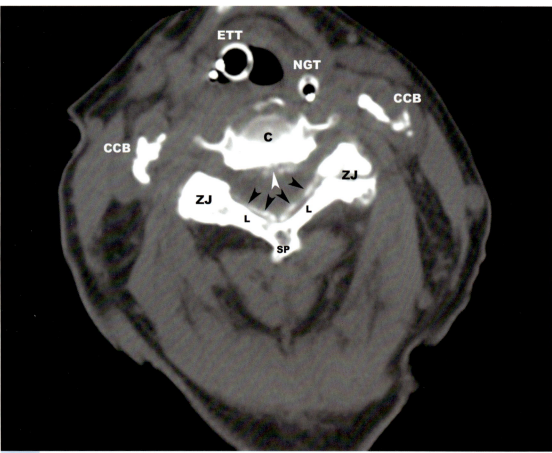

2.15d

FIGURES 2.15c,d (*continued*) (c) Axial CT myelogram at C7 showing the soft tissue density ligamenta flava (LF) and emergence of the intervening interlaminar fat pad (FP). (d) Axial noncontrasted CT image demonstrating heavy calcification of the ligamenta flava (black arrowheads). Ossification of the posterior longitudinal ligament (short white arrow) and heavy calcification of the common carotid bifurcations (CCB) are also present. C—centrum, CCB—common carotid bifurcations, ETT—endotracheal tube, IVF—intervertebral foramen, L—lamina, NGT—nasogastric tube, SC—spinal cord, SP—spinous process, TP—transverse process, ZJ—zygapophyseal joint.

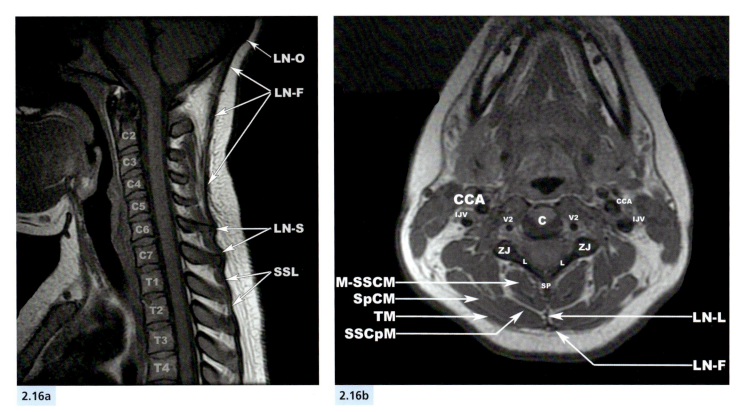

2.16a

2.16b

FIGURES 2.16a,b   The ligamentum nuchae is demonstrated on T1-weighted TSE images. (a) The funicular component (LN-F) is visualized as a craniad extension of the supraspinous ligament (SSL) projecting from the C6 or C7 spinous process (LN-S) to the external occipital protuberance (LN-O). (b) On axial images, the funicular component is typically triangular in shape. The lamellar component (LN-L) is often visible as a thin hypointense band. The funicular component serves as a site of attachment of the aponeuroses of the trapezius (TM), multifidis-semispinalis cervicus (M-SSCM), semispinalis capitis (SSCpM), and splenius capitis (SpCM) muscles. C—centrum, CCA—common carotid artery, IJV—internal jugular vein, L—lamina, SP—spinous process, V2—intraforaminal segment vertebral artery, ZJ—zygapophyseal joint.

The *interspinous ligaments* extend from the inferior margins of the spinous processes above to the superior margins of the spinous processes below in the sagittal plane and from the root to the apex of the spinous processes in the transverse plane. The cervical interspinous ligaments are rudimentary in comparison with the more developed interspinous ligaments in the thoracic and lumbar spine. The rudimentary interspinous ligaments blend with the funicular portion of the ligamentum nuchae discussed in the following.

The *ligamentum nuchae* has two components, the funicular (dorsal) and lamellar (ventral), demonstrated on **Figures 2.16a,b**. The *funicular* component is a thick, fibrous band that extends from the C7 spinous process, less commonly C6, to the external occipital protuberance, forming firm attachments proximally and distally. The funicular component serves as a site of attachment of the aponeuroses of the trapezius, semispinalis, serratus posterior superior, rhomboid minor, and splenius capitis muscles. The trapezius muscles attach along the entire length of the funicular component of the ligamentum nuchae. The *lamellar* component projects anteriorly from the ventral margin of the funicular component to the C1 posterior tubercle and cervical spinous processes and superiorly to attach along the median occipital protuberance from the posterior margin of the foramen magnum to the external occipital protuberance. The most anterior lamellar component blends significantly with the interspinous ligaments. There are well-established connective tissue attachments between the ligamentum nuchae and the posterior dura at the C0–C1 and C1–C2 levels. The ligamentum nuchae functions to limit neck flexion and maintain cervical lordosis.

Anterior subluxation of C2 on C3 is seen in approximately 10%–20% of children ages 1 to 8 years. Factors that contribute to physiologic subluxation in children include horizontal orientation of the zygapophyseal joints, ligamentous laxity, underdeveloped uncovertebral joints, high fulcrum for neck flexion, and relatively large skull. Anterior subluxation of C3 on C4 is less commonly observed, but may also be physiologic. The *Swischuk line* is drawn from the anterior margin of the C1 neural arch to the anterior margin of the C3 neural arch. Physiologic subluxation ("pseudosubluxation") is present when this line passes through the anterior cortex of the C2 neural arch, when this line touches the anterior cortex of the C2 neural arch, or the anterior cortex of the C2 neural arch resides up to 1 mm posterior to this line. If this line passes 2 mm or more anterior to the cortex of the C2 neural arch, pathologic subluxation is assumed. Physiologic subluxation is accentuated in the flexion and resolves in extension (**Figure 2.17**).

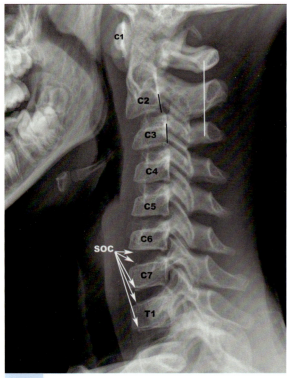

2.17

FIGURE 2.17   Pseudosubluxation in a 7 year-old. There is a 2-mm anterior subluxation of C2 with respect to C3 (black lines). The Swischuk line (white line) is drawn from the inner margin of the C1 neural arch to the inner margin of the C3 neural arch and is normal in this case. The mild kyphosis observed in this case can be a normal finding in this age group. Incidental note is made of the emergence of secondary ossification centers (SOC) at C6, C7, and T1.

ARTERIAL ANATOMY OF THE SUBAXIAL CERVICAL SPINE

The blood supply to the cervical subaxial segments is primarily derived from the vertebral arteries. There are four segments of the vertebral arteries (**Figures 2.18a–c**). The V1 segments extend from the vertebral artery origins to their entrance into the foramina transversaria. The V2 segments travel through the foraminal transversaria, typically from C2 to C6. The V3 segments begin at the point the vertebral arteries exit the C2 foramina transversaria and end at the point they pierce the dura at the foramen magnum. The V4 segments are the intracranial portions of the vertebral arteries.

The vertebral arteries arise from the subclavian arteries greater than 90% of the time. The most common variant origin of the vertebral arteries is from the aortic arch between the left common carotid and left subclavian arteries (**Figures 2.19a,b**). Numerous rare variant origins have been described, comprising less than 1%. The left vertebral artery is typically larger in caliber than the right vertebral artery. About 12% the population has a unilateral hypoplastic vertebral artery that either terminates in the ipsilateral posterior inferior cerebellar artery (**Figures 2.20a–c**) or there is a hypoplastic post-PICA V4 segment (**Figure 2.21**).

The vertebral arteries enter the C6 foramina transversaria the great majority of the time, with exit points at C7 (6%), C5 (4%), and other levels (1%) comprising the remaining cases. The diameter of the foramina transversaria does not have a direct relationship to the size of the vertebral artery contained therein, as small caliber vessels within large foramina are commonly encountered (**Figure 2.22**). However, vertebral artery size does tend to be consistent throughout the course of the vessel on the same side. Tortuosity of the V2 segments is common, including remodeling or erosion of the adjacent bony foramina transversaria (**Figures 2.23a–c**).

The longitudinal arteries of the cervical spine include the vertebral arteries, deep cervical arteries, ascending cervical arteries, and the costocervical trunks. The vertebral arteries give off the segmental branches within the upper cervical segments (**Figure 2.24**). The segmental arteries tend to arise from the deep cervical artery, ascending cervical artery, and costocervical trunk in the lower cervical segments. However, a rich anastamotic network is the rule in the cervical spine, making the cervical spinal cord relatively resistant to infarction. The segmental arteries from vertebral artery origin arise on both sides of the midline and give off anterior and posterior rami. The posterior rami give off spinal arterial and muscular branches.

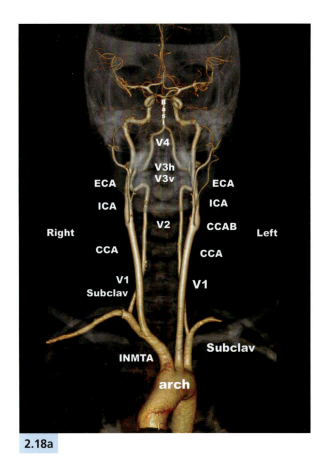

2.18a

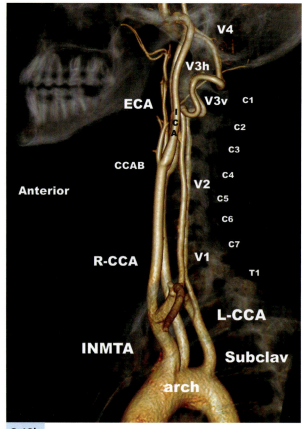

2.18b

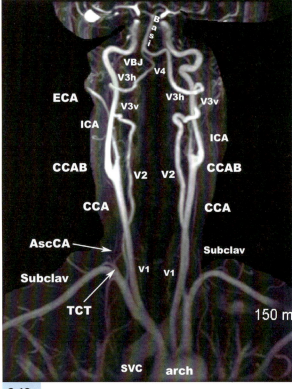

2.18c

FIGURES 2.18a–c (a) Frontal projection surface rendered computed tomography angiography (CTA) image demonstrating the vertebral artery segments (V1–V4). (b) Lateral projection surface rendered CTA image showing the course of the V1–V4 segments. (c) Anterior maximum intensity projection image from a contrast enhanced magnetic resonance angiography (MRA) of the neck demonstrates the origins and course of the vertebral arteries (V1–V4). The origin of the right ascending cervical artery (AscCA) from the thyrocervical trunk (TCT) is well visualized. arch—aortic arch, Basi—basilar artery, CCA—common carotid artery (L—left, R—right), CCAB—common carotid artery bifurcation, ECA—external carotid artery, ICA—internal carotid artery, INMTA—innominate artery, Subclav—subclavian artery, SVC—superior vena cava, V3h—horizontal portion V3 segment of vertebral artery, V3v—vertical portion V3 segment of vertebral artery, VBJ—vertebrobasilar junction.

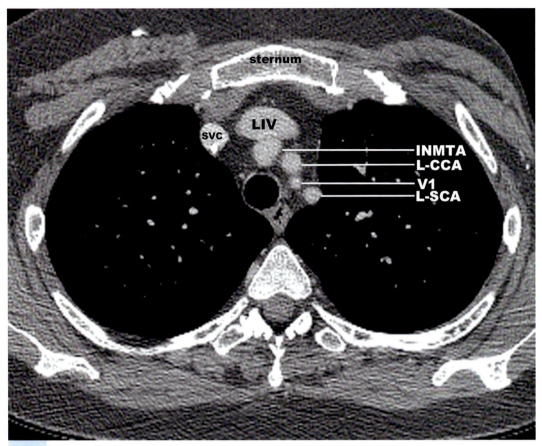

2.19a

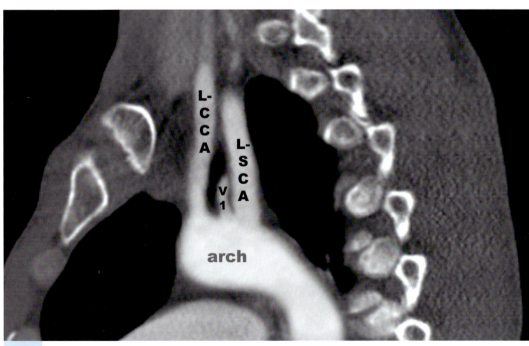

2.19b

FIGURES 2.19a,b   Origin of the left vertebral artery (V1) from the aortic arch (arch) between the left common carotid artery (L-CCA) and the left subclavian artery (L-SCA) demonstrated on (a) axial CTA and (b) sagittal oblique CTA images. INMTA—innominate artery, LIV—left innominate vein, SVC—superior vena cava.

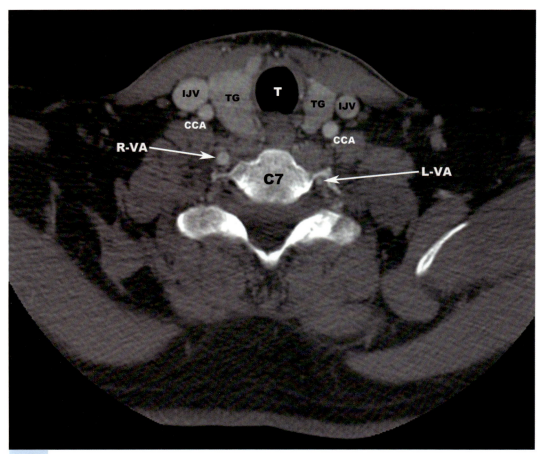

2.20a

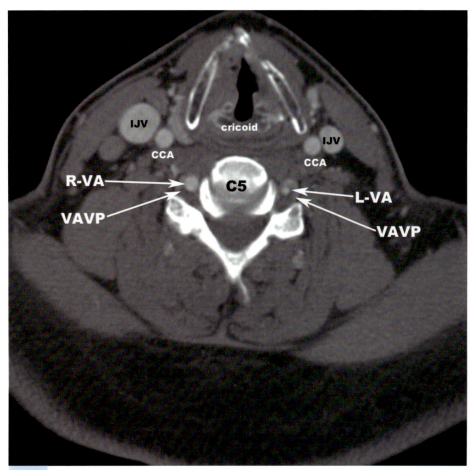

2.20b

FIGURES 2.20a–c Hypoplastic left vertebral artery (L-VA) that ends in the left posterior inferior cerebellar artery (PICA). (a) Axial CTA image at C7 showing the hypoplastic left vertebral artery (L-VA) entering the left C7 transverse foramen, a normal anatomic variant. The dominant right vertebral artery (R-VA) is located ventral to the foramen and will enter the right C6 transverse foramen (not shown). (b) At C5, the vertebral arteries are both located within the foramina transversaria and are surrounded by the vertebral artery venous plexuses (VAVP). CCA—common carotid artery, IJV—internal jugular vein, T—trachea, TG—thyroid gland, VA—vertebral artery (L—left, R—right).

(continued)

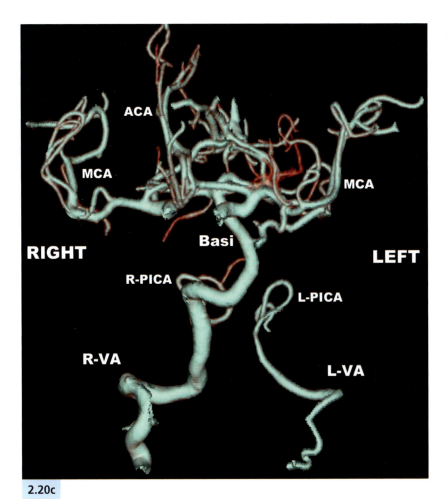

2.20c

FIGURE 2.20c   (*continued*) (c) Surface rendered 3D image shows the hypoplastic left vertebral artery terminating in the left posterior inferior cerebellar artery (L-PICA). ACA—anterior cerebral artery, Basi—basilar artery, MCA—middle cerebral artery, PICA—posterior inferior cerebellar artery (L—left, R—right), VA—vertebral artery (L—left, R—right).

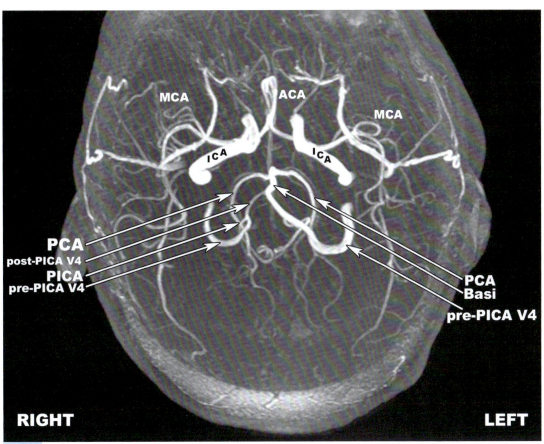

2.21

FIGURE 2.21   Hypoplastic right-sided post-PICA V4 segment demonstrated on an axial maximum intensity projection MRA image. The majority of the flow from the nondominant right vertebral artery is directed to the right posterior inferior cerebellar artery (PICA). ACA—anterior cerebral artery, Basi—basilar artery, ICA—internal carotid artery, MCA—middle cerebral artery, PCA—posterior cerebral artery, PICA—posterior inferior cerebellar artery.

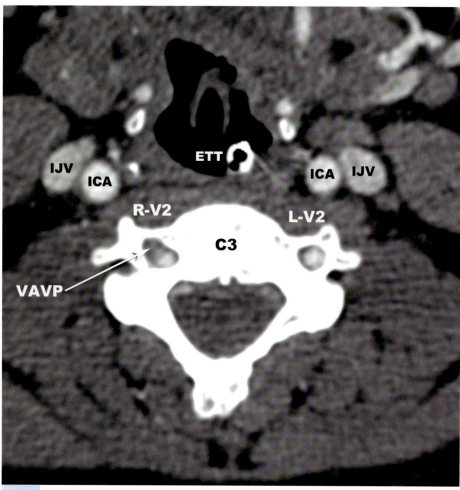

FIGURE 2.22 The size of the foramina transversaria does not necessarily reflect the caliber of the vertebral artery. The right transverse foramen is larger in size than the left, even though the left vertebral artery is dominant. This has to do with right V2 tortuosity and a somewhat prominent vertebral artery venous plexus (VAVP). ETT—endotracheal tube, ICA—internal carotid artery, IJV—internal jugular vein, V2—intraforaminal segment of the vertebral artery (L—left, R—right).

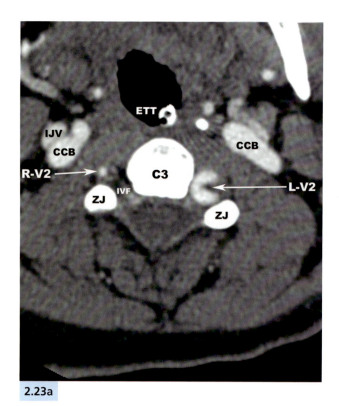

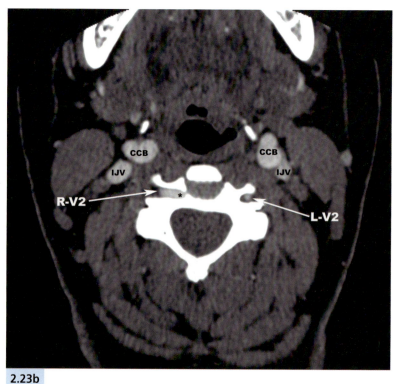

FIGURES 2.23a–c Variant anatomy of the V2 segments. (a) Axial CTA showing tortuosity of the left V2 segment (L-V2) with projection into the left C3–C4 intervertebral foramen (IVF). (b) Axial CTA demonstrates a tortuous right V2 segment (R-V2) that significantly remodels the C4 centrum (asterisk). CCB—common carotid bifurcation, ETT—endotracheal tube, IJV—internal jugular vein, L-V2—Left V2 segment, R-V2—right V2 segment, ZJ—zygapophyseal joint.

(continued)

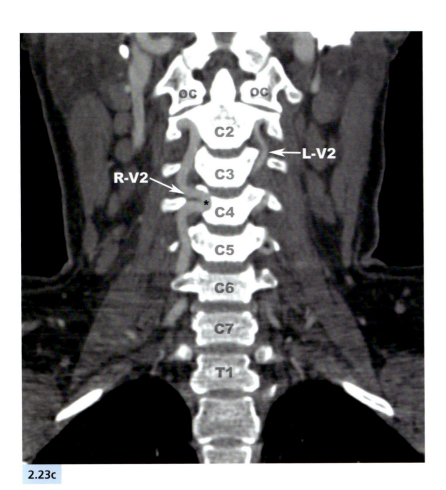

2.23c

FIGURE 2.23c *(continued)* (c) Coronal planar reformatted CTA images demonstrate a tortuous right V2 segment (R-V2) that significantly remodels the C4 centrum (asterisk). L-V2—Left V2 segment, R-V2—right V2 segment, OC—occipital condyles.

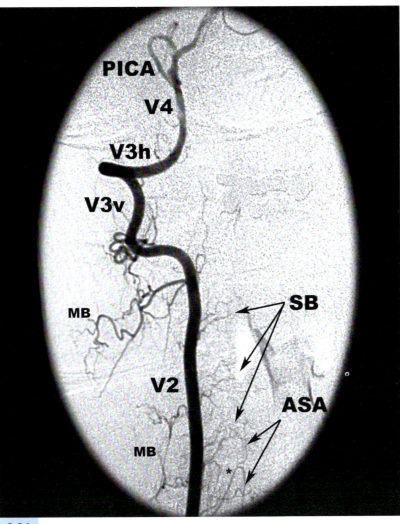

2.24

FIGURE 2.24   Digital subtraction angiogram of the right vertebral artery showing multiple segmental branches (SB) arising from the V2 segment. The most inferior segmental branch displayed gives rise to a radiculomedullary artery (asterisk) that supplies the anterior spinal artery (ASA). MB—muscular branches, PICA—posterior inferior cerebellar artery, V2—intraforaminal segment of vertebral artery, V3h—horizontal portion V3 segment of vertebral artery, V3v—vertical portion V3 segment of vertebral artery, V4—intradural segment of vertebral artery.

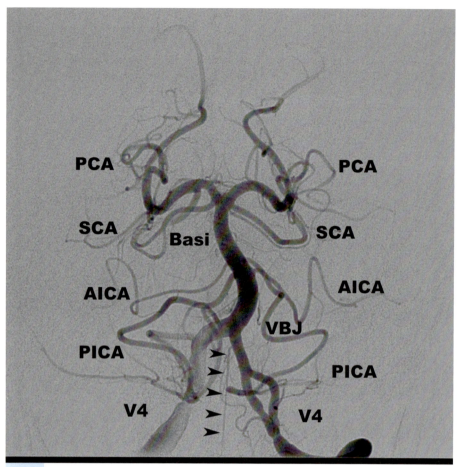

FIGURE 2.25 Digital subtraction angiographic image obtained following a selective left vertebral artery injection shows the anterior spinal artery (black arrowheads) arising from the left post-PICA V4 segment just proximal to the vertebrobasilar junction (VBJ) and retrograde filling of the right vertebral (V4) and posterior inferior cerebellar arteries (PICA). AICA—anterior inferior cerebellar artery, Basi—basilar artery, PCA—posterior cerebral artery, SCA—superior cerebellar artery.

2.25

The spinal branches course through the neural foramina and branch into anterior and posterior radicular arteries. The radicular arteries may supply the nerve roots, dura mater, spinal ganglia, spinal cord, or combinations thereof. The radicular arteries that supply the spinal cord are referred to as *radiculomedullary arteries* and tend to travel with the ventral roots. Radiculomedullary arteries are more equally distributed in the cervical region, without the left-sidedness that is typical of the thoracic and lumbar segments. The anterior spinal artery in the cervical spine consists of anterior radiculomedullary arteries in series, ranging in number from zero to six. The dominant cervical radiculomedullary artery has been termed the *cervical radiculomedullary artery of Lazorthes* (Figure 2.24). A variable number of posterior radiculomedullary arteries make up the posterior spinal arteries.

The origins of the anterior and posterior spinal arteries are discussed in Chapter 1. The origin of the anterior spinal artery is frequently observed on cerebral angiograms, generally arising from two small branches of the distal vertebral arteries (**Figure 2.25**). The anterior spinal artery resides in the anterior median fissure and supplies the anterior two-thirds of the spinal cord. The paired posterior spinal arteries are positioned lateral to the posterior median sulcus (medial to the dorsal root entry zones) and supply the posterior one-third of the spinal cord. The central arteries branch from the anterior spinal arteries and penetrate deeply into the anterior median fissure to supply the central cord. The anterior and posterior spinal arteries contribute to a network of arteries that encircle the spinal cord, the *pial arterial plexus* or *vasa coronae*.

VENOUS ANATOMY OF THE SUBAXIAL CERVICAL SPINE

Venous drainage of the subaxial cervical spine and spinal cord is carried out through a heavily interconnected venous network that has three main divisions: intrinsic, extrinsic, and extradural. The *intrinsic system* includes the venous network that drains the spinal cord central gray matter and peripheral white matter. The pia mater marks the border of the *extrinsic system*, which includes the coronal venous plexus and radiculomedullary veins. The *extradural system* includes the anterior internal vertebral venous plexus, posterior internal vertebral venous plexus, anterior external vertebral venous plexus, and posterior external vertebral venous plexus.

The anterior sulcal vein is located in the anterior median fissure of the spinal cord. The posterior sulcal vein is located in the posterior sulcus. The anterior and posterior central veins drain the central gray matter. The white matter is drained by small caliber radial veins within the pia that form a network called the *coronal venous plexus*. Transmedullary anastomotic veins are larger in caliber than the sulcal veins and project through the substance of the spinal cord, connecting ventral and dorsal surfaces. Some of the larger caliber longitudinally oriented veins within the coronal plexus form a variable number of anterior and posterior median and lateral spinal veins (**Figure 2.26a**).

The anterior and posterior radiculomedullary veins drain the spinal cord and spinal nerve roots and function to connect the extrinsic and extradural systems. The radiculomedullary

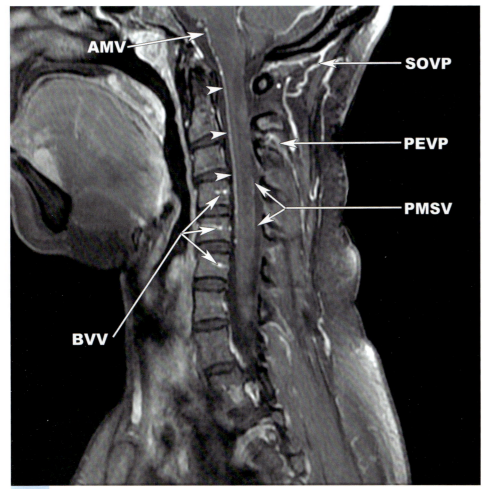

2.26a

FIGURES 2.26a–e   (a) Sagittal post contrast T1-weighted TSE image demonstrating the anterior median spinal vein (white arrows) continuing cranially as the anterior medullary vein (AMV). (b) Axial post contrast T1-weighted TSE image demonstrating adequate visibility of the anterior median spinal vein (AMSV) and posterior median spinal vein (PMSV). (c) Axial fat saturated post contrast T1-weighted image demonstrating the anterior and posterior radiculomedullary veins (ARV, PRV). BVV—basivertebral veins, PEVP—posterior external vertebral venous plexus, PMSV—posterior median spinal vein, SOVP—suboccipital venous plexus.   *(continued)*

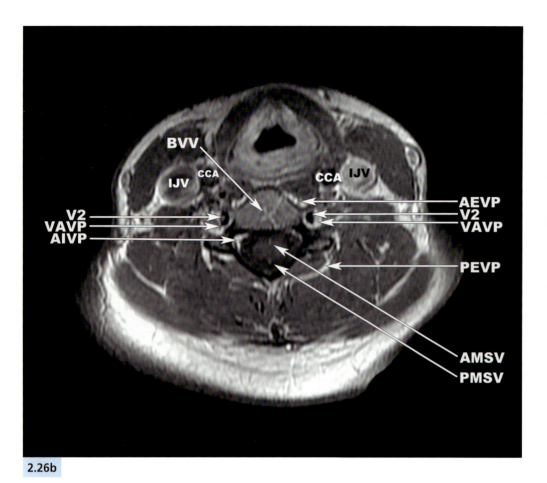

2.26b

FIGURES 2.26b,c *(continued)* AEVP—anterior external vertebral venous plexus, AIVP—anterior internal vertebral venous plexus, AMSV—anterior median spinal vein, ARV—anterior radiculomedullary vein, BVV—basivertebral veins, CCA—common carotid artery, IJV—internal jugular vein, PEVP—posterior external vertebral venous plexus, PMSV—posterior median spinal vein, PRV—posterior radiculomedullary vein, V2—intraforaminal segment of the vertebral artery, VAVP—vertebral artery venous plexus.

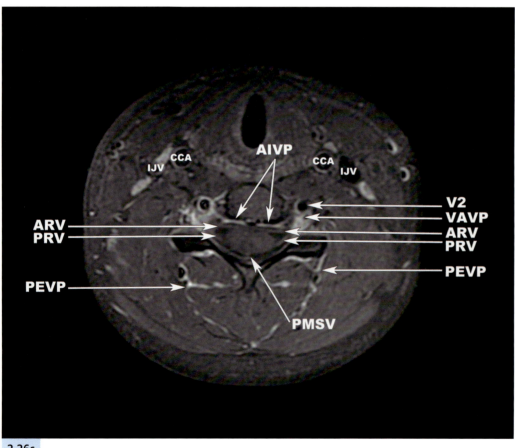

2.26c

(continued)

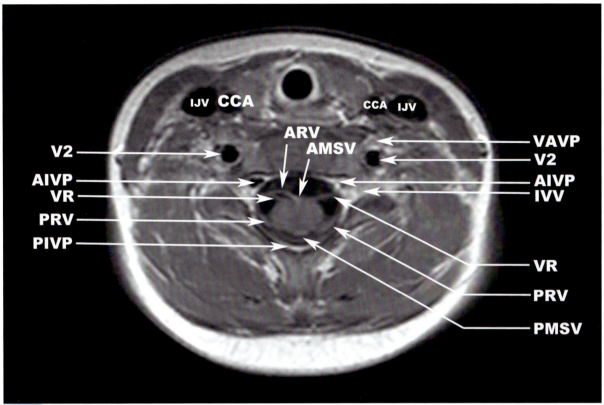

2.26d

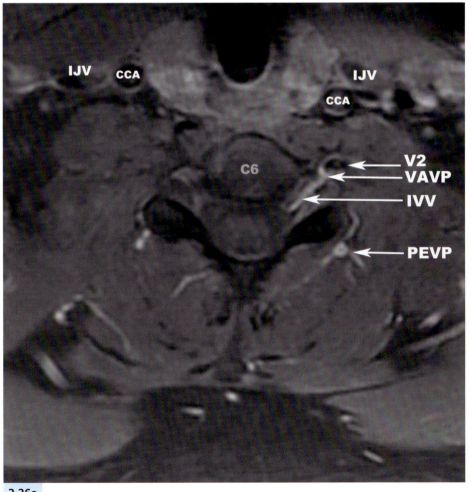

2.26e

FIGURES 2.26d,e (*continued*)
(d) Axial post contrast T1-weighted image showing the right anterior radiculomedullary vein (ARV) arising from the anterior median spinal vein (AMSV) and a distinct structure from the adjacent ventral root (VR). (e) Fat saturated post contrast T1-weighted image demonstrating a left intervertebral vein (IVV) draining into the vertebral artery venous plexus (VAVP). AIVP—anterior internal vertebral venous plexus, AMSV—anterior median spinal vein, ARV—anterior radiculomedullary veins, CCA—common carotid artery, IJV—internal jugular vein, IVV—intervertebral vein, PEVP—posterior external vertebral venous plexus, PIVP—posterior internal vertebral venous plexus, PMSV—posterior median spinal vein, PRV—posterior radiculomedullary vein, VAVP—vertebral artery venous plexus, VR—ventral root.

veins are equipped with a complex valveless system that prevents reflux into the intrinsic and extrinsic venous systems. The radiculomedullary veins and anterior and posterior external vertebral venous plexuses drain into the intervertebral veins (**Figures 2.26b–e**).

The anterior internal vertebral venous plexus resides within two layers of the posterior longitudinal ligament, separated by the dorsomedian septum. It is generally composed of two large, longitudinally oriented veins on either side of the posterior longitudinal ligament (**Figures 2.27a,b**). The anterior internal vertebral venous plexus is typically less prominent

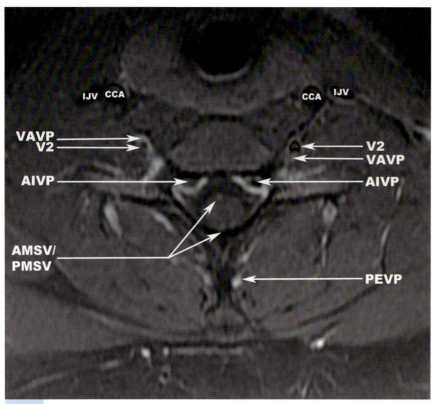

2.27a

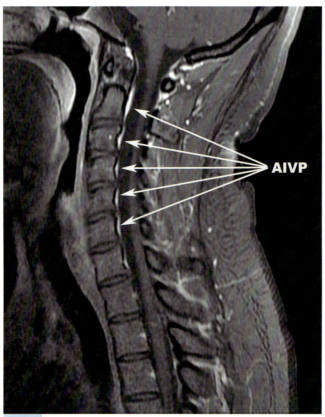

2.27b

FIGURES 2.27a,b   Axial (a) and parasagittal (b) post contrast T1-weighted images displaying the anterior internal vertebral venous plexus (AIVP). AMSV—anterior median spinal vein, CCA—common carotid artery, IJV—internal jugular vein, PEVP—posterior external vertebral venous plexus, PMSV—posterior median spinal vein, V2—intraforaminal segment of the vertebral artery, VAVP—vertebral artery venous plexus.

at the level of the intervertebral discs and courses medially at the pedicle level, where it connects through transversely oriented venous anastamoses to the basivertebral veins, the valved system that provides the primary drainage of the vertebral bodies (Figure 2.26a,b). The minor venous drainage of the vertebral bodies occurs through small peripheral tributaries that communicate directly with the anterior external vertebral venous plexus. The anterior internal vertebral venous plexus also anastamoses with the posterior internal vertebral venous plexus and anterior external vertebral venous plexus (**Figure 2.28**).

The posterior internal vertebral venous plexus is generally smaller in size than the anterior internal vertebral venous plexus and is composed of longitudinally oriented veins traversing the dorsal epidural space that tend to be more laterally located in the cervical spinal canal. In the thoracic and lumbar spinal canal, this plexus is embedded within epidural fat. However, there is little epidural fat within the cervical spinal canal other than a scant dorsal epidural fat pad at C7. The posterior internal vertebral venous plexus receives small draining branches from the lateral masses, lamina, and spinous processes. It also connects with the posterior external vertebral venous plexus via small perforating veins through the ligamenta flava.

The anterior external vertebral venous plexus is located anterior the vertebral bodies and has extensive connections with the intervertebral and basivertebral veins. The posterior external vertebral venous plexus is located dorsal to the spine and drains the paravertebral muscles and the posterior elements (Figure 2.28). It is best developed in the cervical region and has extensive connections with the posterior internal vertebral venous plexus (through the ligamenta flava) and intervertebral veins. Bicuspid valves are variably present within the veins comprising the posterior external vertebral venous plexus.

The intervertebral veins connect the internal and external vertebral venous plexuses and primarily drain into the vertebral veins. There is also venous drainage into the deep cervical and jugular veins. The vertebral veins arise from the suboccipital venous plexus and enter the foramina transversaria at the level of the atlas. The vertebral veins traverse

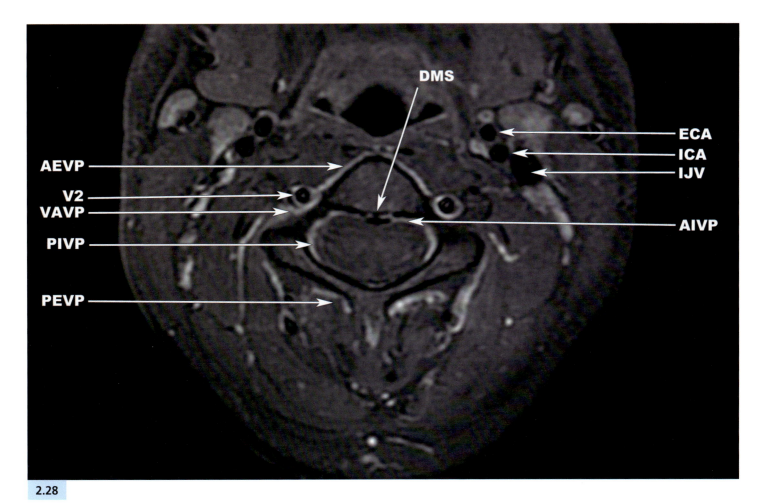

2.28

FIGURE 2.28   The vertebral venous plexuses. There are extensive anastomotic connections between the anterior external vertebral venous plexus (AEVP), anterior internal vertebral venous plexus (AIVP), vertebral artery venous plexus (VAVP), posterior internal vertebral venous plexus (PIVP), and posterior external vertebral venous plexus (PEVP). The anterior internal vertebral venous plexus resides within two layers of the posterior longitudinal ligament, separated by the dorsomedian septum (DMS). ECA—external carotid artery, ICA—internal carotid artery, IJV—internal jugular vein, V2—intraforaminal segment of the vertebral artery.

the C1–C6 foramina transversaria as a single vessel, two vessels, or as a dense plexus (**Figures 2.29a,b**). The distal vertebral veins display significant variability. Most commonly, the vertebral veins exit the foramina transversaria at C6 (range C4–C7) through a single foramen (versus two or more), as a single vessel (versus two or more), descends ventral to the subclavian artery (versus dorsal or both), and drain into the upper (versus lower) portion of the brachiocephalic veins.

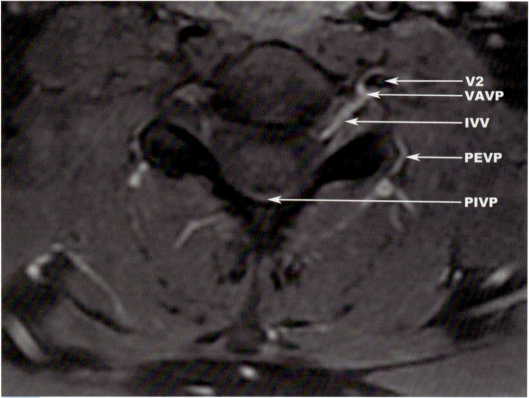

2.29a

FIGURES 2.29a,b Variation of the intervertebral vein (IVV) displayed on T1-weighted fat saturated post contrast images as (a) a single vessel or (b) a dense plexus. PEVP—posterior external vertebral venous plexus, PIVP—posterior internal vertebral venous plexus, V2—intraforaminal segment of the vertebral artery, VAVP—vertebral artery venous plexus.

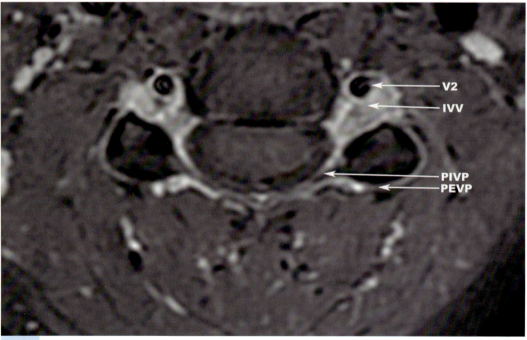

2.29b

MENINGES AND SPACES OF THE SUBAXIAL CERVICAL SPINE

The spinal cord is surrounded by three meninges: pia mater, arachnoid mater, and dura mater. The *pia mater* is a vascularized membrane that is tightly adherent to the spinal cord, envelopes the anterior spinal artery, projects into the ventral median fissure (linea splendans), and forms the *denticulate ligaments*. The denticulate ligaments are longitudinally oriented, discontinuous ligaments that extend from the lateral margins of the spinal cord to the lateral margins of the spinal dura mater and arachnoid between the ventral and dorsal nerve roots. Pia mater also covers the nerve rootlets and roots. In rare instances, pathologic processes (eg, hemorrhage, abscess) disrupt the astrocytic footplates that firmly connect the pia mater to cord parenchyma. Although likely technically incorrect, pathologic processes in this space are commonly referred to as residing within the "subpial space."

The *arachnoid mater* is composed of two layers, a loose inner layer and a compact outer layer. The loose inner layer is composed of arachnoid trabeculations which form a loose collagenous network that connects the pia mater and the outer layer of arachnoid. This space is referred to as the *subarachnoid space* and is where the cerebrospinal fluid is found (**Figures 2.30a–d**). This layer forms a mechanical suspension system for the neural elements and the collagen content of the spinal arachnoid is more prominent than that found in the cranial arachnoid.

The *dura mater* is the outermost layer of the meninges that is made up of three distinct components, the innermost dural border cells, the meningeal dura, and the outer dural border layer. The dural border cells form a structurally weak interface between the outer layer of arachnoid mater and the meningeal layer of the dura mater through which pathologic processes can dissect (eg, blood, injectates). Although a misnomer, this is commonly referred to as the "subdural space" (**Figures 2.31a–c**). The meningeal dura is the thickest layer, is highly vascular, and has sparse innervation. The endosteal layer of the cranial dura mater continues as the spinal periosteum. The spinal dura mater attaches firmly to the foramen magnum,

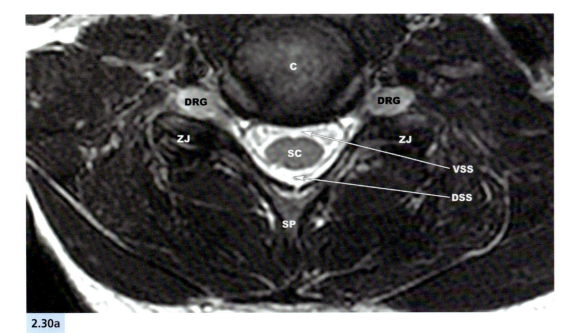

2.30a

FIGURES 2.30a–d   Subarachnoid spaces of the subaxial cervical spine. (a) Axial T2-weighted TSE image demonstrating the ventral (VSS) and dorsal subarachnoid spaces (DSS) surrounding the spinal cord (SC). (b) T2-weighted TSE image demonstrating the appearance of the subarachnoid spaces in the sagittal plane. (c) Axial CT myelogram image in soft tissue algorithm displaying the relationship of the subarachnoid spaces with the epidural fat pads (EFP) and ligamenta flava (LF). (d) Axial image from a CT myelogram in bone algorithm showing contrast opacification of the subarachnoid spaces and outline of the ventral (VR) and dorsal roots (DR). Each set of ventral and dorsal roots exit the subarachnoid space through a dural sleeve (DS). C—centrum, DRG—dorsal root ganglion, SP—spinous process, ZJ—zygapophyseal joint.

(continued)

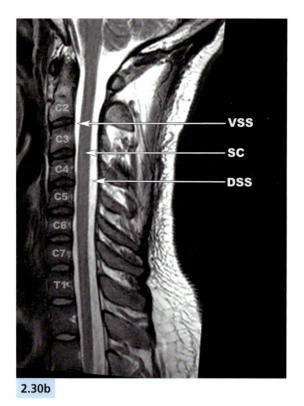

2.30b

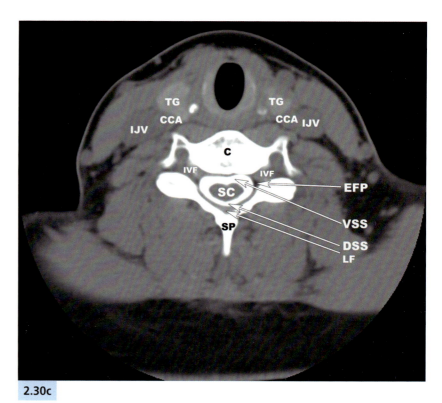

2.30c

2.30d

FIGURES 2.30b–d (*continued*) C—centrum, CCA—common carotid artery, DR—dorsal root, DS—dural sleeve, DSS—dorsal subarachnoid spaces, EFP—epidural fat pads, IJV—internal jugular vein, IVF—intervertebral foramen, LF— ligamenta flava, SC—spinal cord, SP—spinous process, TG—thyroid gland, VR—ventral roots, VSS—ventral subarachnoid spaces.

posterior margins of the C2–C3 vertebral bodies, and the posterior longitudinal ligament. The dura and arachnoid also surround the exiting ventral and dorsal nerve roots along the lateral aspect of the spinal canal, extending toward the neural foramina. The dura blends with the epineurium and the arachnoid blends with the perineurium where the ventral and dorsal nerve roots join to form the spinal nerves.

The *epidural space* lies between the outer dural layer and the periosteum lining the spinal canal (**Figure 2.32**). The anterior boundary includes the dorsal margin of the posterior longitudinal ligament, dorsal periostium of the vertebral bodies, and dorsal annulus of the intervertebral discs. The lateral boundary includes the periostium covering the uncovertebral joints, pedicles, transverse processes, and articular processes. The posterior boundary includes

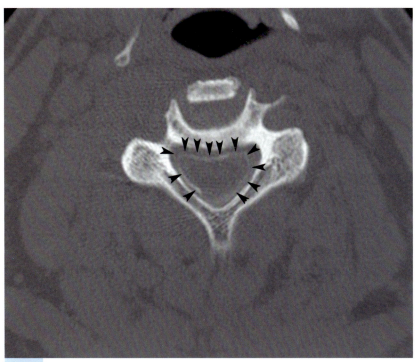

2.31a

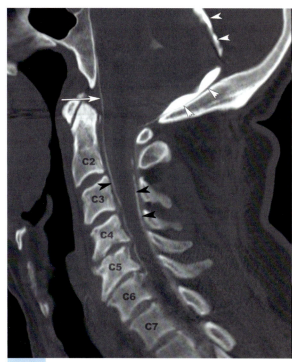

2.31b

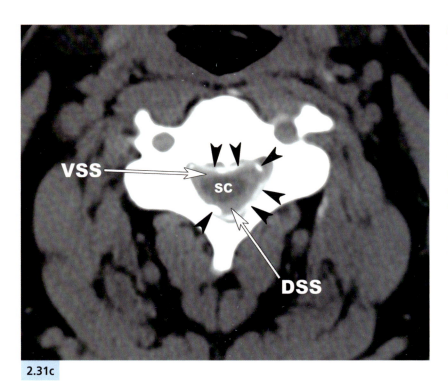

2.31c

FIGURES 2.31a–c   (a) Axial CT myelogram demonstrating dissection of intrathecally administered contrast between outer layer of arachnoid mater and the meningeal layer of the dura mater or the "subdural space" (black arrowheads). (b) Sagittal reformatted image from a CT myelogram showing communication of the "subdural" injection (black arrowheads) with the subdural spaces along the tectorial membrane (white arrow), posterior fossa and tentorial leaflets (white arrowheads). (c) Delayed images from the same patient display filling of the ventral (VSS) and dorsal subarachnoid spaces (DSS) in addition to more concentrated contrast in the "subdural space" (black arrowheads). SC—spinal cord.

the periostium covering the vertebral laminae, the ventral margin of the ligamenta flava, and the ventral periostium of the spinous process roots. The epidural space of the cervical spinal canal contains loose areolar connective tissue, the internal vertebral venous plexuses, arteries, lymphatics, and spinal nerve roots within the intervertebral foramina. There is a paucity of epidural fat within the cervical spinal canal, except for small triangular interlaminar fat pads at C7 and less commonly at C6 (**Figures 2.33a,b**).

Steroids can be injected into the epidural space through an interlaminar or a transforaminal approach for pain relief in the clinical setting. The epidural location of the needle can be confirmed by injecting a small amount of contrast into the epidural space (**Figure 2.34**).

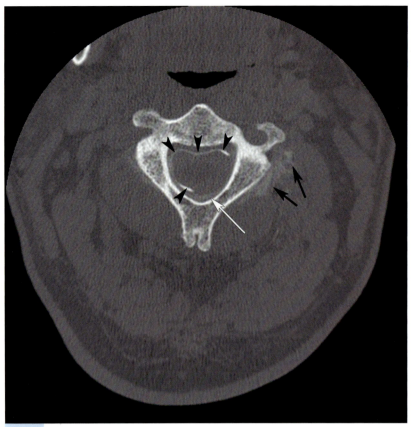

FIGURE 2.32 The dorsal epidural space (white arrow) is distinguished from the "subdural space" (black arrowheads) by its more dorsal location and less concentrated contrast on this axial image from a CT myelogram. Contrast within the epidural space has escaped through the left C2–C3 intervertebral foramen (not shown) and can be seen outside of the spinal canal on the left (black arrows).

2.32

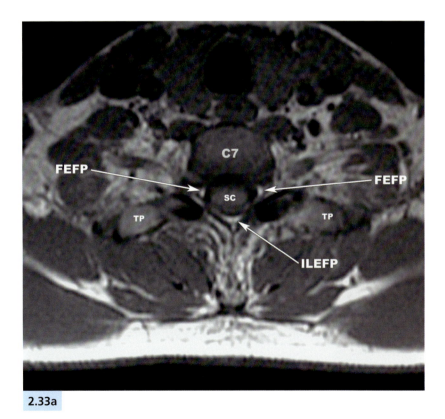

2.33a

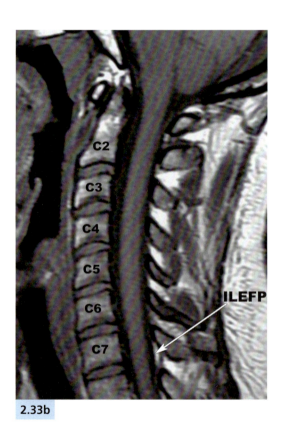

2.33b

FIGURES 2.33a,b The epidural fat pads at C7. (a) Axial and (b) sagittal T1-weighted image showing the triangular interlaminar fat pad (ILEFP) and the crescent-shaped foraminal epidural fat pads (FEFP). SC—spinal cord, TP—transverse process.

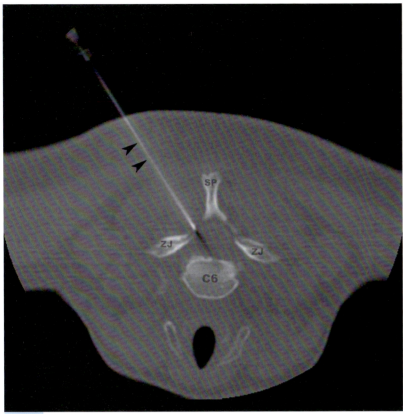

2.34a

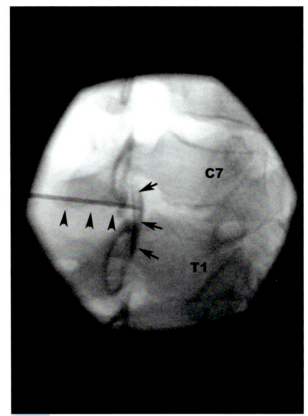

2.34c

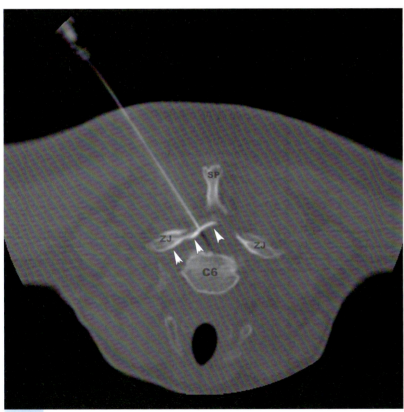

2.34b

FIGURES 2.34a–c   Epidural steroid injections.
(a) CT-guided epidural steroid injection via a C6–C7 interlaminar approach. The spinal needle (black arrowheads) is advanced to the dorsal epidural space through the C6–C7 interlaminar space. (b) A small amount of contrast (white arrowheads) is injected to confirm the epidural location of the needle tip. (c) Lateral oblique fluoroscopic image from a fluoroscopically guided epidural steroid injection displaying the posterolateral interlaminar approach of the needle (black arrowheads) and the epidural location of injected contrast (black arrows) at the level of C7–T1. SP—spinous process, ZJ— zygapophyseal joint. (Figures 2.34a,b, courtesy of Dr. Sumir Patel)

NEURAL ANATOMY OF THE SUBAXIAL CERVICAL SPINE

The cervical spine cord has a circular elliptical shape at C1–C2, increases in transverse dimension to form a broader and larger ellipse at C4–C5, then gradually returns to a circular elliptical shape in the upper thoracic segments. The increase in transverse dimension between C3 and T2 is referred to as the *cervical enlargement* and corresponds to increased numbers of efferent and afferent neurons associated with the upper extremities. Because the spinal canal within the subaxial cervical segments is relatively constant in diameter, the subarachnoid spaces around the cervical enlargement are smaller relative to those of the upper cervical and mid to lower thoracic segments (**Figure 2.35**).

The outer contour of the cervical spinal cord is formed by a deep *ventral median fissure* and a shallow *dorsal median sulcus*. A short distance lateral to the dorsal median sulcus is a shallow groove called the *dorsal intermediate sulcus*, rarely seen on imaging. The *dorsolateral sulcus* corresponds to the dorsal root entry zone. Located just lateral to the ventral median fissure is the *ventrolateral sulcus* which corresponds to the ventral root entry zone. The anterior spinal artery courses in the ventral median fissure. The posterior spinal arteries course just medial to the dorsolateral sulci. Spinal cord surface anatomy is summarized in **Figure 2.36**.

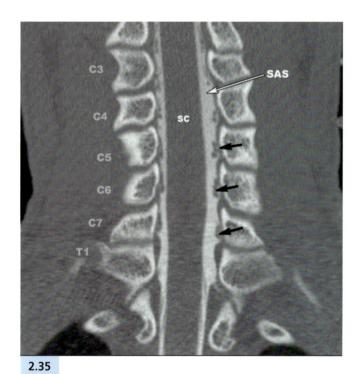

2.35

FIGURE 2.35 The cervical enlargement. Coronal curved reformatted CT image following injection of contrast into the subarachnoid space (CT myelography) demonstrates a progressive increase in the transverse dimension of the spinal cord (SC) from C4 to C7, with a corresponding progressive decrease in the size of the subarachnoid spaces (SAS). Nerve roots (black arrows) within the subarachnoid space can be seen along the lateral margin of the spinal canal. SC—spinal cord.

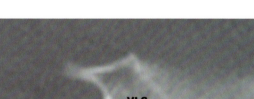

2.36

FIGURE 2.36 Axial image from a cervical CT myelogram displays the surface anatomy of the subaxial cervical spinal cord. The root entry zones of the ventral (VR) and dorsal roots (DR) mark the positions of the ventrolateral (VLS) and dorsolateral sulci (DLS). The ventral median fissure (VMF) and dorsal median sulcus (DMS) are seen as shallow ventral and dorsal grooves, respectively.

In contradistinction to the cerebrum, the white matter of the spinal cord is located at the periphery. The central gray matter has a butterfly or H-shape formed by two ventral horns, two dorsal horns, and the gray commissure. The ventral horns are prominent C4–C7 and contain the cell bodies for motor neurons that form the ventral roots. These neurons coalesce into multiple rootlets that exit the cord (ventral root entry zone) at the ventrolateral sulci. The dorsal horns receive second order afferents from the dorsal root ganglia. The dorsal root entry zones are the dorsolateral sulci. The internal organization of the spinal cord gray matter has been further subdivided into 10 layers called the *Rexed laminae*. The Rexed lamina are arranged in numerical order from lamina I in the tip of the dorsal horns to lamina IX in the ventral horn. Lamina X comprises the ventral and dorsal gray matter commissures surrounding the central canal of the spinal cord. The central canal is an ependyma-lined extension of the fourth ventricle that obliterates with increasing age. The central canal is located between the anterior and posterior gray commissures. Spinal cord internal anatomy is summarized in **Figure 2.37**.

The white matter of the cervical spinal cord is disproportionate relative to cord gray matter and can be subdivided into the ventral, dorsal, and lateral funiculi. Each funiculus contains multiple fiber tracts that are either ascending (sensory), descending (motor), or transverse. The ventral funiculi contain mainly descending tracts, including the medial reticulospinal tracts, anterior corticospinal tracts, tectospinal tracts, and vestibulospinal tracts. The ventral funiculi or *dorsal columns* contain ascending tracts, including the fasciculus gracilis and fasciculus cuneatus. *Lissauer's tracts* are thin columns of white matter that are situated between the dorsal horns and the surface of the cord at the dorsal root entry zones. The lateral funiculi contain both ascending and descending tracts. Ascending tracts within the lateral funiculi include the anterior spinocerebellar tracts, lateral spinothalamic tracts, and posterior spinocerebellar tracts. Descending tracts within the lateral funiculi include the rubrospinal tracts, lateral corticospinal tracts, and lateral reticulospinal tracts.

Individual fiber tracts are generally not visible on standard imaging studies, with the exception of some of the larger caliber tracts with the use of diffusion tensor imaging. However, knowledge of the expected location of the major ascending and descending tracts can be useful when lesions are encountered and correlation with neurological deficits is required. **Figure 2.38** demonstrates the typical location of the major ascending and descending tracts.

Multiple rootlets arise from the ventrolateral (6–8) and dorsolateral sulci (2–13) that coalesce to form the ventral and dorsal roots, respectively. On axial images, the ventral and dorsal roots in the subaxial segments course ventrolaterally at about a 45 degree angle into

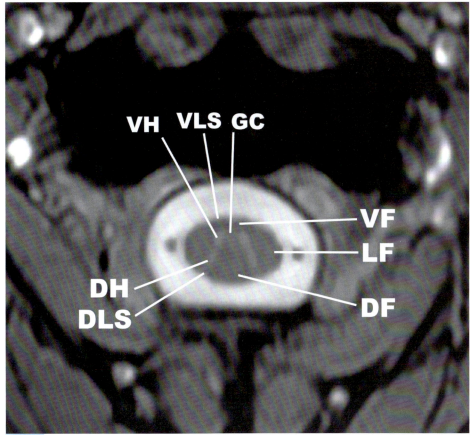

FIGURE 2.37   White and gray matter organization of the spinal cord. The ventral (VF), lateral (LF), and dorsal funiculi (DF) are displayed on the right of the image. Gray matter structures include the gray commissure (GC), ventral horn (VH), and dorsal horn (DH) are shown on the left side of the image. DLS—dorsolateral sulcus, VLS—ventral lateral sulcus.

2.37

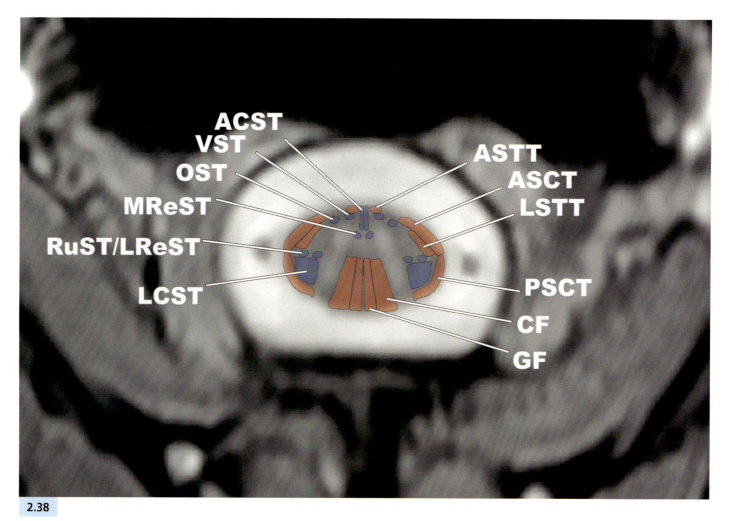

2.38

FIGURE 2.38   The expected positions of the ascending (red) and descending (blue) tracts are superimposed upon an axial multi-fast field echo (m-FFE) image of the cervical spinal cord. ACST—anterior corticospinal tract, ASCT—anterior spinocerebellar tract, ASTT—anterior spinothalamic tract, CF—cuneate fasciculus, GF—gracile fasciculus, LCST—lateral corticospinal tract, LSTT—lateral spinothalamic tract, MReST—medial reticulospinal tract, OST—olivospinal tract, PSCT—posterior spinothalamic tract, RuST/LReST—rubrospinal tract/lateral reticulospinal tract, VST—vestibulospinal tract.

the neural foramina (Figure 2.36). The C3–C7 nerve roots travel caudad one vertebral segment from their root entry zones to their exit through the intervertebral foramina (**Figure 2.39**). For example, the C4 nerve root entry zones are located at the C3 vertebral level and they exit through the C4–C5 intervertebral foramina. The C8 nerve roots exit the cord at the C6 vertebral level and exit through the C7–T1 intervertebral foramina (**Figure 2.40**). The more caudal cervical nerve roots arise closer to the midline of the spinal cord.

The dorsal root ganglia are found along the lateral margin of the neural foramina and are visualized as ovoid enlargements. The dorsal root ganglia contain the cell bodies of the sensory fibers. The dorsal root ganglia lack a blood-nerve barrier and enhance avidly following iodinated and gadolinium contrast administration (**Figure 2.41**). Just distal to the dorsal root ganglia, the ventral and dorsal roots coalesce to form mixed spinal nerves. The spinal nerves exit the neural foramina and divide into ventral and dorsal rami.

The innervation of the spine can be roughly divided into two compartments, ventral and dorsal. The ventral compartment is innervated by the sinuvertebral nerves and branches of the ventral rami and includes the intervertebral discs, ventral dura mater, nerve roots, and longitudinal ligaments. The dorsal compartment is innervated by the dorsal rami and mixed spinal nerves and includes the zygapophyseal joints, posterior ligamentous complex, and dorsal paraspinal musculature.

The arrangement of the cervical nerve roots differs from that seen in the thoracic, lumbar, and sacral levels. The C3–C7 spinal nerves exit the neural foramina above their corresponding level. For example, the C3 spinal nerves exit the C2–C3 neural foramina. The C8 spinal nerves exit the C7–T1 neural foramina.

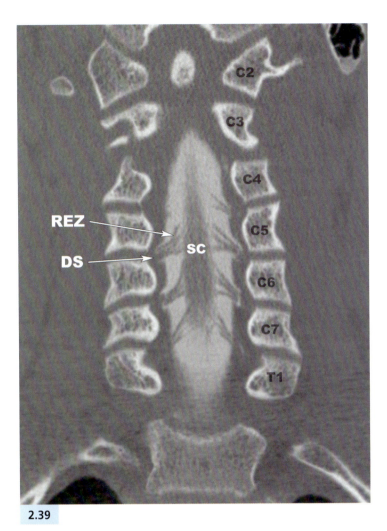

2.39

FIGURE 2.39   The C3–C7 nerve root entry zones (REZ) are located one segment above their points of exit through the dural sleeves (DS). SC—spinal cord.

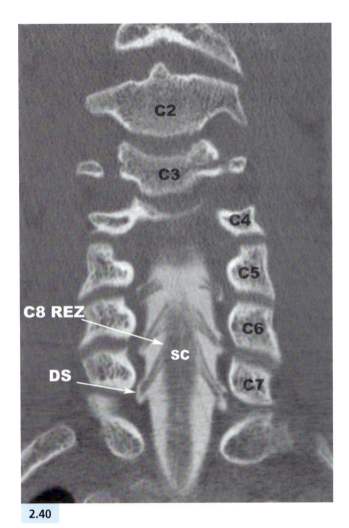

2.40

FIGURE 2.40   The C8 nerve root entry zones (C8 REZ) are located at the C6 level. The C8 nerve roots course inferiorly to exit through the dural sleeves (DS) at C7–T1. SC—spinal cord.

FIGURE 2.41   Fat saturated post contrast T1-weighted image at C5–C6 demonstrating the avid enhancement of the dorsal root ganglia (white arrows). ICA—internal carotid artery, IJV—internal jugular vein, VA—vertebral artery.

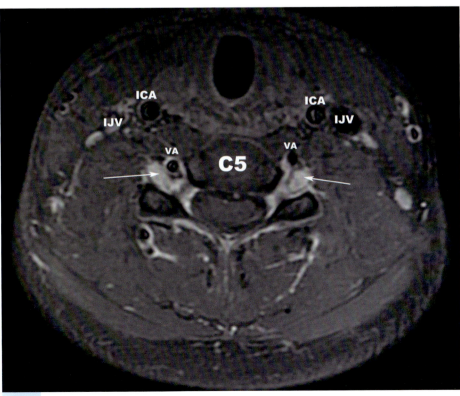

2.41

GALLERY OF ANATOMIC VARIANTS AND VARIOUS CONGENITAL ANOMALIES

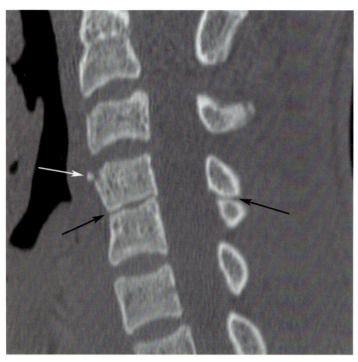

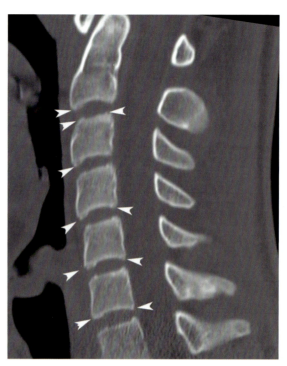

IMAGE 1   Sagittal reformatted CT image showing a C4 limbus vertebra (white arrow) and partial fusion of the C4–C5 vertebral bodies and posterior elements (black arrows).

IMAGE 2   Sagittal reformatted CT image demonstrating incomplete ossification of the ring apophyses (white arrowheads).

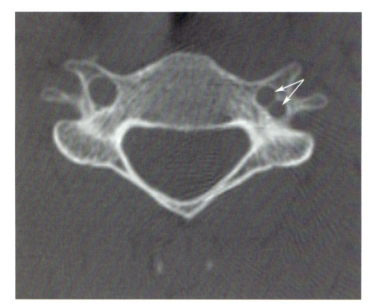

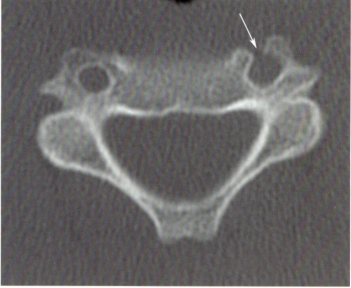

IMAGE 3   Axial CT image displaying a duplicated left foramen transversarium (white arrows).

IMAGE 4   Axial CT image showing incomplete ossification of the left costal element, exposing the left foramen transversarium ventrally (white arrow).

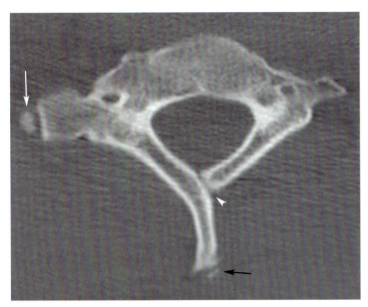

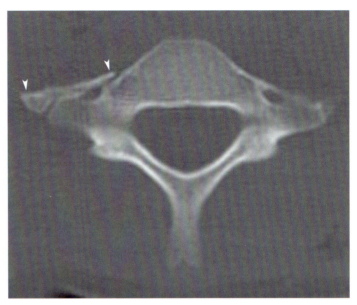

IMAGE 5   Axial CT image of C7 demonstrating nonfusion of the right transverse process secondary ossification center (white arrow), nonfusion of a spinous process secondary ossification center (black arrow), and nonfusion of the left lamina with the spinous process (white arrowhead).

IMAGE 6   Axial CT image displaying nonfusion of the ventral bar on the right (white arrowheads).

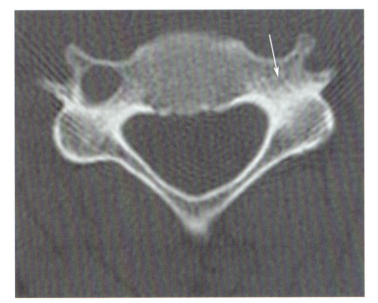

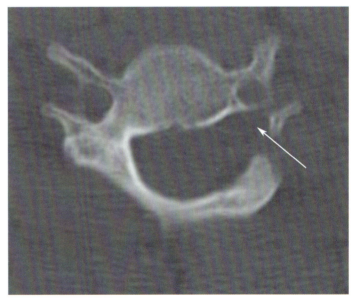

IMAGE 7   Axial CT image showing an absent left foramen transversarium (white arrow).

IMAGE 8   Axial CT image demonstrating congenital absence of the left pedicle (white arrow).

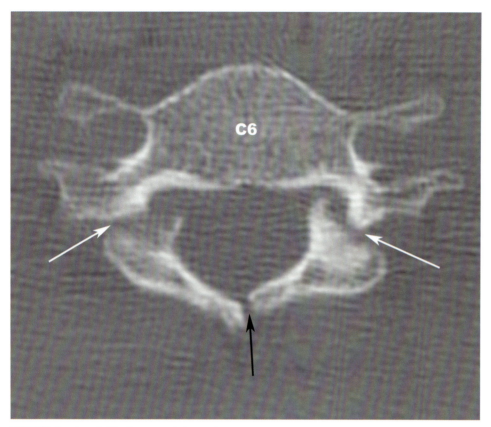

IMAGE 9 Axial CT showing bilateral C4 pars interarticularis defects (white arrows) and a bifid spinous process (black arrow).

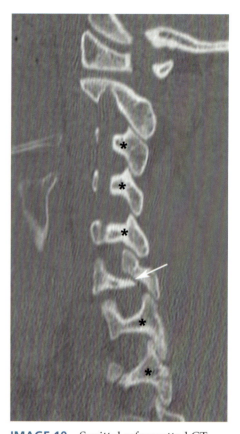

IMAGE 10 Sagittal reformatted CT image displaying nonfusion of the right C6 pedicle with the right pars interarticularis. The normal pattern of fusion (asterisks) is shown for comparison. The reader may also notice the dysplastic appearance of the right C6 superior and inferior articular processes.

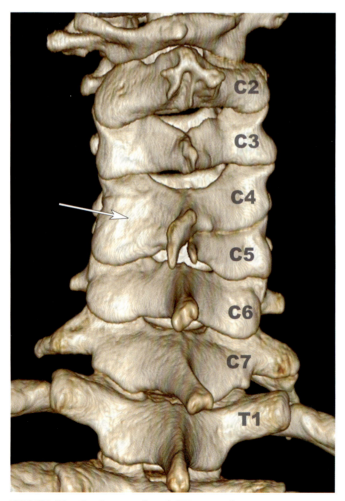

IMAGE 11 Surface rendered CT image from a posterior projection shows nonsegmentation of the left C4 and C5 lamina and articular processes (white arrow).

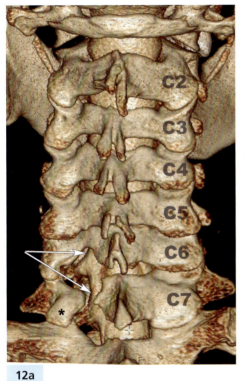

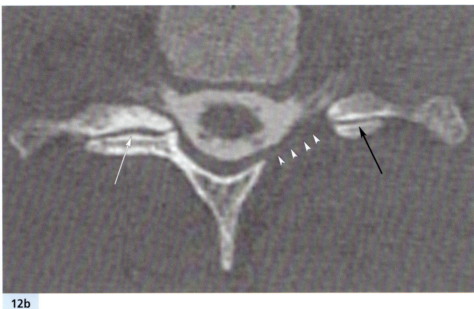

IMAGES 12a,b   Hypoplastic left C7–T1 zygapophyseal joint. (a) Surface rendered image from a CT myelogram captured from a posterior projection showing a hypoplasia of the left C7–T1 zygapophyseal joint (*). The patient has undergone a left C6 laminotomy (top white arrow) and left C7 laminectomy (bottom white arrow). (b) Axial image from a CT myelogram demonstrating the significant asymmetry in the size of the left (black arrow) and right (white arrow) zygapophyseal joints. The left-sided laminectomy is better visualized (white arrowheads).

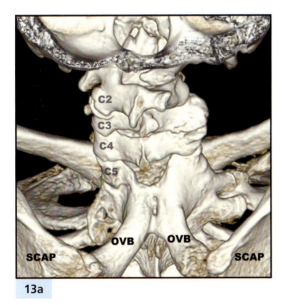

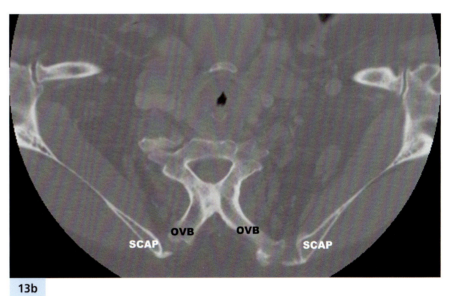

IMAGES 13a,b   Omovertebral bones. Surface rendered (a) and axial (b) CT images from a posterior projection displays bilateral omovertebral bones (OVB), projecting from the C5 spinous processes to high-riding scapulae (SCAP). There are segmentation anomalies of the C5 and C6 posterior elements.

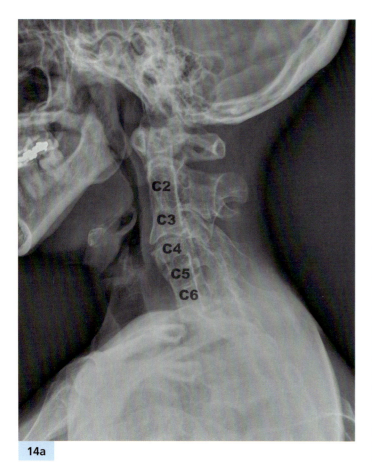

14a

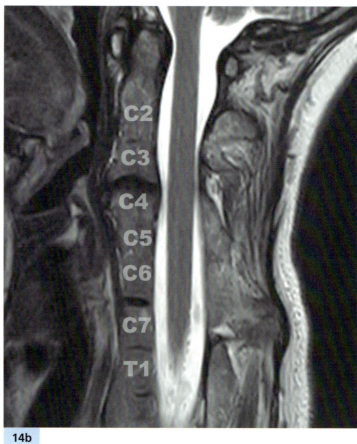

14b

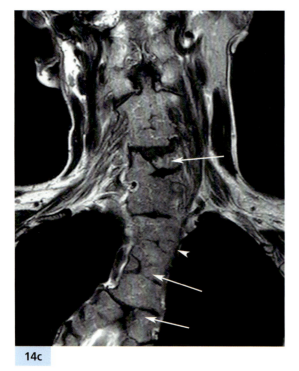

14c

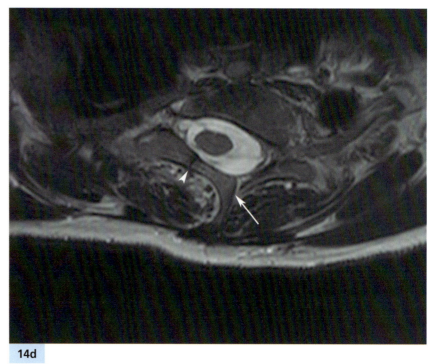

14d

IMAGES 14a–d The Klippel–Feil syndrome is characterized by congenital fusion of any two cervical segments and is demonstrated on (a) lateral x-ray and (b) sagittal T2-weighted TSE MR images. (c) Coronal T2-weighted TSE MR image demonstrates the presence of butterfly vertebrae (white arrows) and a left-sided hemivertebra (white arrowhead). (d) Axial T2-weighted TSE MR image from the same patient displaying coexisting nonfusion of the left lamina with the spinous process (white arrow) and incomplete fusion of the right lamina (white arrowhead).

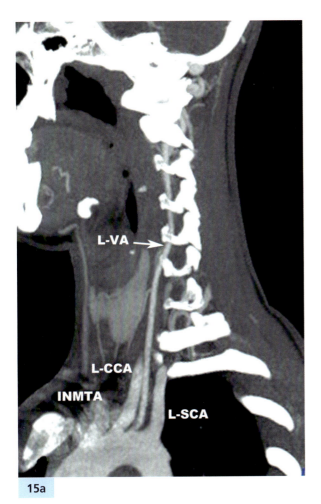

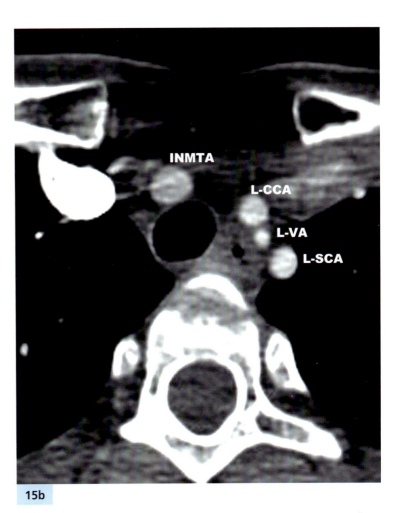

IMAGES 15a,b   Sagittal oblique maximum intensity projection CTA image (a) and axial CTA image (b) demonstrating origin of the left vertebral artery (L-VA) from the aortic arch between the left common carotid artery (L-CCA) and the left subclavian artery (L-SCA), the second most common origin of the left vertebral artery. The left vertebral artery enters the C5 foramen transversarium (white arrow). INMTA—innominate artery.

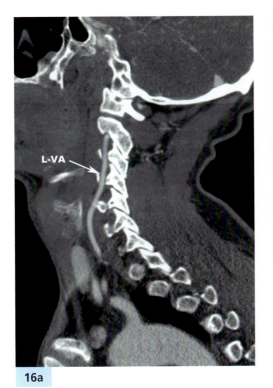

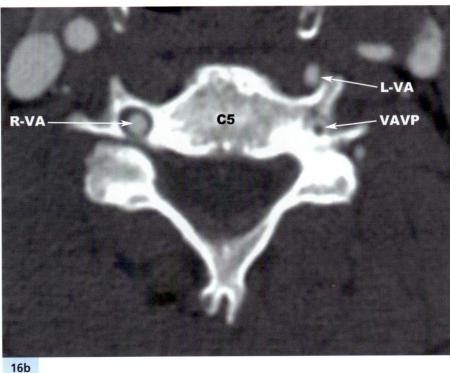

IMAGES 16a,b   (a) Sagittal oblique CTA image showing the left vertebral artery (L-VA) entering the left C4 foramen transversarium (white arrow). (b) Axial CTA image at C5 displays a small caliber left foramen transversarium that houses only the vertebral artery venous plexus (VAVP), while the L-VA is positioned in the vertebral groove prior to entering the C4 foramen transversarium. The right vertebral artery (R-VA) at this level is located within the foramen transversarium.

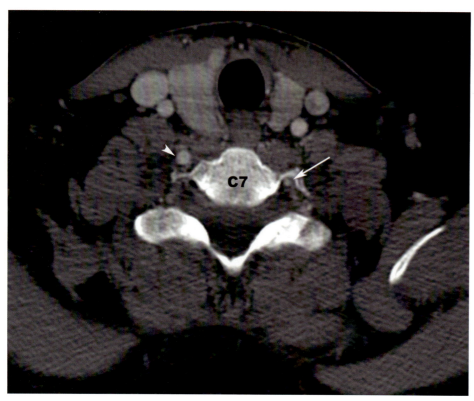

IMAGE 17 Axial CTA image demonstrates a nondominant left vertebral artery that enters the C7 foramen transversarium (white arrow). The dominant right vertebral artery (white arrowhead) is located within the vertebral groove prior to its entry at C6.

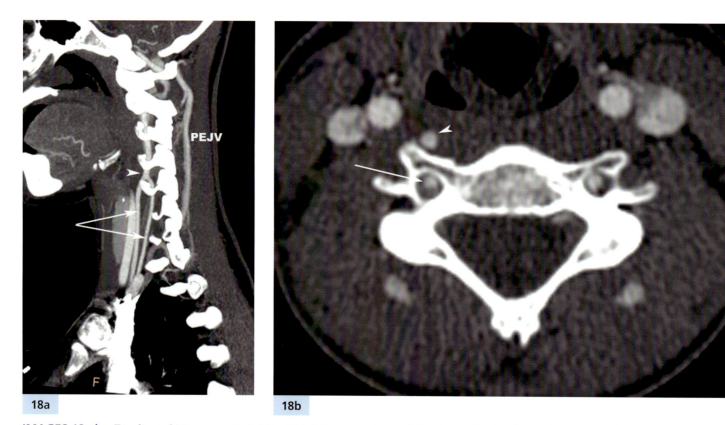

IMAGES 18a,b Duplicated V1 segments. (a) Sagittal oblique maximum intensity projection image from a CTA demonstrating two right V1 segments that both arise from the subclavian artery. The posteriorly located V1 segment enters the C5 foramen transversarium (lower white arrow) and the anterior V1 enters the C4 foramen transversarium (upper white arrow). A single V2 segment is present C2–C4 (white arrowhead). (b) Axial CTA image at C5 shows the posterior V1 segment within the right foramen transversarium (white arrow) and the anterior V1 segment adjacent to the anterior tubercle (white arrowhead). PEJV—posterior external jugular vein.

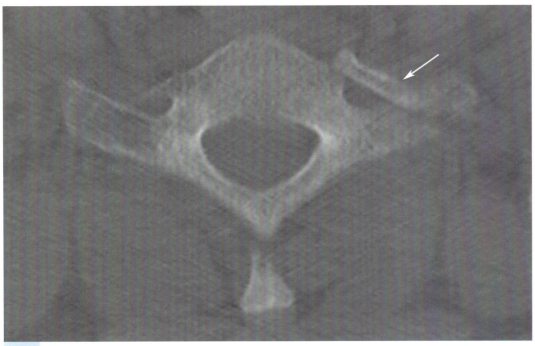

19a

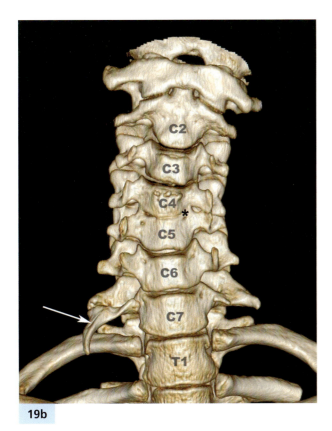

19b

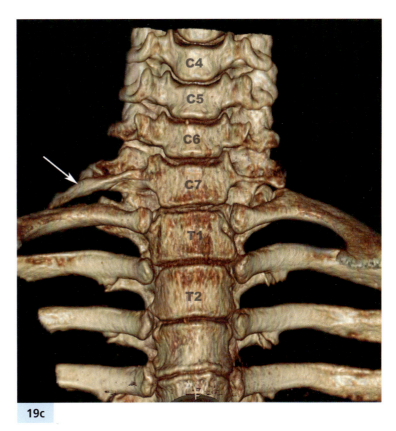

19c

IMAGES 19a–c   Unilateral cervical ribs. (a) Axial CT image showing a small left-sided C7 rib (arrow). (b) Surface rendered CT image from a frontal projection showing a small right C7 rib. There is partial fusion of the C4 and C5 vertebral bodies (asterisk) that is associated with a right convex cervical scoliosis. (c) Surface rendered CT image from a frontal projection showing a right-sided C7 rib that has a more elongated configuration.

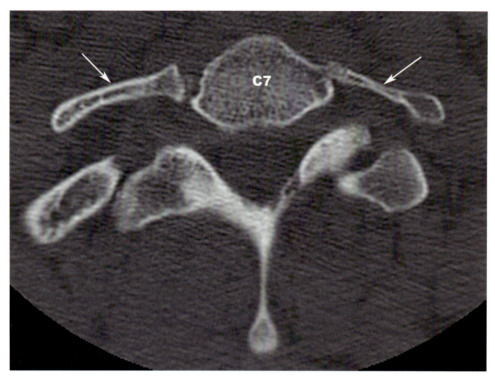

IMAGE 20 Axial CT image showing small, floating C7 ribs bilaterally (white arrows).

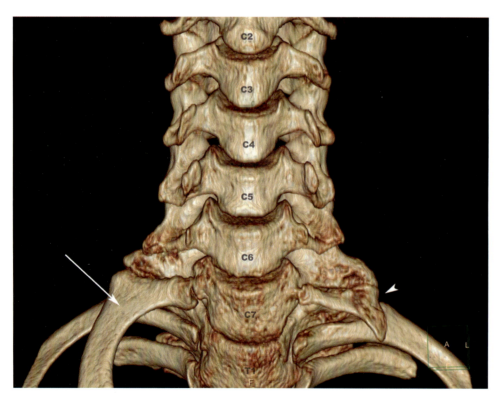

IMAGE 21 Surface rendered CT image from a frontal projection showing a small, floating left C7 rib (white arrowhead) and a full right C7 rib (white arrow) that articulates with the sternum (not shown).

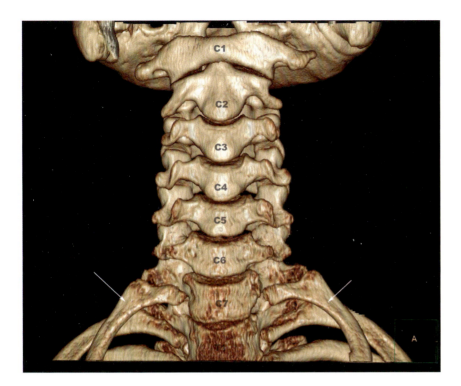

IMAGE 22   Surface rendered CT image from a frontal projection displaying full C7 ribs bilaterally (white arrows) that articulate with the sternum (not shown).

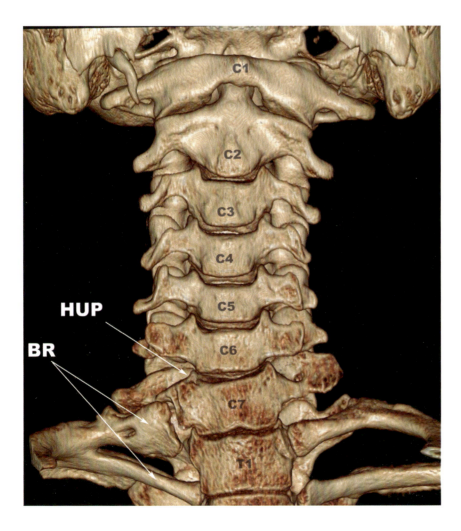

IMAGE 23   Surface rendered CT image from a frontal projection demonstrating a bifid T1 rib (BR) that articulates with C7 (upper arrow) and T1 (lower arrow). The ipsilateral C7 uncinate process is hypoplastic (HUP).

SUGGESTED READINGS

Abrams HL. The vertebral and azygous venous systems, and some variations in systemic venous return. *Radiology.* 1957;69:508–526.

Bland J. *Disorders of the Cervical Spine.* Philadelphia: W. B. Saunders; 1987.

Bogduk N. The innervation of the vertebral column. *Aust J Physio.* 1985;31(3):89–94.

Boreadis AG, Gershon-Cohen J. Luschka joints of the cervical spine. *Radiology.* 1956;66(2):181–187.

Brismee JM, Sizer PS Jr, Dedrick GS, et al. Immunohistochemical and histological study of human uncovertebral joints: a preliminary investigation. *Spine.* 2009;34:1257–1263.

Catell HS, Filtzer DL. Pseudosubluxation and other normal variations in the cervical spine in children. *J Bone Joint Surg Am.* 1965;47:1295–1309.

Cramer GD, Darby SA. *Clinical Anatomy of the Spine, Spinal Cord, and Ans.* 3rd ed. St. Louis: Elsevier, 2014.

Dean NA, Mitchell BS. Anatomic relation between the nuchal ligament (ligamentum nuchae) and the spinal dura mater in the craniocervical region. *Clin Anat.* 2002;15:182–185.

Demondion X, Lefebvre G, Fisch O, et al. Radiographic anatomy of the intervertebral cervical and lumbar foramina (vessels and variants). *Diagn Interv Imaging.* 2012;93:690–697.

Dilenge D. The physiologic role of the miningorachidian plexus. In: Theron J, Moret J, eds. *Spinal Phlebography. Lumbar and Cervical Techniques.* Berlin: Springer-Verlag: 3–23.

Forsberg DA, Martinez S, Volger III JB, et al. Cervical spondylolysis: imaging findings in 12 patients. *Am J Roentgenol.* 1990;154:751–755.

Gabrielsen TO. Size of vertebral artery and of foramen transversarium of axis. An anatomic study. *Acta Radiol Diagn.* 1969;9:285–291.

Ghanem I, El Hage S, Rachkidi R, et al. Pediatric cervical spine instability. *J Child Orthop.* 2008;2:71–84.

Griessenauer CJ, Raborn J, Foreman P, et al. Venous drainage of the spine and spinal cord: a comprehensive review of its history, embryology, anatomy, physiology, and pathology. *Clin Anat.* 2014. doi:1002/ca.22354

Hartman J. Anatomy and clinical significance of the uncinate process and uncovertebral joint: a comprehensive review. Clin Anat. 2014;27:431–440.

Hayashi K, Yabuki T, Kurokawa T, et al. The anterior and posterior longitudinal ligament of the lower cervical spine. *J Anat.* 1977;124(3):633–636.

Humphreys BK, Kenin S, Hubbard BB, Cramer GD. Investigation of connective tissue attachments to the cervical spinal dura mater. *Clin Anat.* 2003;16:152–159.

Johnson GM, Zhang M, Jones DG. The fine connective tissue architecture of the human ligamentum nuchae. *Spine.* 2000;25(1):5–9.

Kadri PAS, Al-Mefty O. Anatomy of the nuchal ligament and its surgical applications. *Neurosurgery.* 2007;61(5 suppl 2):301–304.

Karatas A, Caglar S, Savas A, Erdogan A. Microsurgical anatomy of the dorsal cervical rootlets and dorsal root entry zones. *Acta Neurochir (Wien).* 2005;147(2):195–199.

Kim JH, Lee CW, Chun KS, et al. Morphometric relationship between the cervicothoracic cord segments and vertebral bodies. *J Korean Neurosurg Soc.* 2012;52:384–390.

Martirosyan NL, Feuerstein JS, Theodore N, et al. Blood supply and vascular reactivity of the spinal cord under normal and pathological conditions. *J Neurosurg Spine.* 2011;15:238–251.

Mercer S, Bogduk N. The ligaments and annulus fibrosus of human adult cervical intervertebral discs. *Spine (Phila Pa 1976).* 1999;24(7):619–626.

Mercer S, Jull GA. Morphology of the cervical intervertebral disc: implications for McKenzie's model of the disc derangement syndrome. *Man Therap.* 1996;2:76–81.

Miyake H, Kiyosue H, Tanoue S, et al. Termination of the vertebral veins: evaluation by multidetector row computed tomography. *Clin Anat.* 2010;23:662–672.

Pal GP, Routal RV, Saggu SK. The orientation of the articular facets of the zygapophyseal joints at the cervical and upper thoracic region. *J Anat.* 2001;198:431–441.

Panjabi MM, Oxland T, Takata K, et al. Articular facets of the human spine. *Spine.* 1993;18:1298–1310.

Przybylski, GJ, Carlin GJ, Patel PR, Woo SL. Human anterior and posterior cervical longitudinal ligaments possess similar tensile properties. *J Orthop Res.* 1996;14(6):1005–1008.

Sanelli PC, Tong S, Gonzalez RG, Eskey CJ. Normal variation of vertebral artery on CT angiography and its implications for diagnosis of acquired pathology. *J Comp Assist Tomog.* 2002;26(3):462–470.

Scott JE, Bosworth TR, Cribb AM, Taylor JR. The chemical morphology of age-related changes in human intervertebral disc glycosaminoglycans from cervical, thoracic, and lumbar nucleus pulposus and anulus fibrosis. *J Anat.* 1994;184:73–82.

Shaw M, Burnett H, Wilson A, Chan O. Pseudosubluxation of C2 on C3 in polytraumatized children—prevalence and significance. *Clin Radiol.* 1999;54:377–380.

Sherman JL, Nassaux PY, Citrin CM. Measurements of the normal cervical spinal cord on MR imaging. *Am J Neuroradiol.* 1990;11:369–372.

Stringer MD, Restieaux M, Fisher AL, Crosado B. The vertebral venous plexuses: the internal veins are muscular and external veins have valves. *Clin Anat.* 2012; 25:609–618.

Swischuk LE. Anterior displacement of C2 in children: physiologic or pathologic. A helpful differentiating line. *Radiology.* 1977;122:759–763.

Taylor JR, Twomey LT. Vertebral column development and its relation to adult pathology. *Aust J Physiother*. 1985;31(3):83–88.

Tonetti J, Peoc'h M, Merloz P, et al. Elastic reinforcement and thickness of the joint capsules of the lower cervical spine. *Surg Radiol Anat*. 1999;21:35–39.

Yasui K, Hashizume Y, Yoshida M, et al. Age-related morphologic changes of the central canal of the human spinal cord. *Acta Neuropathol*. 1999;97:253–259.

Yoganandan N, Pintar FA, Lew SM, et al. Quantitative analyses of pediatric cervical spine ossification patterns using computed tomography. *Ann Adv Automot Med.* 2011;55:159–168.

The Thoracic Spine

The thoracic spine is the longest portion of the spine, containing 12 segments. The thoracic kyphosis is one of the primary curves of the spine, forming during fetal development along with the sacral kyphosis. The unique anatomy of the thoracic segments results in relative immobility in comparison to the cervical and lumbar segments.

DEVELOPMENTAL ANATOMY OF THE THORACIC SPINE

The thoracic segments are formed from the centrum, and right and left neural arches. The neurocentral synchondroses are located between the central and neural arches. The posterior synchondroses are located between the dorsal tips of the neural arches (**Figure 3.1**). The posterior synchondroses close within 2 to 3 postnatal months. The neurocentral synchondroses of the thoracic segments close later than the cervical and lumbar segments and close in a rostral to caudal fashion beginning around 5 to 6 years of age. It is not uncommon to see partially unfused thoracic neurocentral synchondroses in adults.

There are five typical secondary ossification centers found within each thoracic segment, including ring apophyses along the superior and inferior margins of the vertebral body, the tip of each transverse process, and the tip of the spinous process. Additional secondary ossification centers can be found along the articular and nonarticular surfaces of the transverse processes, upper costal demifacets, and lower costal demifacets (discussed in the following). Complete fusion of the secondary ossification centers can occur as early as 15 years of age. Incomplete fusion of the secondary ossification centers may be seen in the early part of the third decade. Complete fusion is usually present by the mid-20s. Fusion of the neurocentral synchondroses in the thoracic segments may be incomplete in adulthood. The typical appearance of the ossification centers of the typical thoracic vertebrae at various ages is summarized in **Figures 3.2a–p**.

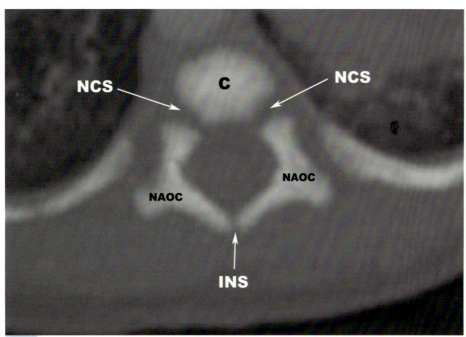

3.1

FIGURE 3.1   The typical thoracic vertebrae are derived from three primary ossification centers, a centrum (C) and two neural arches. The neurocentral synchondroses (NCS) are located between the C and the neural arch ossification centers (NAOC). The intraneural synchondrosis (INS) is located between the NAOC posteriorly.

Newborn

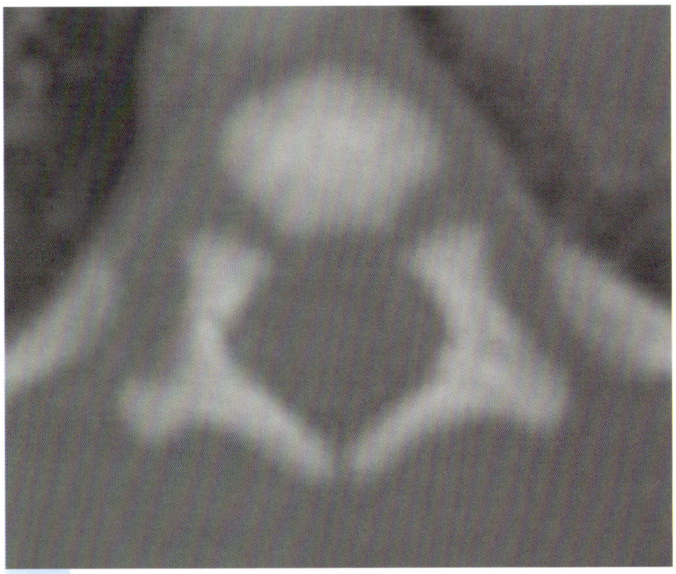

3 months

3.2a

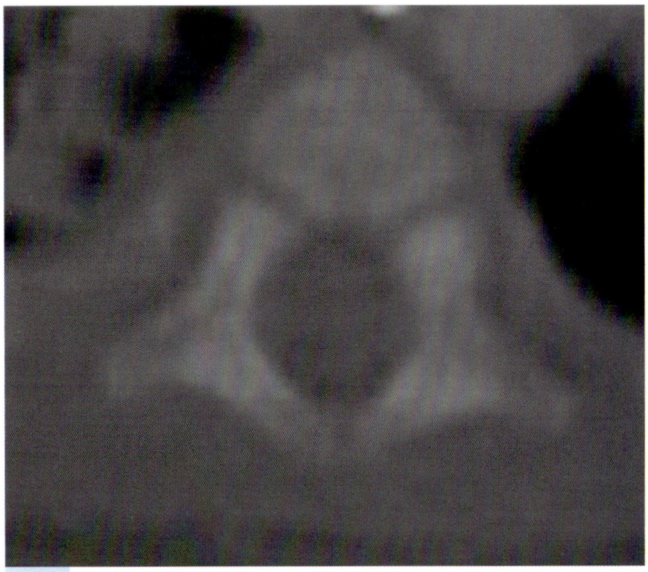

3.2c

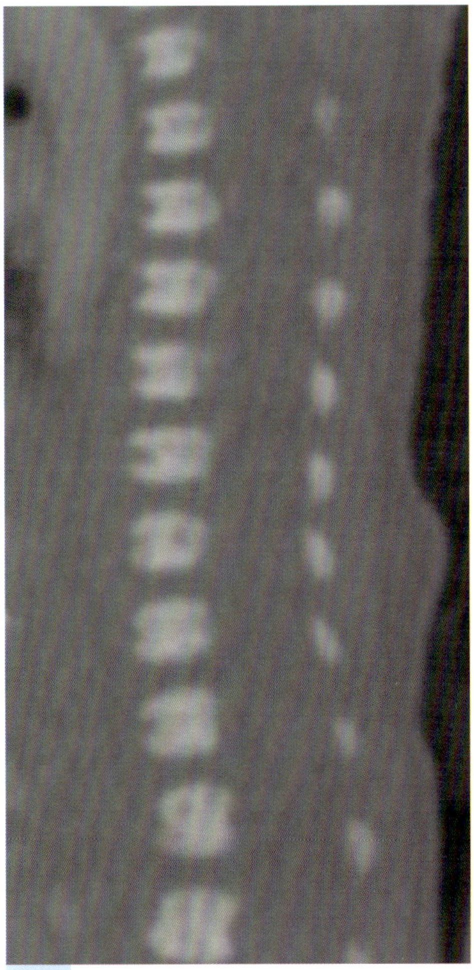

3.2b

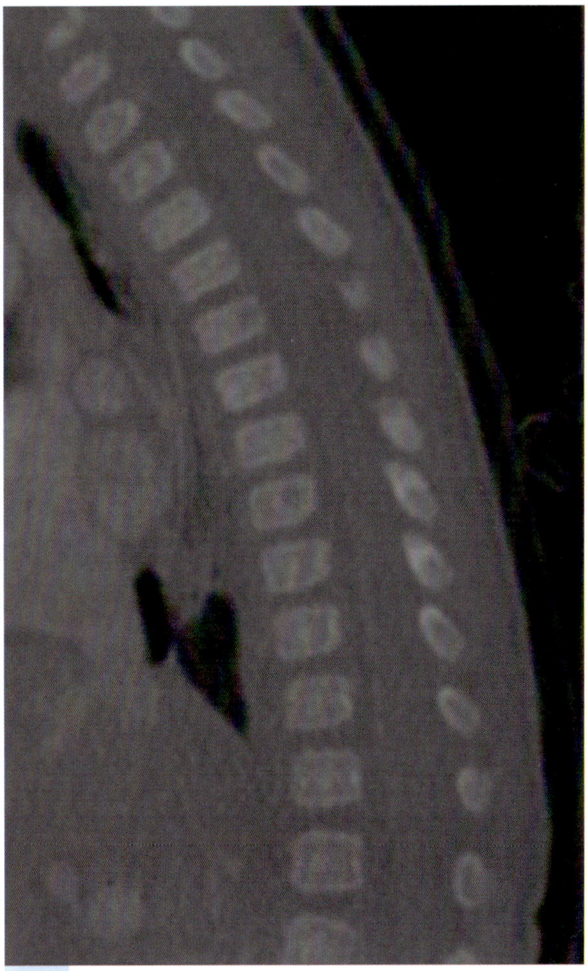

3.2d

FIGURES 3.2a–p   The appearance of the primary ossification centers of the typical thoracic vertebrae at various ages on CT: (a,b)—newborn, (c,d)—3 months, (e,f)—12 months, (g,h)—2 years, (i,j)—3 years, (k,l)—5 years, (m,n)—10 years, (o,p)—18 years.

(continued)

1 year

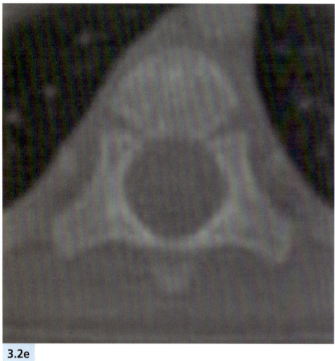

3.2e

2 years

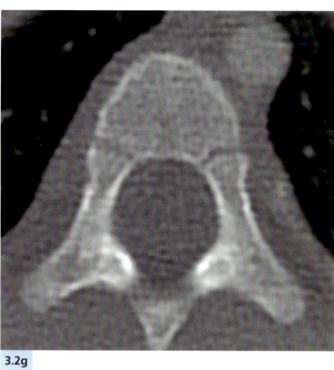

3.2g

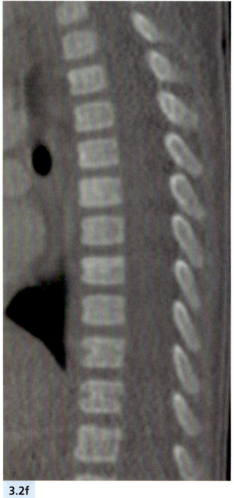

3.2f

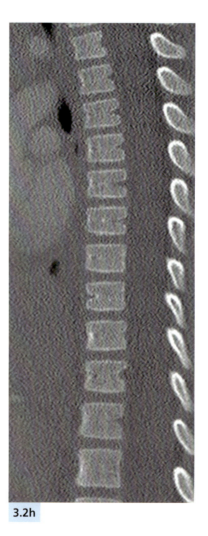

3.2h

FIGURES 3.2e–h

(continued)

3 years

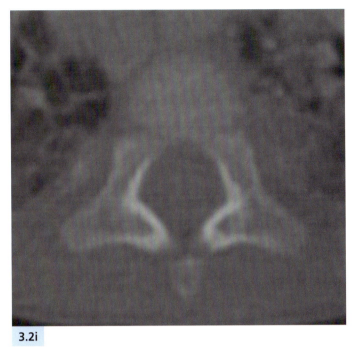

3.2i

5 years

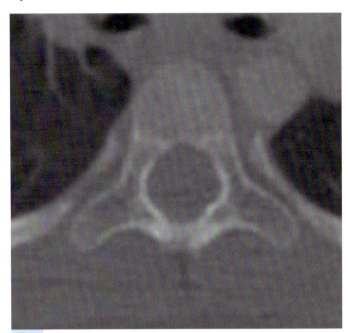

3.2k

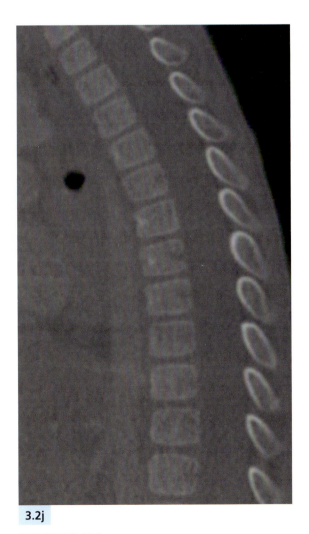

3.2j

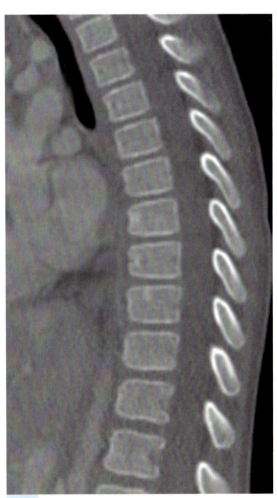

3.2l

FIGURES 3.2i–l

(continued)

10 years

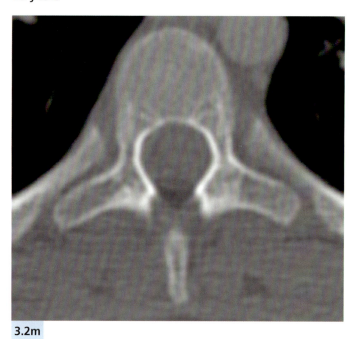

3.2m

18 years

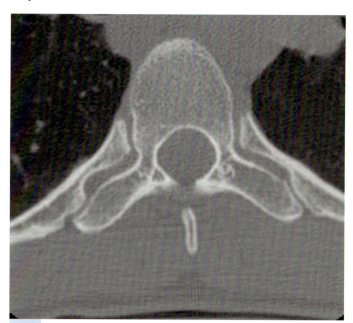

3.2o

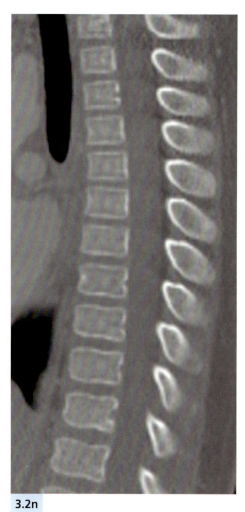

3.2n

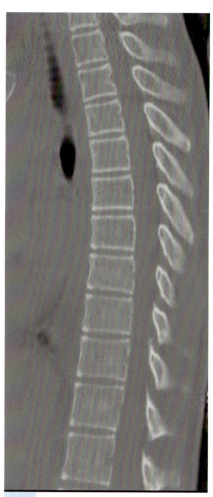

3.2p

FIGURES 3.2m–p

MULTIMODALITY ATLAS IMAGES OF THE THORACIC SPINE

The primary modalities used to image the thoracic spine are plain films, computed tomography (CT), and magnetic resonance imaging (MRI). The basic anatomy of the thoracic segments is presented in **Figures 3.3a–zz** in order to provide a foundation for the more detailed anatomic descriptions to follow.

■ PLAIN FILMS (FIGURES 3.3a–3.3b)

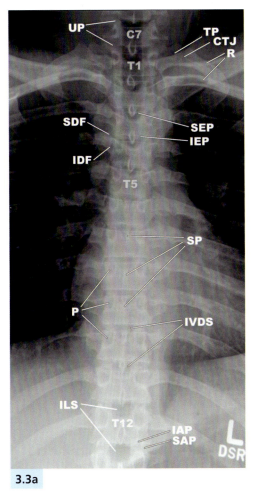

3.3a

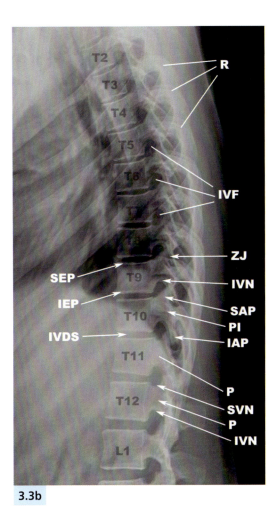

3.3b

FIGURES 3.3a–zz   Multimodal image gallery demonstrating the anatomy of the thoracic spine on plain films (a,b), CT (c–l), and MR (m—zz).

KEY						
CTJ	costotransverse joint	IVN	inferior vertebral notch	SP	spinous process
IAP	inferior articular process	P	pedicle	SVN	superior vertebral notch
IDF	inferior demifacet	PI	pars interarticularis	TP	transverse process
IEP	inferior endplate	R	rib	UP	uncinate process
ILS	interlaminar space	SAP	superior articular process	ZJ	zygapophyseal joint
IVDS	intervertebral disc space	SDF	superior demifacet		
IVF	intervertebral foramen	SEP	superior endplate		

(continued)

■ CT (FIGURES 3.3c–3.3l)

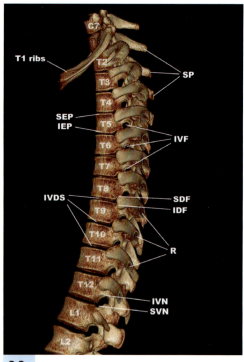

3.3c

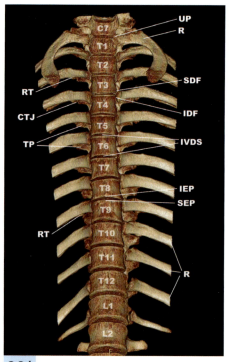

3.3d

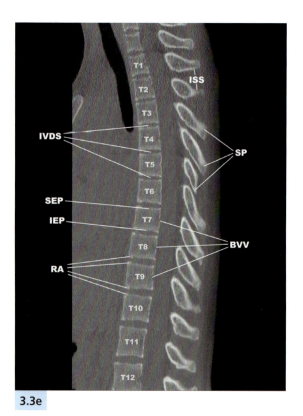

3.3e

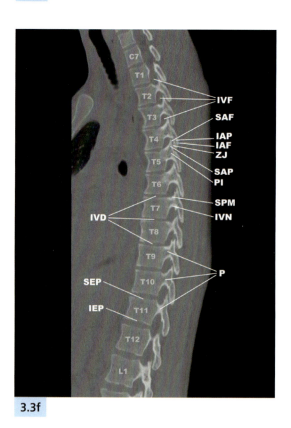

3.3f

FIGURES 3.3c–f

KEY

BVV	basivertebral vein	IVF	intervertebral foramen	SDF	superior demifacet
CTJ	costotransverse joint	IVN	inferior vertebral notch	SEP	superior endplate
IAF	inferior articular facet	P	pedicle	SP	spinous process
IAP	inferior articular process	PI	pars interarticularis	SPM	superior pedicle margin
IDF	inferior demifacet	R	rib	SVN	superior vertebral notch
IEP	inferior endplate	RA	ring apophyses	TP	transverse process
ISS	interspinous space	RT	rib tubercle	UP	uncinate process
IVD	intervertebral disc	SAF	superior articular facet	ZJ	zygapophyseal joint
IVDS	intervertebral disc space	SAP	superior articular process		

(continued)

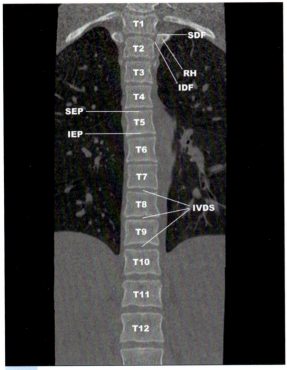

3.3g

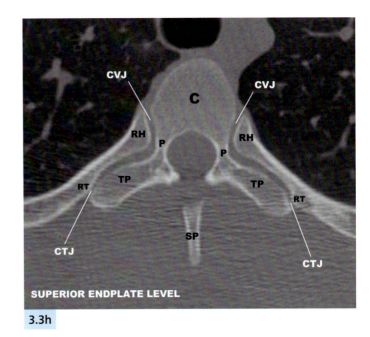

SUPERIOR ENDPLATE LEVEL

3.3h

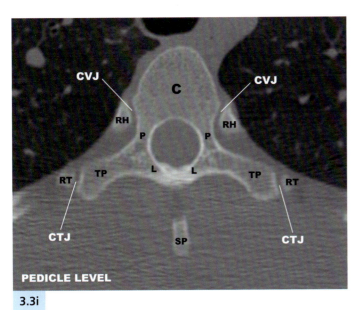

PEDICLE LEVEL

3.3i

LOWER PEDICLE LEVEL

3.3j

FIGURES 3.3g–j

KEY					
C	centrum	IVDS	intervertebral disc space	SDF	superior demifacet
CTJ	costotransverse joint	L	lamina	SEP	superior endplate
CVJ	costovertebral joint	P	pedicle	SP	spinous process
IDF	inferior demifacet	RH	rib head	TP	transverse process
IEP	inferior endplate	RT	rib tubercle		

(continued)

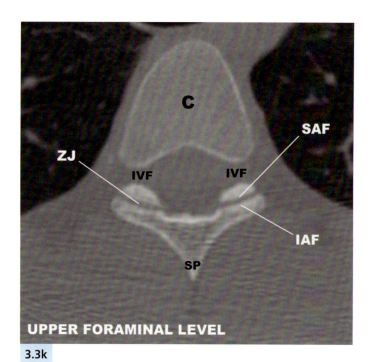

UPPER FORAMINAL LEVEL

3.3k

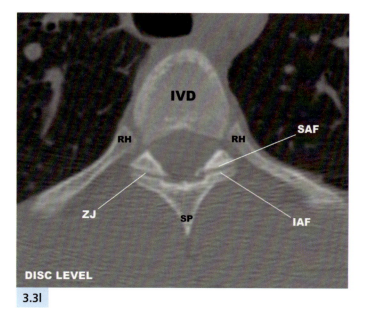

DISC LEVEL

3.3l

FIGURES 3.3k,l

(continued)

■ MR (FIGURES 3.3m–3.3zz)

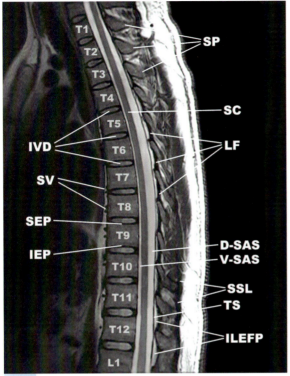

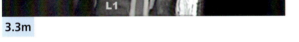

3.3m

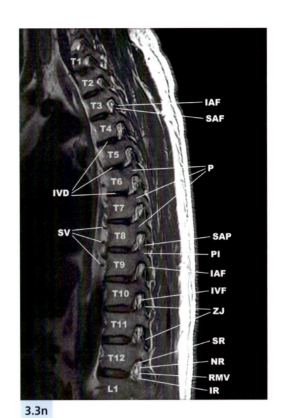

3.3n

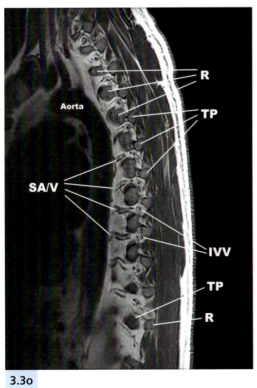

3.3o

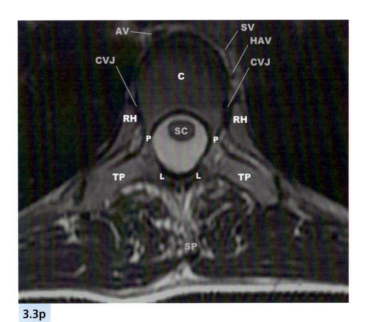

3.3p

FIGURES 3.3m–p

KEY							
AV	azygous vein	**L**	lamina	**SAS**	subarachnoid space (V - ventral, D - dorsal)		
C	centrum	**LF**	ligamentum flavum				
CVJ	costovertebral joint	**NR**	nerve roots	**SC**	spinal cord		
HAV	hemiazygos vein	**P**	pedicle	**SEP**	superior endplate		
IAF	inferior articular facet	**PI**	pars interarticularis	**SP**	spinous process		
IEP	inferior endplate	**R**	rib	**SR**	superior recess		
ILEFP	interlaminar epidural fat pad	**RH**	rib head	**SSL**	supraspinous ligament		
IR	inferior recess	**RMV**	radiculomedullary veins	**SV**	segmental vein		
IVD	intervertebral disc	**SA/V**	segmental arteries/veins	**TP**	transverse process		
IVF	intervertebral foramen	**SAF**	superior articular facet	**TS**	thecal sac		
IVV	intervertebral vein	**SAP**	superior articular process	**ZJ**	zygapophyseal joint		

(continued)

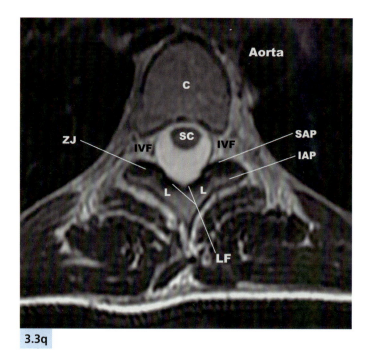

3.3q

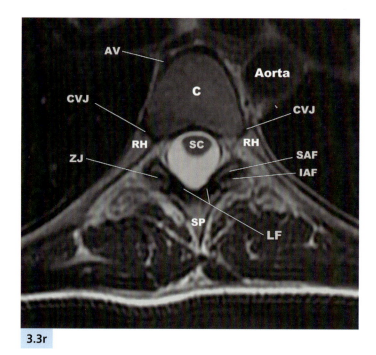

3.3r

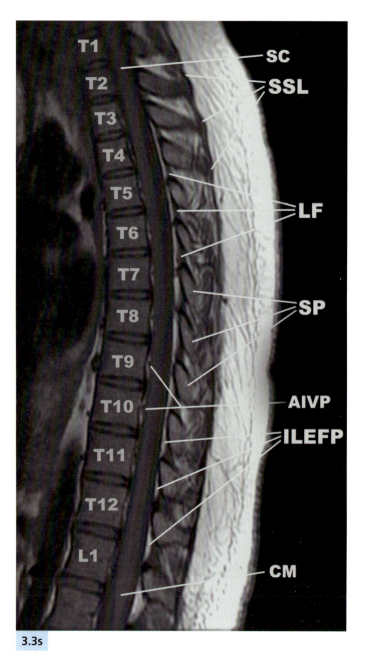

3.3s

KEY			
AIVP	anterior internal vertebral venous plexus	**L**	lamina
		LF	ligamentum flavum
AV	azygous vein	**RH**	rib head
C	centrum	**SAF**	superior articular facet
CM	conus medullaris		
CVJ	costovertebral joint	**SAP**	superior articular process
IAF	inferior articular facet		
IAP	inferior articular process	**SC**	spinal cord
		SP	spinous process
ILEFP	interlaminar epidural fat pad	**SSL**	supraspinous ligament
		ZJ	zygapophyseal joint
IVF	intervertebral foramen		

FIGURES 3.3q–s

(*continued*)

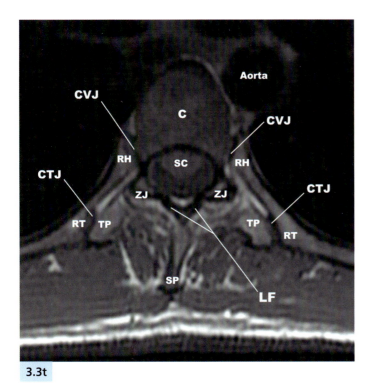

3.3t

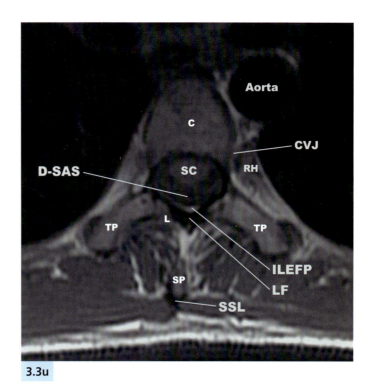

3.3u

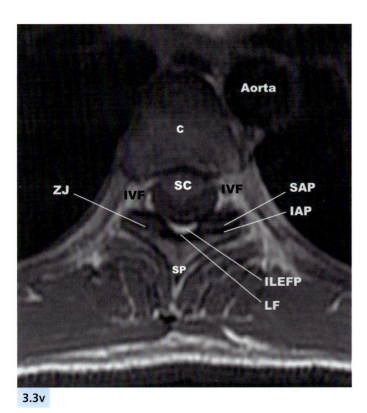

3.3v

FIGURES 3.3t–v

KEY			
C	centrum	RT	rib tubercle
CTJ	costotransverse joint	SAP	superior articular
CVJ	costovertebral joint		process
IAP	inferior articular	SAS	subarachnoid space
	process		(V - ventral, D - dorsal)
ILEFP	interlaminar epidural	SC	spinal cord
	fat pad	SP	spinous process
IVF	intervertebral foramen	SSL	supraspinous ligament
L	lamina	TP	transverse process
LF	ligamentum flavum	ZJ	zygapophyseal joint
RH	rib head		

(continued)

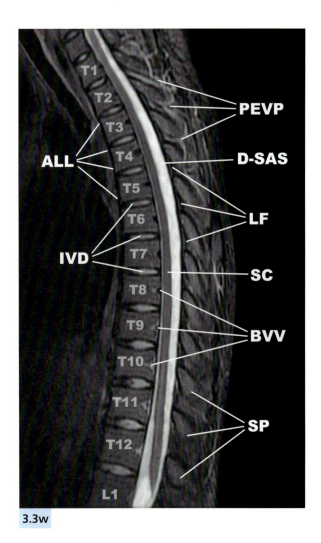

3.3w

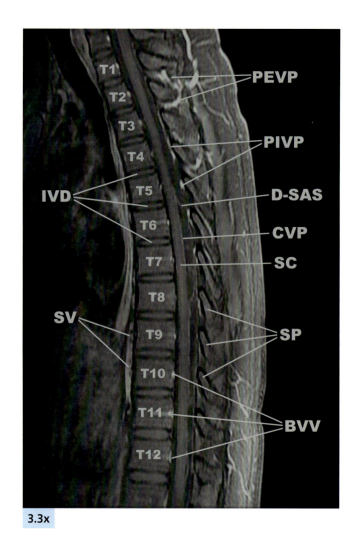

3.3x

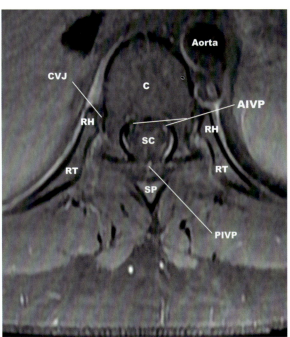

3.3y

KEY			
ALL	anterior longitudinal ligament	PEVP	posterior external vertebral venous plexus
AIVP	anterior internal vertebral venous plexus	PIVP	posterior internal vertebral venous plexus
BVV	basivertebral vein	RH	rib head
C	centrum	RT	rib tubercle
CVJ	costovertebral joint	SAS	subarachnoid space (V - ventral, D - dorsal)
CVP	coronal venous plexus	SC	spinal cord
IVD	intervertebral disc	SP	spinous process
LF	ligamentum flavum	SV	segmental vein

FIGURES 3.3w–y

(*continued*)

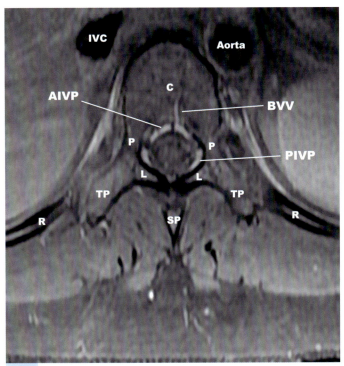

3.3z

KEY

AIVP	anterior internal vertebral venous plexus	**P**	pedicle
		PIVP	posterior internal vertebral venous plexus
BVV	basivertebral vein	**R**	rib
C	centrum	**SC**	spinal cord
IVC	inferior vena cava	**SP**	spinous process
IVF	intervertebral foramen	**SVC**	superior vena cava
IVV	intervertebral vein	**TP**	transverse process
L	lamina		

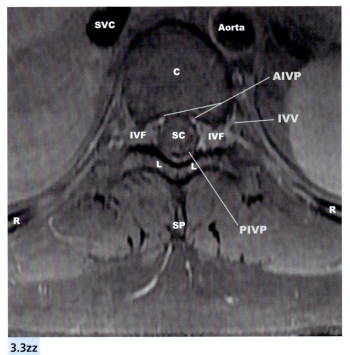

3.3zz

FIGURES 3.3z–zz

OSTEOLOGY OF THE THORACIC SEGMENTS

The "typical" thoracic segments are T2–T8. The T1 vertebral body has transitional features, including uncinate processes and a more "cervical" configuration of the vertebral body (**Figure 3.4**). The T9–T12 segments progressively reveal lumbar transitional features.

The thoracic kyphosis results from the wedge-shaped configuration of the thoracic vertebral bodies, which increases T1–T8. In general, the bone mineral content, trabecular density, volume, and compressive strength of the thoracic vertebral bodies all increase T1–T12. As viewed in the coronal plane, the lateral widths of the thoracic vertebral bodies at the superior endplates are smaller than the lateral widths of the vertebral bodies at the inferior endplates, resulting in a trapezoidal configuration. The lateral width of the thoracic vertebral bodies is greater than the anterior-posterior dimension. In the axial plane, the typical thoracic vertebral bodies have a dorsal midline concavity that produces an upside-down heart configuration (**Figure 3.5**). There is a shallow contour deformity along the anterolateral margin of the vertebral bodies to the left of midline, adjacent to the aorta. Attachments to the thoracic vertebral bodies include the anterior longitudinal ligament and longus coli muscles (T1–T3) anteriorly, psoas major and minor muscles (T12) laterally, and posterior longitudinal ligament posteriorly.

The pedicles of the thoracic spine arise from a more superior position on the vertebral bodies and are significantly longer and broader than the cervical pedicles. The T1 pedicles display deep superior vertebral notches. The pedicles of the typical thoracic segments do not have a superior vertebral notches, but have deep inferior vertebral notches (**Figure 3.6**). Superior vertebral notches are frequently found T10–T12 (**Figures 3.3b,c,f**). The thoracic pedicles are narrow in the transverse plane and broad in the sagittal plane, forming an ovoid shape as viewed in the coronal and coronal oblique planes (**Figure 3.7a**). The T4–T5 pedicles are the narrowest in the transverse plane and increase in size caudally. There is a smooth tapering of the pedicles within the middle one third that is referred to as the isthmus. The thoracic pedicles are primarily composed of cancellous bone. The cortical bone is thicker on the medial margins and thinner on the lateral margins. The thoracic pedicles are oriented slightly anteromedial to posterolateral in the transverse plane and anteroinferior to posterosuperior in the sagittal plane. The size and configuration of the thoracic pedicles allows safe access to the thoracic vertebral bodies for percutaneous biopsy (**Figure 3.7b**) or augmentation (**Figures 3.7c–f**).

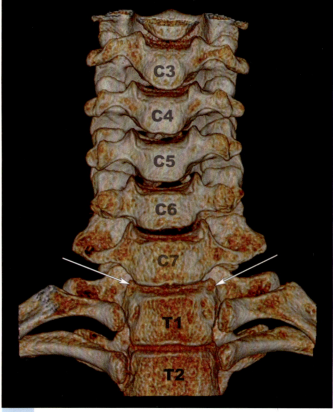

FIGURE 3.4 Surface rendered CT from a frontal projection demonstrates the transitional features of T1, including small uncinate processes (arrows) and a more "cervical" configuration of the vertebral body as compared with the more trapezoidal shape of the T2 vertebral body.

3.4

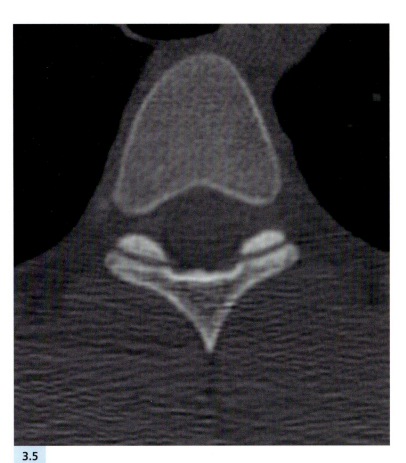

3.5

FIGURE 3.5   Axial CT image showing the upside-down heart configuration of the typical thoracic vertebral body.

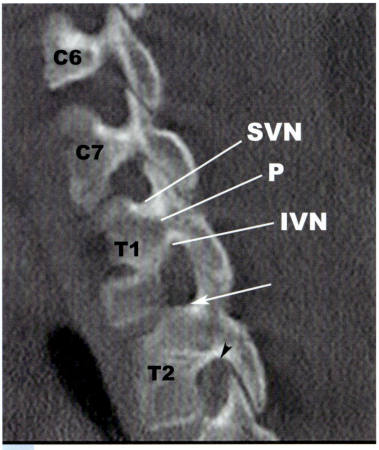

3.6

FIGURE 3.6   Sagittal reformatted CT image demonstrating a deep superior vertebral notch (SVN) along the superior margin of the T1 pedicle (P). There is no SVN at T2 (white arrow). There are deep inferior vertebral notches at T1 (IVN) and T2 (black arrowhead).

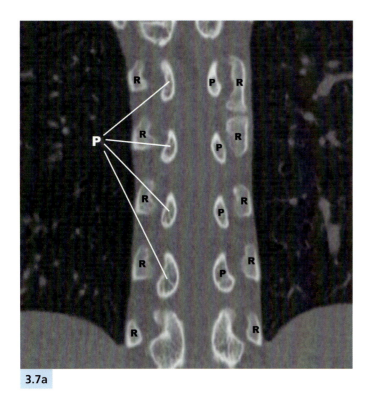

3.7a

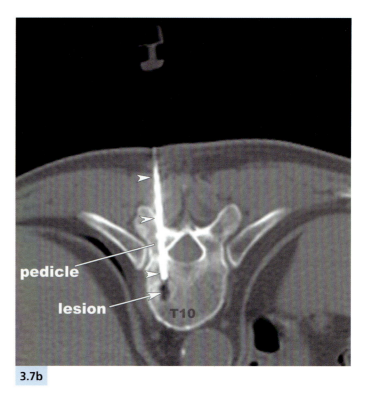

3.7b

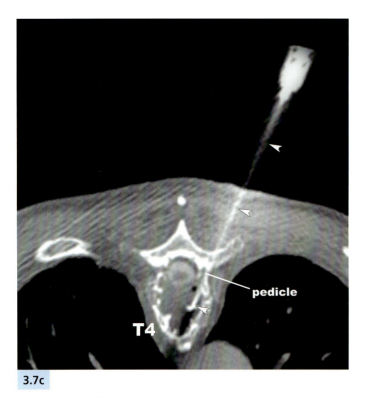

3.7c

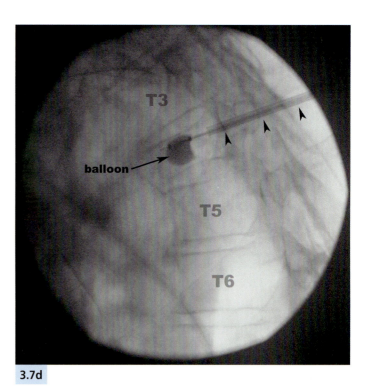

3.7d

FIGURES 3.7a–f (a) Curved coronal reformatted CT image displaying the ovoid shape of the typical thoracic pedicles (P).
(b) Axial CT fluoroscopy image showing a right T10 transpedicular approach bone biopsy needle (arrowheads) entering a lytic lesion in the T10 vertebral body. (c) Positioning of a needle (arrowheads) through the left T4 pedicle with the use of CT fluoroscopy during kyphoplasty. (d) Inflation of the kyphoplasty balloon within the T4 vertebral body under lateral fluoroscopic guidance. The arrowheads indicate the position of the needle within the pedicle. Injection of methyl methacrylate (cement) into the cavity formed by the balloon is demonstrated with (e) lateral fluoroscopy and (f) axial CT fluoroscopy. R—ribs.

(continued)

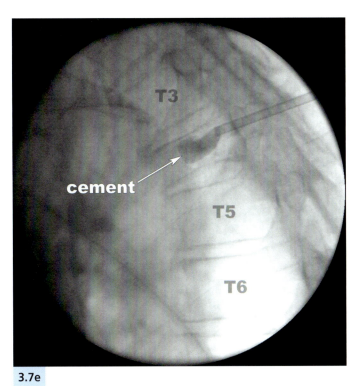

3.7e

FIGURES 3.7e,f

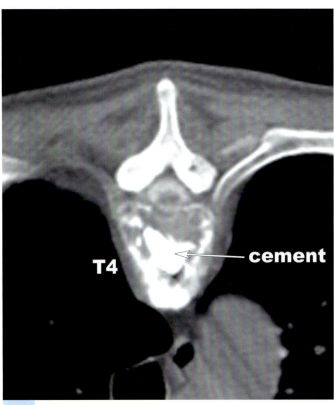

3.7f

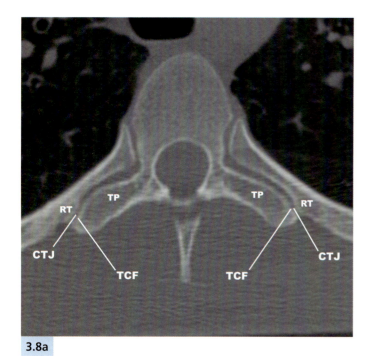

3.8a

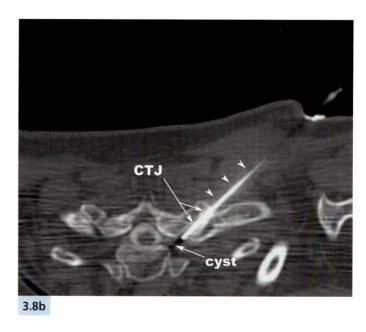

3.8b

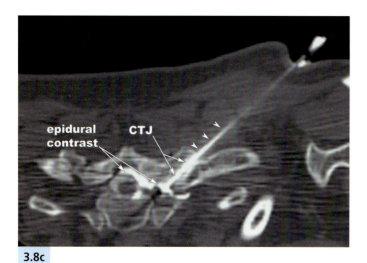

3.8c

FIGURES 3.8a–c (a) The transverse costal facets (TCF) arise along the lateral margins of the transverse processes (TP), face anterolaterally, and articulate with small facets arising from the rib tubercles (RT) to form the costotransverse joints (CTJ). (b) Axial mage from a CT-guided blood patch of a leaking meningeal cyst demonstrating percutaneous needle (arrowheads) access into the left T1–T2 intervertebral foramen through the costovertebral joint (CTJ). (c) Contrast is injected to confirm needle positioning that shows the outline the cyst within the intervertebral foramen and tracks into the dorsal epidural space.

The transverse processes assume a more posterior position in the thoracic segments, located posterior to the zygapophyseal joints, neural foramina, and pedicles. The thoracic transverse processes are broader than the cervical transverse processes and are posterolaterally oriented (Figures 3.3h,p,u,z). They decrease in length from T1 to T12. There are small facets located along the anterior margins of the transverse processes that are called the *transverse costal facets*. These facets face slightly anterolaterally (T1–T5) or anterosuperolaterally (T6–T12) and articulate with tubercles arising from the ribs of the same segment, forming the costotransverse joints (**Figure 3.8**).

The superior articular processes of the thoracic segments arise at the junction of the pedicles and laminae and are vertically oriented. The superior articular facets are oriented posteriorly and slightly superolaterally. The inferior articular processes arise from the laminae (**Figure 3.9**). The inferior articular facets face anteriorly and slightly inferomedially.

The thoracic lamina are thick anteriorly to posteriorly, elongated craniad to caudad, and short in the transverse dimension. Elongation of the thoracic laminae affords greater protection of the spinal canal contents and results in narrowing of the interlaminar spaces in the thoracic region (**Figures 3.10a,b**). Laminar length decreases T1–T5 and increases T5–T12. Careful inspection of the thoracic segments frequently reveals tiny spicules of bone or calcium arising from the anterior and inferior margins of the lamina at the lateral attachment sites of the ligamenta flava, called *paraarticular processes* (**Figure 3.11**). They are most commonly found in the lower thoracic segments, are typically bilateral, and are considered normal imaging findings.

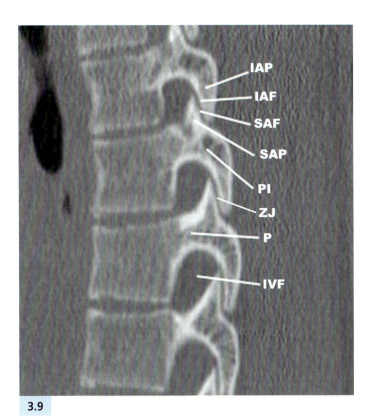

3.9

FIGURE 3.9   Sagittal reformatted CT image demonstrating the superior (SAP) and inferior (IAP) articular processes arising from the pars interarticularis (PI). The superior articular facets (SAF) are located on the dorsal surface of the SAP. The inferior articular facets (IAF) arise on the ventral surface of the inferior articular processes (IAPs). IVF—intervertebral foramen, P—pedicle, ZJ—zygapophyseal joint.

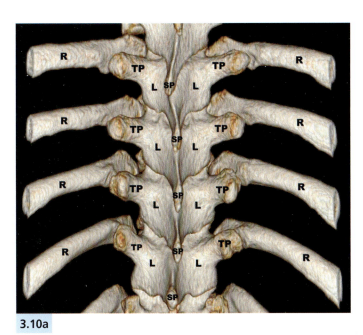

3.10a

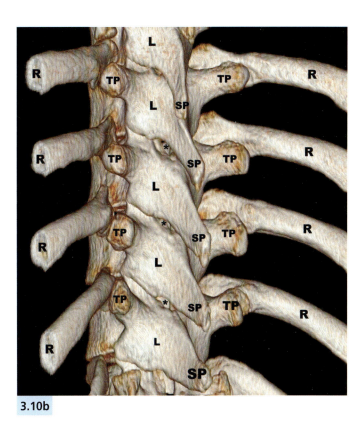

3.10b

FIGURES 3.10a,b   Surface rendered CT images from posterior (a) and posterolateral oblique (b) projections display the elongated laminae (L) of the typical thoracic segments. The interlaminar spaces (ILS) (asterisks) are correspondingly narrow. R—rib, SP—spinous process, TP—transverse process.

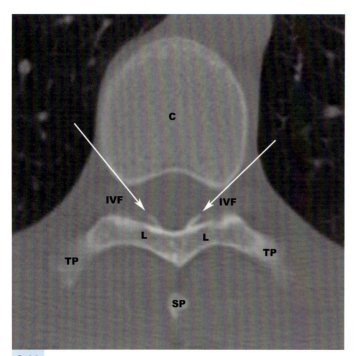

FIGURE 3.11 Axial CT image showing two, fine bony spicules arising from the ventral margins of the laminae (L), referred to as paraarticular processes (white arrows). C—centrum, IVF—intervertebral foramen, SP—spinous process, TP—transverse process.

3.11

The thoracic spinous processes have an elongated rectangular shape, similar to the C7 spinous process. The T1–T4 spinous processes are oriented in the horizontal plane. The T5–T8 spinous processes are oriented inferiorly. The T9–T12 spinous processes take on features of the lumbar spinous processes, such as a more square configuration and orientation in the horizontal plane (**Figures 3.12a,b**). The posterior margins serve as attachment points for the supraspinous ligaments. The superior and inferior margins are the attachment points for the interspinous ligaments. Muscles that attach to the thoracic spinous processes include the trapezius, latissimus dorsi, rhomboid major and minor, serratus posterior superior and inferior, erector spinae and transversospinalis.

The thoracic vertebrae at the cervicothoracic and thoracolumbar transitions differ from the "typical" thoracic segments that have been described in the preceding paragraphs. The T1 retains certain cervical vertebral features, including uncovertebral joints, superior vertebral notches, and a rectangular shape. The lower thoracic segments progressively take on lumbar features. The T10 segment typically has oval facets that articulate with the T10 rib heads and variable facets on the transverse processes that articulate with the anterior tubercles of the T10 ribs. The T11 segment has facets arising from the pedicles that articulate with the T11 ribs. There are generally no facets arising from the T11 vertebra that articulate with the T11 ribs. The T12 segment has small processes that are homologues of the transverse processes, mammillary, and accessory processes (**Figures 3.13a–c**).

The boundaries of the thoracic spinal canal include the vertebral body anteriorly, pedicles anterolaterally, laminae posterolaterally, and spinous processes posteriorly. The width of the thoracic spinal canal decreases from T1 to T6 and increases from T7 to T12. The length increases from T1 to T5 and decreases from T6 to T12. This results in a more rounded configuration of the thoracic spinal canal than the cervical and lumbar regions. The caliber of the thoracic spinal canal is smaller than the cervical and lumbar spinal canal.

The thoracic intervertebral foramina are formed by the inferior vertebral notch of the pedicle superiorly, posterolateral margin of the vertebral body anterosuperiorly, demifacets and rib head anteroinferiorly, superior vertebral notch inferiorly, and the superior articular process posteriorly (**Figure 3.14**). The intervertebral foramina of the thoracic spine are oriented laterally, like those of the upper lumbar segments.

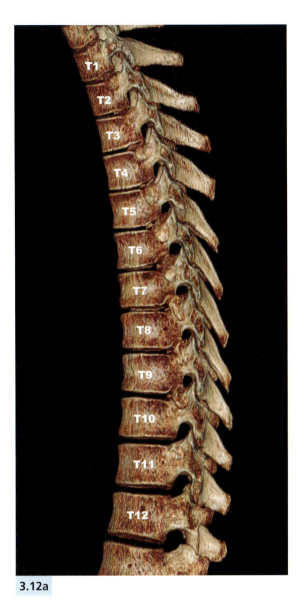

3.12a

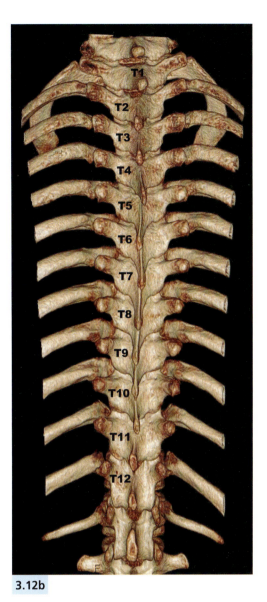

3.12b

FIGURES 3.12a,b   Surface rendered CT reformatted images in the (a) lateral and (b) posterior projections display the typical horizontal orientation of the T1–T4 spinous processes (SP) and inferior orientation of the T5–T8 SPs. The T9–T12 SPs progressively take on a squared, "lumbar" appearance.

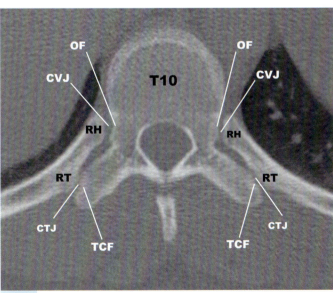

3.13a

FIGURES 3.13a–c   Axial maximum intensity projection CT images at (a) T10, (b) T11, and (c) T12 demonstrating the typical progression to "lumbar" features. The T10 rib heads (RH) articulate with a single oval-shaped facet (OF) and there are variable costotransverse joints (CTJ). Small articular facets (AF) arise from the lateral margins of the pedicle (P) and articulate with rib heads (RH) to form the costovertebral joints (CVJ). There are no CTJ at T11, the transverse costal facets (TCF) are absent and rib tubercles (RT) may be absent (left) or rudimentary (right). The T12 vertebra has rudimentary transverse processes (TP) and mammillary processes (MP).

(continued)

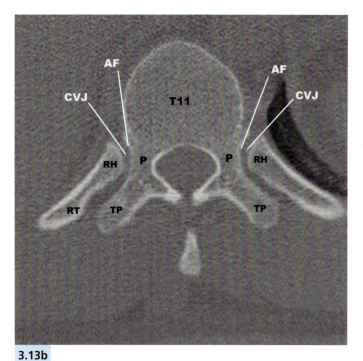

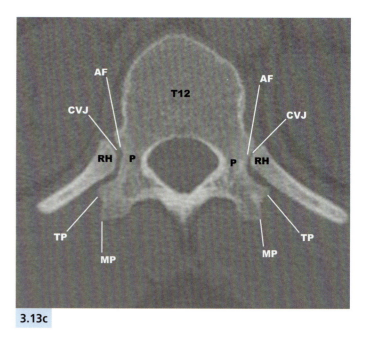

FIGURES 3.13b,c (*continued*) AF—articular facets, CVJ—costovertebral joints, MP—mammillary processes, P—pedicle, RH—rib heads, RT—rib tubercles, TP—transverse processes.

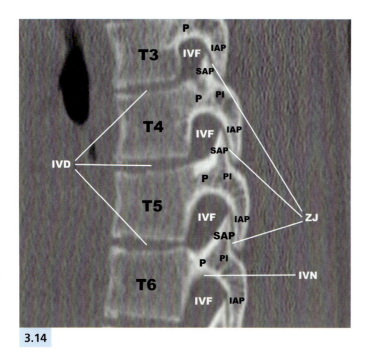

FIGURE 3.14 Sagittal CT image displaying the osteology of the intervertebral foramen (IVF). The anterior wall is formed by the posterior margin of the vertebral body rostrally and dorsal margin of the intervertebral disc (IVD) caudally. The inferior wall is formed by the rostral margin of the pedicle (P). The posterior wall is made up of the inferior articular process (IAP) superiorly and the superior articular process (SAP) inferiorly. The superior wall is formed by the inferior vertebral notch (IVN) of the pedicle. PI—pars interarticularis, ZJ—zygapophyseal joint.

THE INTERVERTEBRAL DISCS OF THE THORACIC SPINE

The thoracic intervertebral discs are similar in height anteriorly and posteriorly, unlike the cervical and lumbar intervertebral discs. The thoracic kyphosis is primarily determined by the shape of the vertebral bodies, rather than the intervertebral discs (Figure 3.3m,s,w). The thoracic intervertebral discs are narrower superiorly to inferiorly than the cervical and lumbar discs and increase in height T1–T12. Viewed in the coronal plane, the thoracic intervertebral discs have an inverted trapezoidal shape.

THE ZYGAPOPHYSEAL (FACET) JOINTS

As is the case in the rest of the spine, the zygapophyseal joints are composed of opposing articular cartilages lining the superior and inferior facets that are surrounded by a synovium-lined fibrous capsule. The zygapophyseal joints function to transmit compressive loads, resist shearing forces, and prevent excessive segmental translation and distraction.

The zygapophyseal joints are formed by articular facets arising from superior and inferior articular processes of adjacent segments (Figures 3.3k,q,v, 3.9, and 3.14). Like the articular facets of the subaxial cervical segments, the typical thoracic articular facets are relatively flat. The articular processes of the thoracic segments are more vertically oriented than the cervical articular processes. Viewed in the axial and sagittal planes, the superior articular processes are positioned anterior to the inferior articular processes. The superior articular facets are oriented posteriorly and slightly superolaterally. The inferior articular facets are oriented anteriorly and slightly inferomedially. This orientation allows for ample rotation while restricting flexion, extension, and lateral bending. The tensile strength of the capsular ligaments is greatest at the cervicothoracic and thoracolumbar junctions.

The orientation of the articular facets transitions at the thoracolumbar junction from the more coronally oriented thoracic type facets to the posterolaterally oriented lumbar type facets. This transition is most commonly abrupt (94%) and occurs at the T12 level (76%). Figures 3.15a,b display the most commonly encountered thoracolumbar facet transition, with the superior articular facets of T12 facing posteriorly and slightly superomedially and the T12 inferior articular facets facing anterolaterally.

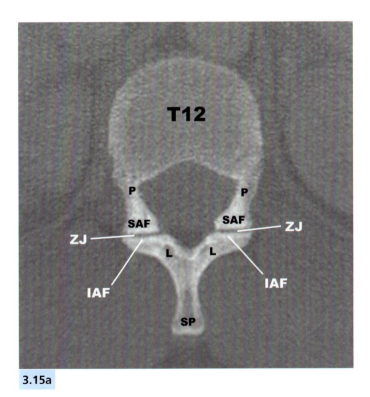 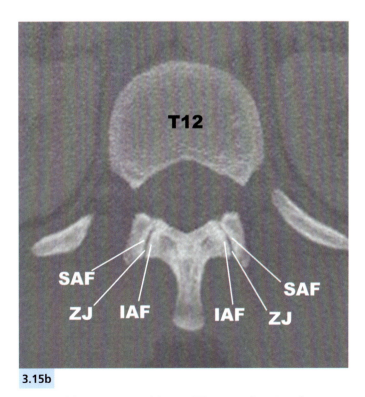

3.15a   3.15b

FIGURES 3.15a,b   The typical thoracolumbar facet transition occurs at T12. (a) Transverse oblique CT image showing the posteromedial orientation of the T12 superior facets (SAF). The T11 inferior articular facets (IAF), lamina (L), and spinous process (SP) are visible in this orientation. (b) Transverse oblique maximum intensity projection CT image demonstrating the posteromedial orientation of the T12 IAF. The L1 superior articular facets (SAF) are visible in this view. P—pedicle, ZJ—zygapophyseal joint.

THE COSTOVERTEBRAL AND COSTOTRANSVERSE JOINTS

The typical thoracic vertebrae have two articulations with ribs, the costovertebral and costotransverse joints. These synovial joints contribute added stability to the thoracic segments and serve to limit axial rotation and lateral bending.

The *costovertebral joints* are articulations between rib heads and two adjacent vertebral bodies. Rib heads forming joints with typical thoracic vertebrae have two convex facets that articulate with two concave facets (demifacets) located along the superior endplate of the same segment and the inferior endplate of the segment immediately above (**Figures 3.16a,b**). The *intra-articular ligament* attaches to a thin ridge of bone on the rib head located between the articular facets, the *interarticular crest*, and the adjacent intervertebral disc. Single ovoid facets are typically found at T1, T10, T11, and T12. Demifacets are infrequently encountered at T1 and T10. The intra-articular ligaments, capsular ligaments, and radiate ligaments function to stabilize the costovertebral joints.

The *costotransverse joints* are formed by small facets arising from the posteriorly facing tubercles of the ribs and the facets located along the anterior surface of the transverse processes (Figures 3.3h,p,r,t,y and 3.8a). They are planar type synovial joints that allow a small amount of gliding motion under normal physiological conditions. There are no costotransverse joints at T11 and T12. Ligaments that stabilize the costotransverse joints include the capsular ligament, costotransverse ligament, superior and lateral costovertebral ligaments. Percutaneous access to certain lesions may only be possible by traversing the costotransverse joints (Figures 3.8b,c).

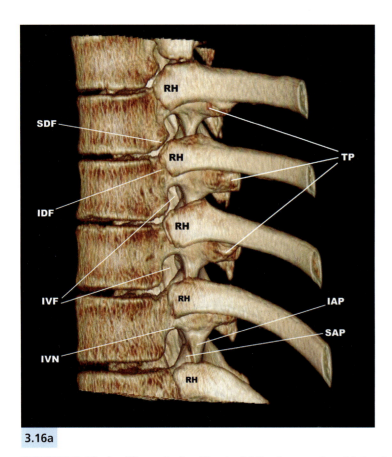

3.16a

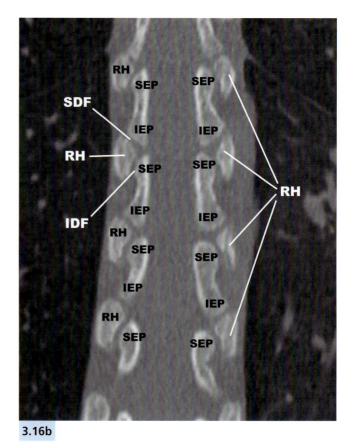

3.16b

FIGURES 3.16a,b Thoracic demifacets. (a) Surface rendered lateral oblique and (b) curved reformatted CT images showing small, concave superior (SDF) and inferior demifacets (IDF) located at the posterolateral margins of adjacent superior (SEP) and inferior endplates (IEP) that articulate with convex facets located on rib heads (RH). IAP—inferior articular process, IVF—intervertebral foramen, IVN—inferior vertebral notch, SAP—superior articular process, TP—transverse process.

LIGAMENTOUS ANATOMY OF THE THORACIC SPINE

The major ligaments of the thoracic spine include the anterior longitudinal ligament, posterior longitudinal ligament, ligamenta flava, interspinous ligaments, and supraspinous ligament. Other notable ligaments found in the thoracic spine include the intra-articular ligaments, capsular ligaments, and radiate ligaments of the costovertebral joints and the costotransverse ligament, superior and lateral costovertebral ligaments of the costotransverse joints.

The *anterior longitudinal ligament* (ALL) is greater in anterior to posterior thickness and thinner in transverse dimension in the thoracic region than the cervical and lumbar regions. Like the cervical and lumbar levels, the anterior to posterior thickness of the ALL is greatest at the vertebral body levels and thinnest at the intervertebral disc levels. The ALL is firmly attached to the anterior superior and anterior inferior endplates and has sparse attachments to the central aspect of the vertebral bodies (**Figures 3.17a–d**). Strong attachments to the intervertebral discs are present in one half of thoracic spines. The tensile strength of the ALL is greatest in the lower thoracic region.

The *posterior longitudinal ligament* (PLL) is located along the anterior margin of the spinal canal and has attachments to the superior and inferior vertebral margins and intervertebral discs (Figures 3.17a,b,e,f). It is broader in the transverse dimension at the level of the intervertebral discs and relatively narrow over the vertebral bodies, giving it a denticulate configuration. The PLL has two layers, superficial and deep. The superficial layer is located posterior to the deep layer, is centrally located, measures 8 to 10 mm in width, and has broad attachments to the intervertebral discs. The deep layer is narrower than the superficial layer (2–3 mm in width), is firmly adherent to the superficial layer at the midline, and also has a denticulate appearance. Fibers of both the superficial and deep layers attach to a midline bony septum at the level of the vertebral bodies.

The *ligamenta flava* ("yellow ligaments") are found throughout the thoracic spinal segments. The ligamenta flava are paired ligaments that are positioned on either side of the midline, extending from the anterior inferior margin of the lamina above to the posterior superior margin of the lamina below (Figures 3.17a,b,g,h). Lateral extensions of the ligamenta flava form the medial capsules of the zygapophyseal joints. The thoracic ligamenta flava are thicker than the cervical ligamenta flava, but not as thick as the lumbar ligamenta flava. Midline gaps in the caudal third of the ligamenta flava are almost always found at T1–T2, are infrequent in the mid-thoracic segments, and increase in frequency T10–T12. It is important to take this into consideration when attempting use the loss of resistance technique for epidural injections in these spinal regions.

The *interspinous ligaments* extend from the inferior margins of the spinous processes above to the superior margins of the spinous processes below in the sagittal plane and from the root to the apex of the spinous processes in the transverse plane. The interspinous ligaments are absent in the upper thoracic spine (T1–T5) and are replaced by loose connective tissue positioned between the multifidus muscles. In the lower thoracic spine (T6–T12), the interspinous ligaments are formed by anterior extensions of the thoracolumbar fascia. The interspinous ligaments increase in thickness and tensile strength in the lower thoracic spine. However, the interspinous ligaments are among the weakest of the spinal ligaments.

The *supraspinous ligament* on imaging appears as a discreet band-like structure (Figures 3.17a,b,g). However, it is formed by a combination of tendinous muscle attachments and fascia. In the upper thoracic spine (T1–T5), the spinal tendinous attachments of the trapezius, rhomboideus major, and splenius cervicis muscles combine with the deep fascia to form the supraspinous ligament. In the power thoracic spine (T6–T12), the posterior layer of the thoracolumbar fascia is the primary contributor to the supraspinous ligament, with a smaller contribution from the trapezius aponeurosis. The supraspinous ligament blends anteriorly with the interspinous ligaments in the lower thoracic spine (T6–T12). The strength of the supraspinous ligament increases from T1 to T12.

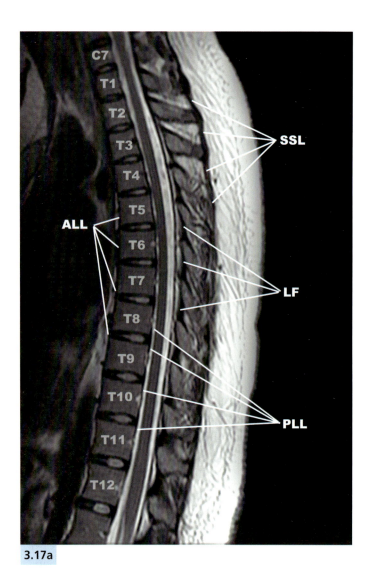

3.17a

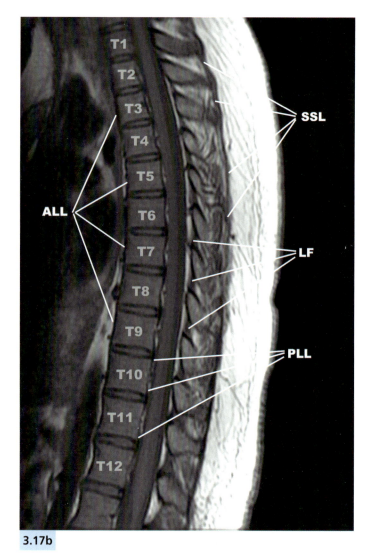

3.17b

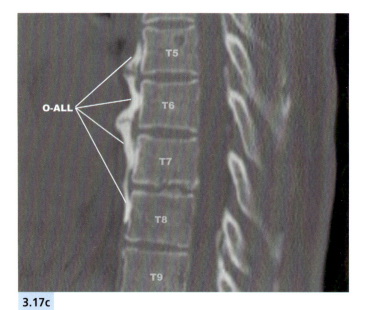

3.17c

FIGURES 3.17a–h Ligamentous anatomy of the thoracic spine. (a) Sagittal T2-weighted and (b) sagittal T1-weighted images demonstrating the anterior longitudinal ligament (ALL), posterior longitudinal ligament (PLL), ligamenta flava (LF), and supraspinous ligaments (SSL). Sagittal (c) and axial (d) CT images showing ossification of the anterior longitudinal ligament (O-ALL). Sagittal (e) and axial (f) CT images showing ossification of the posterior longitudinal ligament (arrows). (g) Sagittal CT image showing ossification of the ligamenta flava (white arrows) and SSL (black arrows). (h) Axial CT image displaying ossification of the ligamenta flava where they form the medial portion of the zygapophyseal joint (ZJ) capsules (white arrows).

(continued)

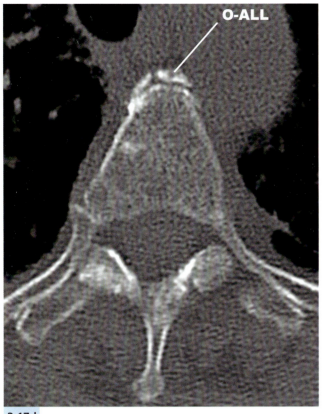

3.17d

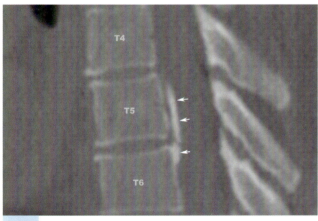

3.17e

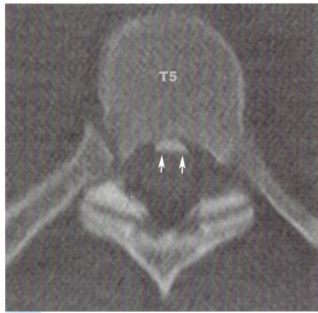

3.17f

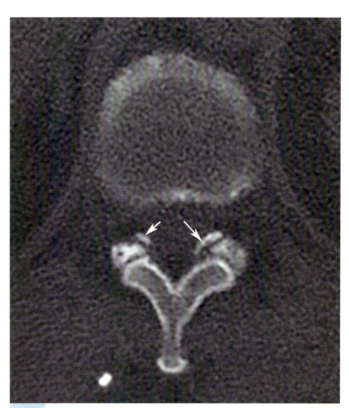

3.17g

3.17h

FIGURES 3.17d–h (*continued*) O-ALL—ossification of the anterior longitudinal ligament.

ARTERIAL ANATOMY OF THE THORACIC SPINE

The longitudinal artery supplying the thoracic spine is the descending thoracic aorta. The descending thoracic aorta is situated to the left of the spine, gradually coursing medially in the lower thoracic region. The segmental arteries of the thoracic spine are nine pairs of *posterior intercostal arteries* and one pair of *subcostal arteries*. Occasionally, multiple adjacent segmental arteries arise from a common origin in the upper thoracic spine, called the *superior (or supreme) intercostal artery*. The superior intercostal arteries may arise from the costocervical trunks, aorta, or the vertebral arteries. There is a rich anastomotic network that includes intersegmental, prevertebral, pretransverse, and posttransverse components.

The intercostal arteries (**Figures 3.18a–d**) branch into anterior and posterior rami. The anterior rami course laterally to supply the tissues of the intercostal spaces, skin, and mammary glands. The anterior rami ultimately anastomose with the superior epigastric and musculophrenic arteries. The posterior rami give off muscular and spinal branches. The *muscular branches* course posteriorly, along the lateral margins of the vertebral bodies and supply the soft tissues along the inferior margins of the neural foramina, inferior aspects of the spinal nerves, intercostal muscles, and soft tissues. The *spinal branches* course through the neural foramina and branch into anterior and posterior radicular arteries.

The radicular arteries may supply the nerve roots, dura mater, spinal ganglia, spinal cord, or various combinations of the above. A variable number of radicular arteries send branches along the anterior and/or posterior nerve roots to supply the spinal cord, called the *radiculomedullary arteries*. Radiculomedullary arteries that supply the anterior spinal artery are called *anterior radiculomedullary* arteries. *Posterior radiculomedullary* arteries supply the posterior spinal arteries. A variable number of radiculomedullary arteries make up the anterior and posterior spinal arteries.

The dominant thoracolumbar anterior radiculomedullary artery supplying the lower spinal cord is the great anterior radiculomedullary artery of Adamkiewicz, or simply the *artery of Adamkiewicz* (AKA). The AKA most commonly arises on the left (65%) between T9–T11 (72%). It may originate as high as T5 or as low as L3. The AKA ascends within the spinal canal and takes a characteristic "hairpin turn" as it joins the anterior spinal artery (**Figures 3.19a,b**).

The anterior and posterior spinal arteries are discussed in Chapter 1. The anterior spinal artery resides in the anterior median fissure and supplies the anterior two-thirds of the spinal cord. The paired posterior spinal arteries are positioned lateral to the posterior median sulcus and supply the posterior one-third of the spinal cord. The central arteries branch from the anterior spinal arteries and penetrate deeply into the anterior median fissure to supply the central cord. The anterior and posterior spinal arteries contribute to a network of arteries that encircle the spinal cord, the pial arterial plexus or vasa coronae.

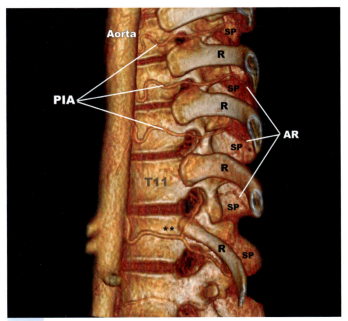

3.18a

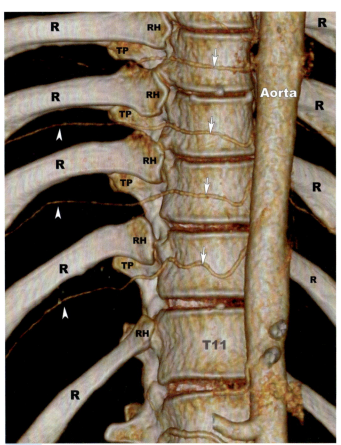

3.18b

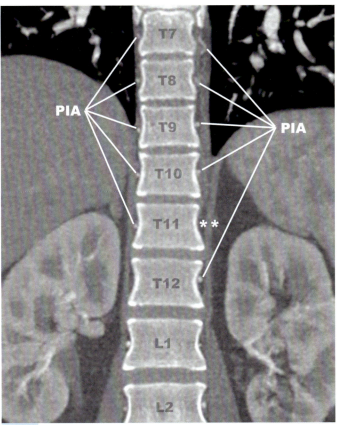

3.18c

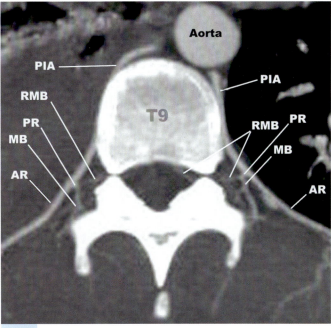

3.18d

FIGURES 3.18a–d   The arterial supply of the thoracic spine. (a) Surface rendered reformatted image from an aortic CT angiogram in lateral oblique orientation demonstrates the typical appearance of the segmental arteries of the thoracic spine, the posterior intercostal arteries (PIA), as they arise from the descending thoracic aorta. The left posterior intercostal artery is absent and the T11 rami are supplied by the left T12 posterior intercostal artery (asterisks). The anterior rami (AR) course within the intercostal spaces. (b) Surface rendered reformatted image from an aortic CT angiogram in anterior projection displays the right PIA (arrows), which are longer than the left PIA as a result of the position of the aorta to the left of midline. The position of the AR (arrowheads) within the intercostal spaces is also demonstrated. (c) Coronal maximum intensity projection image shows the position of the PIA within the concavities along the lateral cortex of the vertebral bodies. The left T11 posterior intercostal artery is absent (asterisks). (d) Axial maximum intensity projection image from an aortic CT angiogram shows the PIA arising from the descending thoracic aorta and giving off the anterior (AR) and posterior rami (PR). The posterior rami give off muscular (MB) and radiculomedullary or radicular branches (RMB). R—rib, RH—rib head, SP—spinous process, TP—transverse process.

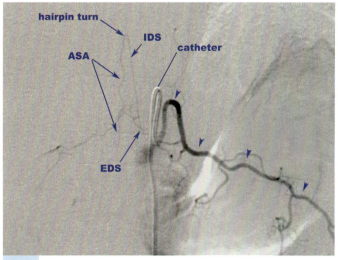

3.19a

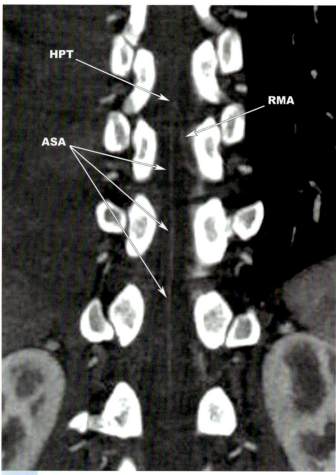

FIGURES 3.19a,b   The artery of Adamkiewicz. (a) Digital subtraction angiographic image obtained during a left T12 segmental artery (subcostal artery = arrowheads) injection demonstrating the extradural (EDS) and intradural segment (IDS) of the radiculomedullary artery of Adamkiewicz (RMA). The intradural segment takes a characteristic hairpin turn at the point it supplies the anterior spinal artery (ASA). (b) Coronal reformatted maximum intensity projection image from a CT angiogram shows the great RMA arising on the left at T9. The characteristic hairpin turn (HPT) is well demonstrated as it supplies the ASA.

3.19b

VENOUS ANATOMY OF THE THORACIC SPINE

Venous drainage of the subaxial thoracic spine and spinal cord is carried out through a heavily interconnected venous network that has three main divisions: intrinsic, extrinsic, and extradural. The *intrinsic system* includes the venous network that drains the spinal cord central gray matter and peripheral white matter. The pia mater marks the border of the *extrinsic system*, which includes the coronal venous plexus and radiculomedullary veins. The *extradural system* includes the anterior internal vertebral venous plexus, posterior internal vertebral venous plexus, anterior external vertebral venous plexus, and posterior external vertebral venous plexus.

The anterior sulcal vein is located in the anterior median fissure of the spinal cord. The posterior sulcal vein is located in the posterior sulcus. The anterior and posterior central veins drain the central gray matter. The white matter is drained by small caliber radial veins within the pia that form the coronal venous plexus. Transmedullary anastomotic veins are larger in caliber than the sulcal veins and project through the substance of the spinal cord, connecting ventral and dorsal surfaces. Some of the larger caliber longitudinally oriented veins within the coronal plexus form a variable number of anterior and posterior median and lateral spinal veins, which drain into the anterior and posterior radiculomedullary veins.

The anterior and posterior radiculomedullary veins drain the spinal cord and spinal nerve roots and function to connect the extrinsic and extradural systems. There is a variable number of anterior and posterior radiculomedullary veins draining the spinal cord. The largest anterior radiculomedullary vein draining the thoracolumbar spinal cord is the great anterior radiculomedullary vein (GARV). On imaging studies, the GARV may be confused with the AKA due to the similarity of the GARVs more obtuse "coat hook" turn to the acute "hairpin turn" of the AKA. Features distinguishing the GARV from the AKA include lower position of the GARV (T11–L3), larger caliber of the GARV, and later contrast opacification of the GARV on multiphase postcontrast imaging. Because it is most commonly found in the lumbar region, the imaging appearance of the GARV is covered in Chapter 4. The radiculomedullary veins and anterior and posterior external vertebral venous plexuses drain into the intervertebral veins.

The anterior internal vertebral venous plexus resides within two layers of the posterior longitudinal ligament (Figures 3.3y,z,zz and **3.20a,b,d**). It is generally composed of two large, longitudinally oriented veins on either side of the posterior longitudinal ligament. The anterior internal vertebral venous plexus is typically less prominent at the level of the intervertebral discs and courses medially at the pedicle level, where it connects through transversely oriented venous anastomoses to the basivertebral veins, the valved system that provides the primary drainage of the vertebral bodies. The minor venous drainage of the vertebral bodies occurs through small peripheral tributaries that communicate directly with the anterior external vertebral venous plexus. The anterior internal vertebral venous plexus also anastomoses with the posterior internal vertebral venous plexus and anterior external vertebral venous plexus (Figures 3.20a,c,d).

The posterior internal vertebral venous plexus is generally smaller in size than the anterior internal vertebral venous plexus and is composed of longitudinally oriented veins traversing the dorsal epidural space that tend to be more laterally located in the cervical spinal canal (Figures 3.4x–z,zz and 3.20a–d). In the thoracic region, this plexus is embedded within an ample epidural fat pad. The posterior internal vertebral venous plexus receives small draining branches from the lateral masses, lamina, and spinous processes. It also connects with the posterior external vertebral venous plexus via small perforating veins through the ligamenta flava.

The anterior external vertebral venous plexus is located anterior the vertebral bodies and has extensive connections with the intervertebral and basivertebral veins. The posterior external vertebral venous plexus is located dorsal to the vertebrae and drains the paravertebral muscles and the posterior elements. It has extensive connections with the posterior internal vertebral venous plexus and intervertebral veins (Figures 3.20a,b,d).

The intervertebral veins connect the internal and external vertebral venous plexuses and primarily drain into the segmental (posterior intercostal) veins (Figures 3.3zz, 3.20a,c,d). The segmental veins subsequently drain into the azygos vein on the right (Figure 3.20c–e) and the hemiazygos and accessory hemiazygos veins on the left. The azygos, hemiazygos, and accessory hemiazygos veins drain into the superior vena cava (Figure 3.20e).

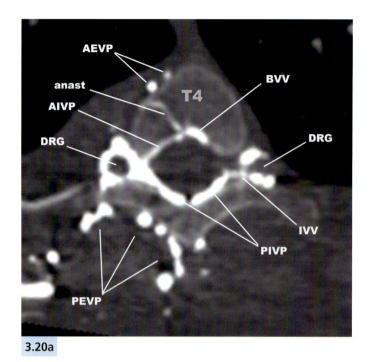

3.20a

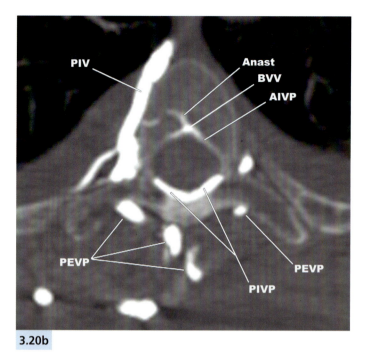

3.20b

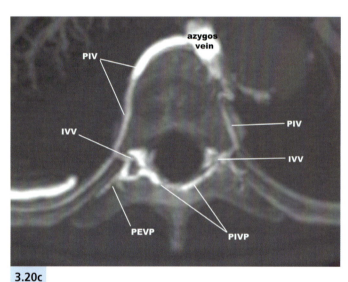

3.20c

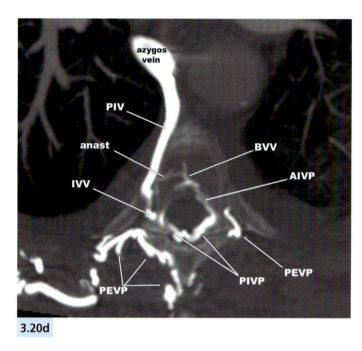

3.20d

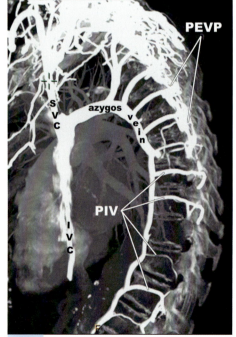

3.20e

FIGURES 3.20a–e   CT angiogram in a patient with an occluded right innominate vein and extensive collateral flow demonstrating the extensive interconnections of the vertebral venous plexuses. (a) Axial image showing one of the anastomotic connections (anast) between the anterior internal (AIVP) and anterior external vertebral venous plexuses (AEVP) through the basivertebral vein (BVV). The intervertebral veins (IVV) connect the anterior (AIVP) and posterior internal vertebral venous plexuses (PIVP) with the external vertebral venous plexuses. There are several connections between the posterior internal (PIVP) and posterior external vertebral venous plexuses (PEVP) that are not shown. (b) Axial image from a contiguous slice showing the right posterior intercostal vein (PIV). (c) and (d) Axial images showing drainage of the PIV draining into the azygos vein. Connections between the PIVP and PEVP, the IVV, and the PIV are visible in this slice. (e) Thick sagittal maximum intensity projection image showing extensive collaterals draining into the PIV. The posterior intercostal veins subsequently drain into the azygos vein and, ultimately, the superior vena cava (SVC). DRG—dorsal root ganglion, IVC—inferior vena cava.

MENINGES AND SPACES OF THE THORACIC SPINE

The spinal meninges and spaces of the thoracic region are largely the same as the meninges of the subaxial cervical segments, which are covered in detail in Chapter 2. The anatomy of the meninges that is unique to the thoracic region will be discussed in this section.

The bony thoracic spinal canal narrows in the mid-thoracic region. However, the subarachnoid spaces remain ample due to a corresponding decrease in the caliber of the mid-thoracic spinal cord. The size of the thoracic subarachnoid spaces varies according to the segmental level and the position of the spinal cord within the thecal sac. The spinal cord is positioned within the central one-third of the spinal canal at the cervicothoracic junction and the ventral and dorsal subarachnoid spaces are similar in size. The ventral subarachnoid space progressively narrows over the apex of the thoracic kyphosis, with a corresponding progressive increase in the size of the dorsal subarachnoid space. Caudal to the apex of the thoracic kyphosis, the spinal cord assumes a progressively more ventral position from craniad to caudad, resulting in progressive widening of the ventral and narrowing of the dorsal subarachnoid spaces. The spinal cord assumes a more dorsal position at the thoracolumbar junction (Figure 3.3m).

In the sitting position with the head down, the denticulate ligaments allow for a small amount of spinal cord translation ventrally. This results in further narrowing of the ventral subarachnoid space and widening of the dorsal subarachnoid space. This concept can be used to guide the approach to patient positioning for spinal anesthesia.

The arachnoid condenses to form incomplete septa within the lower cervical, thoracic, and lumbar subarachnoid spaces. The septa, along with the denticulate ligaments, form partitions in the dorsal and dorsolateral subarachnoid space. The most continuous of these septa extends from the dorsal midline pia mater to the dorsal midline arachnoid mater, called the *septum posticum of Schwalbe*. The septum posticum is best formed in the lower cervical and thoracic spine and is proposed to be the site of origin of intradural extramedullary arachnoid cysts.

The epidural space of the thoracic region is characterized by prominent dorsal fat pads. In the sagittal plane, the thoracic dorsal epidural fat pads have a biconvex to planoconvex configuration. The depth of the thoracic epidural fat pads in the AP dimension is smallest at the disc level and greatest at the pedicle level (**Figure 3.21a**). The shape of the dorsal epidural fat pads in the axial plane gradually transitions from a dorsal convex half ring configuration in the upper and mid-thoracic segments (Figure 3.21b) to the triangular interlaminar fat pad characteristic of the lower thoracic and lumbar segments (Figure 3.21c).

The epidural spaces of the thoracic spine can be accessed via an interlaminar or transforaminal approach in order to inject a variety of substances, such as anesthetics, steroids, autologous blood, fibrin glue, and other substances. Percutaneous access to the epidural space is most commonly achieved with the use of CT (**Figure 3.22a,b**) and fluoroscopy (Figure 3.22c).

The epidural spaces of the thoracic region are partially compartmentalized by the meningovertebral ligaments, similar to the cervical and lumbar regions. The meningovertebral ligaments of the thoracic spine are less prominent and less frequently encountered than the lumbar and cervical regions.

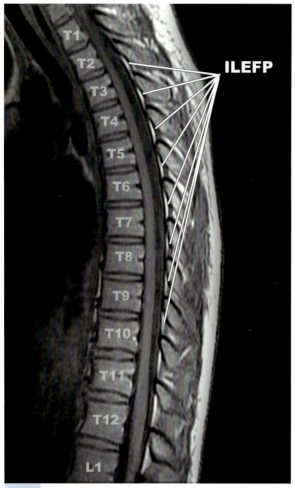

3.21a

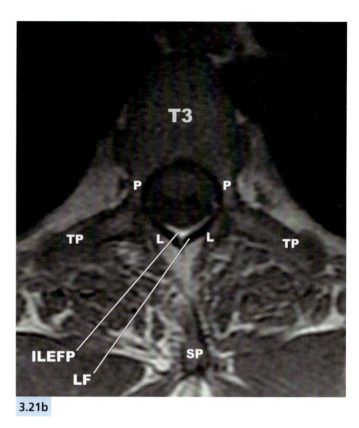

3.21b

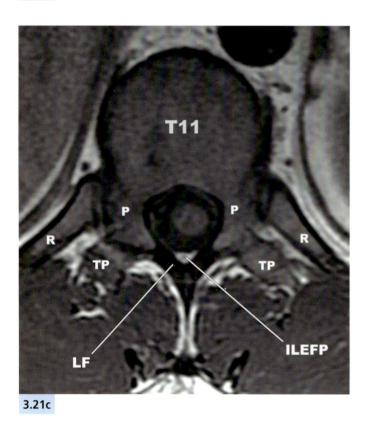

3.21c

FIGURES 3.21a–c   The dorsal epidural fat pads of the thoracic spine. (a) Sagittal T1-weighted MR image demonstrating the planoconvex shape of the thoracic interlaminar epidural fat pads (ILEFP). (b) Axial T1-weighted MR image showing the crescentic shape of the ILEFP at T3. (c) Axial T1-weighted MR image demonstrating the more triangular configuration of the T11 ILEFP. L—lamina, LF—ligamentum flavum, P—pedicle, R—rib, SP—spinous process, TP—transverse process.

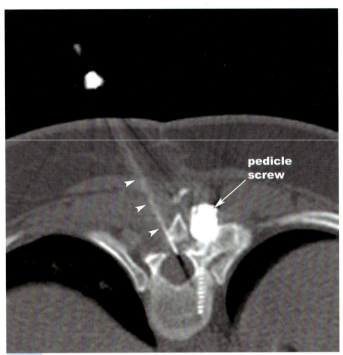

3.22a

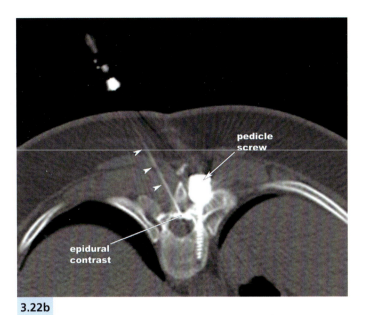

3.22b

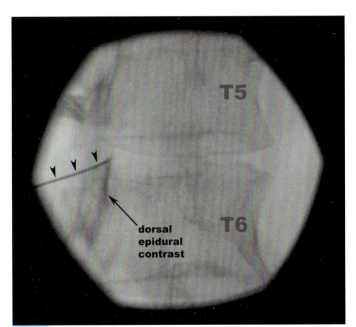

3.22c

FIGURES 3.22a–c   Thoracic interlaminar epidural steroid injections. CT-guided epidural steroid injection showing the needle (arrowheads) positioned along the dorsal margin of the spinal canal just deep to the ligamentum flavum (a) prior to and (b) following contrast administration. The contrast confirms the dorsal epidural location of the needle. (c) Lateral oblique fluoroscopically guided T5–T6 interlaminar epidural steroid injection demonstrating the position of the needle (arrowheads) and confirmation of dorsal epidural positioning by the injection of a small amount of contrast.

NEURAL ANATOMY OF THE THORACIC SPINE

The thoracic spinal cord has a circular elliptical shape in the upper thoracic segments. The caudal-most, tapering portion of the cervical enlargement is found at T1–T2. The transverse diameter of the thoracic spinal cord decreases progressively T1–T7. The transverse diameter of the cord is relatively constant T7–T11, beginning to increase at T12 in association with the lumbar enlargement (**Figure 3.23**). The AP diameter of the spinal cord decreases slightly T1–T7 and increases slightly T8–T12. The length of the thoracic cord segments increases T1–T7 and decreases T8–T12.

As has been stated previously, the central canal of the spinal cord tends to narrow and occlude with increasing age. Stenosis of the central canal is most common from T2 to T8 and occlusion occurs earliest at T6. Next to the L5–S2 segments, the lowest patency rates of the central canal are found in the mid- to lower thoracic spine. In approximately 1.5% of the population, there is persistence of the central canal that is visible on MR examinations. The persistent central canal in these cases is characterized by a filiform or fusiform shape, caliber measuring 2 to 4 mm, and predominantly mid- to lower thoracic cord location (**Figures 3.24a,b**).

The T1 nerve roots arise from the spinal cord at the level of the C7 vertebral body and ultimately exit through the T1–T2 intervertebral foramen. The T2 nerve roots arise from the spinal cord one and one-half vertebral segments above the level of their exit through the intervertebral foramina 75% of the time. The T3–T12 nerve roots arise from the spinal cord two vertebral segments above their eventual exit points through the intervertebral foramina (**Figures 3.25a,b**).

The C8 spinal nerves exit through the C7–T1 neural foramina. From T1–T2 to T12–L1, the exiting spinal nerves are numbered according to the vertebral segment above. For example, the T7 spinal nerves exit the T7–T8 intervertebral foramina.

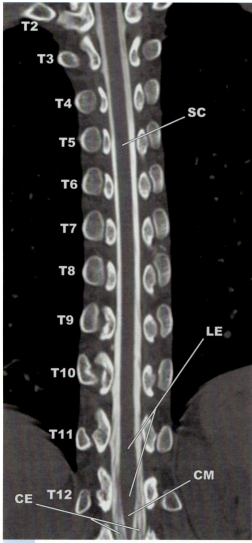

3.23

FIGURE 3.23 Curved reformatted coronal CT myelogram displaying thoracic spinal cord (SC) contour. The transverse diameter of the thoracic SC decreases T1–T7, is relatively constant T7–T11, and increases at the lumbar enlargement (LE). CE—cauda equine, CM—conus medullaris.

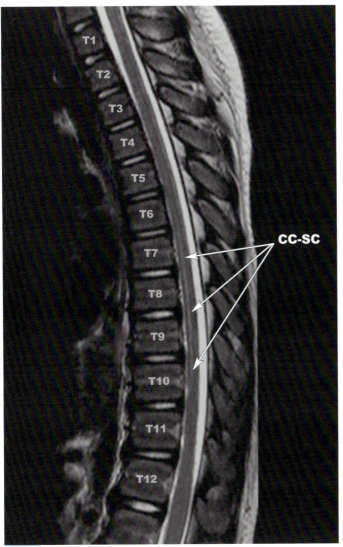

3.24a

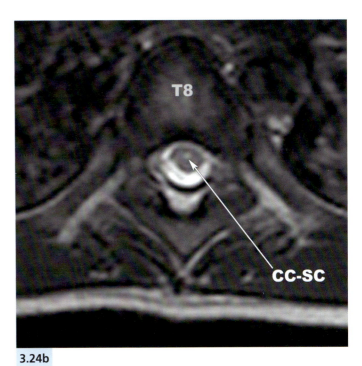

3.24b

FIGURES 3.24a,b   T2-weighted TSE images in the sagittal (a) and axial (b) planes demonstrating persistence of the central canal of the spinal cord (CC-SC) from the T7–T10 levels.

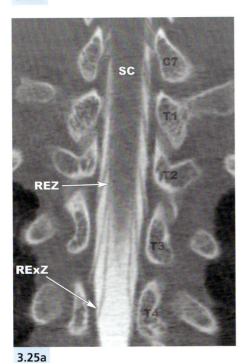

3.25a

3.25b

FIGURES 3.25a,b   (a) Coronal reformatted CT myelogram of the upper thoracic segments displays the difference between cord level and foraminal level. The nerve roots that exit the T4–T5 neural foramen arise from the spinal cord (SC) at T2. The root entry zone (REZ) and root exit zone (RExZ) are well demonstrated. (b) Curved reformatted coronal image from a CT myelogram demonstrating the course of the thoracic nerve roots (NR) inferolaterally under the pedicles, ultimately exiting via a dural sheath (DS). P—pedicle, R—rib, RMV—radiculomedullary vein.

GALLERY OF ANATOMIC VARIANTS AND VARIOUS CONGENITAL ANOMALIES

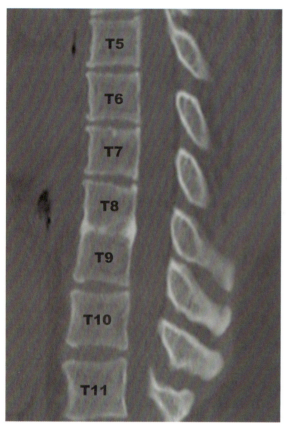

IMAGE 1 Sagittal reformatted CT showing congenital fusion of the T8 and T9 vertebral bodies.

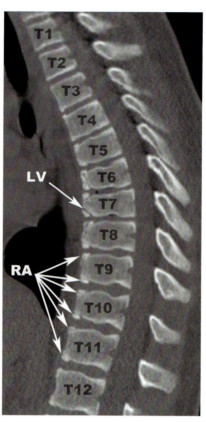

IMAGE 2 Sagittal reformatted CT showing a limbus vertebra (LV) along the anterior inferior endplate (IEP) of T7 in the setting of multiple incompletely fused ring apophyses (RA).

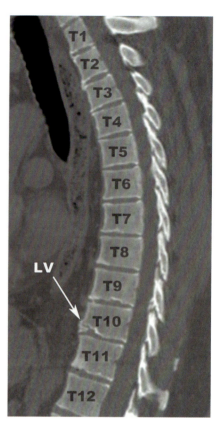

IMAGE 3 Sagittal reformatted CT demonstrating a limbus vertebra (LV) along the anterior inferior endplate of T10.

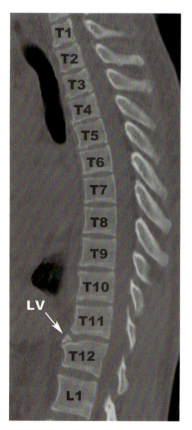

IMAGE 4 Sagittal reformatted CT demonstrating a limbus vertebra (LV) along the anterior superior endplate of T12.

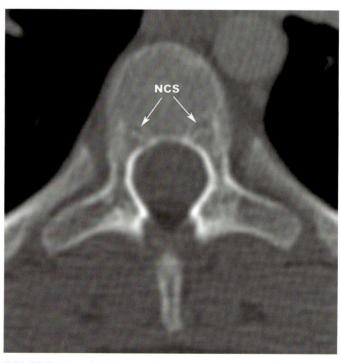

IMAGE 5 Axial CT image displaying incompletely fused neurocentral synchondroses (NCS) bilaterally.

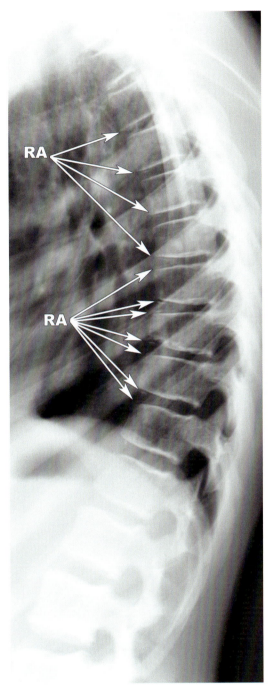

IMAGE 6   Lateral plain radiograph of the thoracic spine showing early ossification of the ring apophyses (RA) in an 8-year old child.

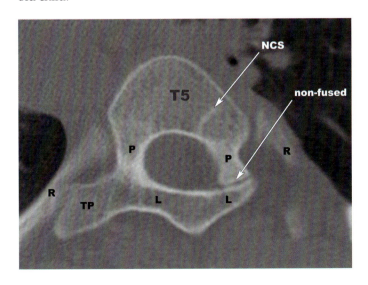

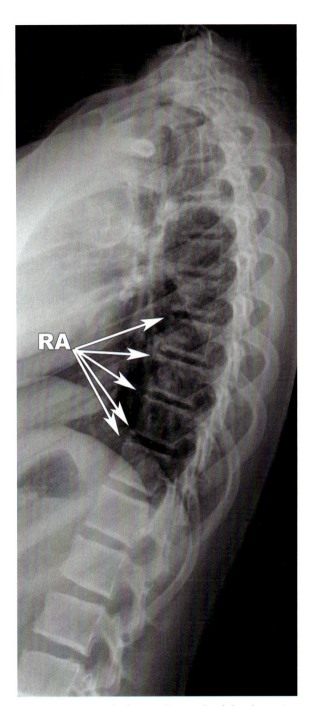

IMAGE 7   Lateral plain radiograph of the thoracic spine demonstrating near complete fusion of the ring apophyses (RA) in a 10-year-old child.

IMAGE 8   Axial CT image showing nonfusion of the left T5 pedicle. L—lamina, NCS—neurocentral synchondrosis, P—pedicle, R—rib, TP—transverse process.

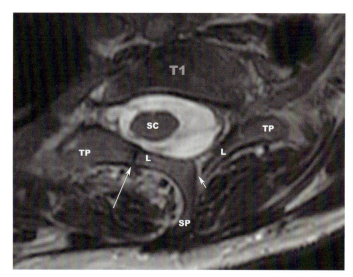

IMAGE 9 Axial T2-weighted MR image demonstrating incomplete fusion of the right lamina (long arrow) and a bifid spinous process (short arrow). L—lamina, SC—spinal cord, SP— spinous processes, TP—transverse processes.

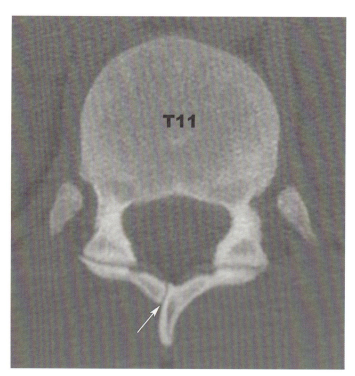

IMAGE 10 Axial maximum intensity projection image at T11 showing incomplete fusion at the spinolaminar junction on the right (arrow).

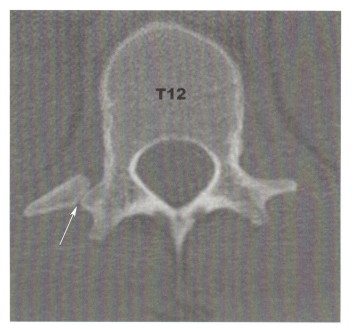

IMAGE 11 Axial CT image showing an enlarged, nonfused right transverse process (arrow). The T12 vertebra has a typical lumbar configuration.

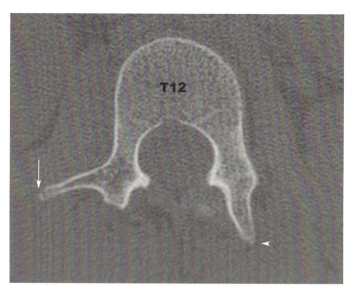

IMAGE 12 Axial CT image demonstrating nonfused secondary ossification centers at the tip of the right transverse process (arrow) and the left mammillary process (arrowhead).

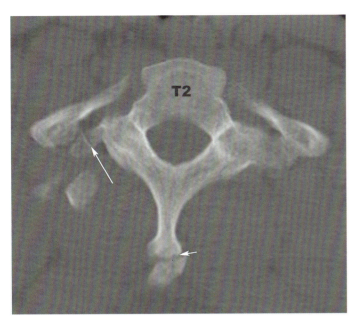

IMAGE 13   Axial maximum intensity projection CT image showing nonfusion of the left T2 transverse process (long arrow) and the spinous process (short arrow).

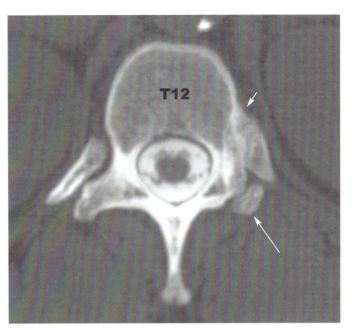

IMAGE 14   Axial image from a CT myelogram showing a dysplastic left transverse process (long arrow) and an anomalous left costovertebral articulation (short arrow).

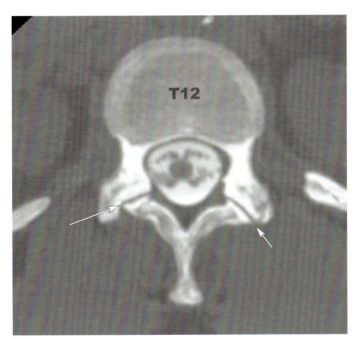

IMAGE 15   Axial maximum intensity projection CT image showing facet tropism, with a posterolaterally oriented left zygapophyseal joint (ZJ) (short arrow) and a more coronally oriented right ZJ (long arrow).

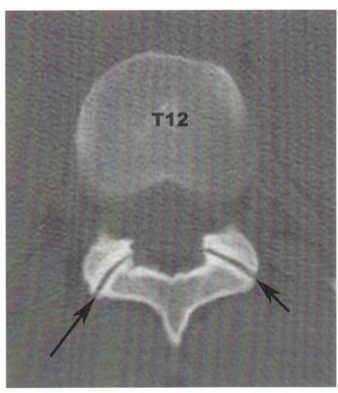

IMAGE 16   Axial CT image showing facet tropism, with a posterolaterally oriented right zygapophyseal joint (long arrow) and more coronally oriented left zygapophyseal joint (short arrow).

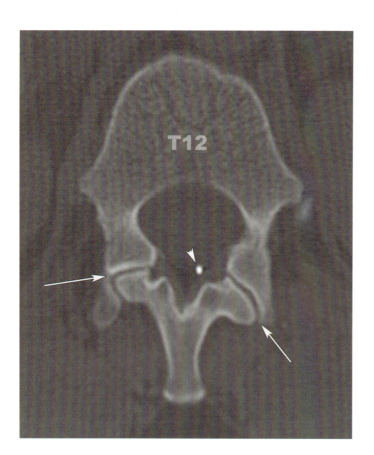

IMAGE 17   Axial CT image displaying a more extreme example of facet tropism (long arrows). The arrowhead identifies the position of a spinal cord stimulator device.

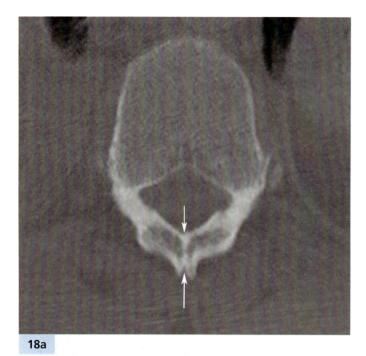

18a

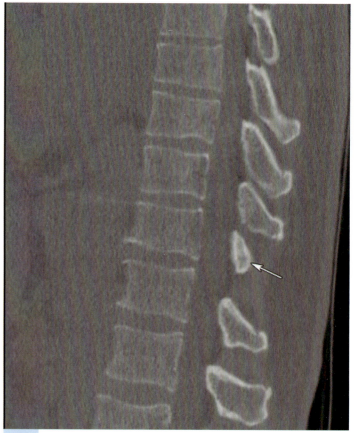

18b

IMAGES 18a,b   (a) Axial CT image demonstrates spinous process hypoplasia, (arrows) with a bifid configuration that is more typical of the subaxial cervical segments. (b) Sagittal CT image from the same patient shows the blunted, hypoplastic spinous process (arrow).

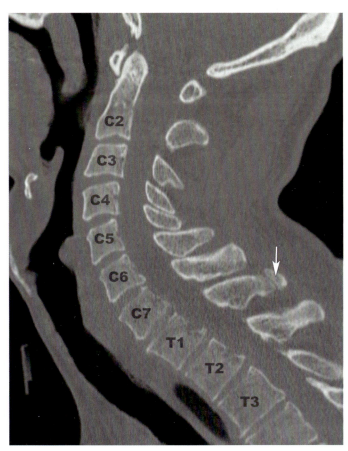

IMAGE 19   Sagittal CT image demonstrates nonfusion of the T1 spinous process secondary ossification center (arrow).

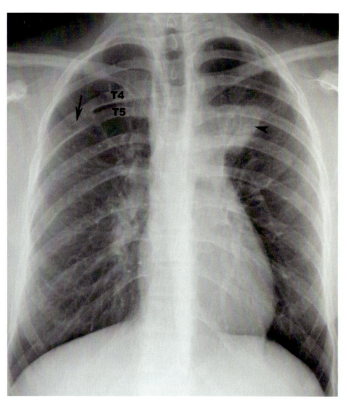

IMAGE 21   AP plain radiograph of the chest shows dorsal fusion (black arrow) of the right T4 and T5 ribs in a patient treated for pulmonary abscess (black arrowhead)

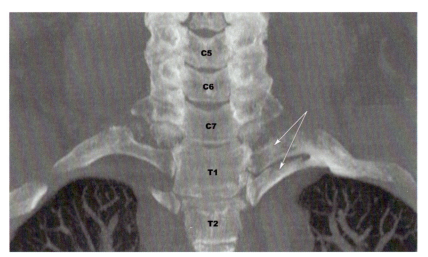

IMAGE 20   Coronal maximum intensity projection CT image shows a bifid left T1 rib (arrows).

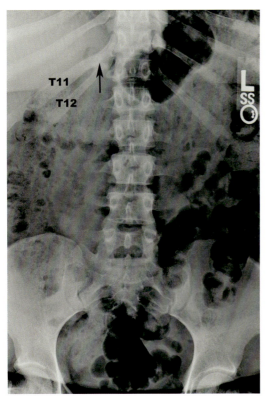

IMAGE 22   AP plain radiograph of the lumbar spine demonstrating fusion of the right T11 and T12 rib heads (arrow).

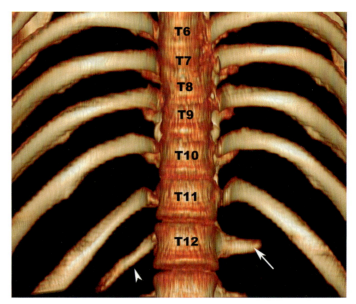

IMAGE 23   Surface rendered reformatted image of the thoracic spine from an anterior projection displays a hypoplastic right T12 rib (arrowhead) and a broad, nonfused left T12 transverse process (arrow).

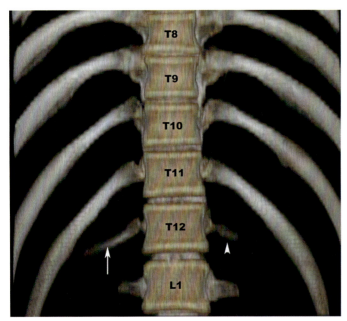

IMAGE 24   Surface rendered reformatted image of the thoracic spine from an anterior projection displays a hypoplastic right T12 rib (arrow) and a thin, nonfused left T12 transverse process (arrowhead).

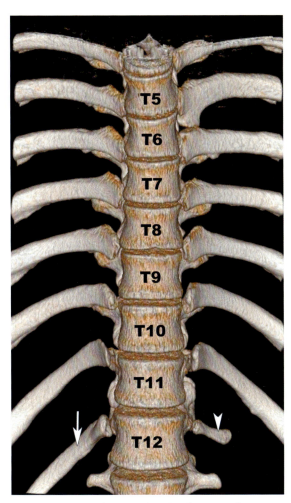

IMAGE 25   Surface rendered reformatted image of the thoracic spine from an anterior projection displays a large, floating right T12 rib (arrow) and a hypoplastic left T12 rib (arrowhead).

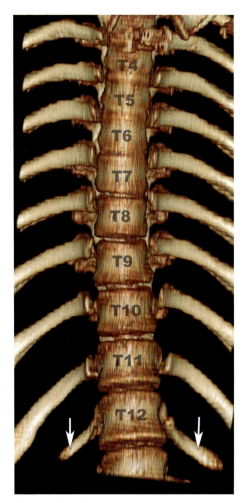

IMAGE 26   Surface rendered reformatted image of the thoracic spine from an anterior projection displays hypoplastic T12 ribs bilaterally (arrows).

SUGGESTED READINGS

Abrams HL. The vertebral and azygous venous systems, and some variations in systemic venous return. *Radiology*. 1957;69:508–526.

Albert M, Mulhern D, Torpey MA, et al. Age estimation using thoracic and first two lumbar vertebral ring epiphyseal union. *J Forensic Sci*. 2010;55(2):287–294.

Alleyne CH, Cawley CM, Shengelaia GG, et al. Microsurgical anatomy of the artery of Adamkiewicz and its segmental artery. *J Neurosurg*. 1998;89:791–795.

Bagnall KM, Harris PF, Jones PRM. A radiographic study of the human fetal spine 1. The development of the secondary cervical curvature. *J Anat*. 1977;123(3):777–782.

Bagnall KM, Harris PF, Jones PRM. A radiographic study of the human fetal spine 2. The sequence of development of ossification centres in the vertebral column. *J Anat*. 1977;124(3):791–802.

Bagnall KM, Harris PF, Jones PRM. A radiographic study of the human fetal spine 3. Longitudinal growth. *J Anat*. 1979;128(4):777–787.

Bley TA, Duffek CC, Francois CJ, et al. Presurgical localization of the artery of Adamiewicz with time-resolved 3.0-T MR angiography. *Radiology*. 2010;255(3):873–881.

Bogduk N. The innervation of the vertebral column. *Aust J Physio*. 1985;31(3):89–94.

Cardoso HFV, Rios L. Age estimation from stages of epiphyseal union in the presacral vertebrae. *Am J Phys Anthrop*. 2011;144(2):238–247.

Cramer G, et al. Identification of the anterior longitudinal ligament on cadaveric spine and comparison with appearance on MRI. Proc 1996 Internat Conf Spinal Manipulation (ICSM); October 17–19, 1996:151–152; Bournemouth, England.

Cramer G, Susan D, Darby A. *Clinical Anatomy of the Spine, Spinal Cord, and Ans*. 3rd ed. St. Louis, MO: Elsevier; 2014.

De Andres J, Reina MA, Maches F, et al. Epidural fat: considerations for minimally invasive spinal injection and surgical therapies. *J Neurosurg Rev*. 2011;1(S1):45–53.

Di Chiro G, Timins EL. Supine myelography and the septum posticum. *Radiology*. 1974;111:319–327.

Edelson JG, Nathan H. Stages in the natural history of the vertebral end-plates. *Spine*. 1988;13(1):21–26.

Gailloud P. The artery of von Haller: a constant anterior radiculomedullary artery at the upper thoracic level. *Neurosurgery*. 2013;73:1034–1043.

Griessenauer CJ, Raborn J, Foreman P, et al. Venous drainage of the spine and spinal cord: a comprehensive review of its history, embryology, anatomy, physiology, and pathology. *Clin Anat*. 2014; doi:1002/ca.22354

Jaumard NV, Welch WC, Winkelstein BA. Spinal facet joint biomechanics and mechanotransduction in normal, injury and degenerative conditions. *J Biomech Eng*. 2011;133(7):71010-NaN.

Johnson GM, Zhang M. Regional differences within the human supraspinous and interspinous ligaments: a sheet plastination study. *Eur Spine J*. 2002;11:382–388.

Kim JH, Lee CW, Chun KS, et al. Morphometric relationship between the cervicothoracic cord segments and vertebral bodies. *J Korean Neurosurg Soc*. 2012;52:384–390.

Ko HY, Park JH, Shin YB, et al. Gross quantitative measurements of the spinal cord segments in human. *Spinal Cord*. 2004;42:35–40.

Kothe R, O'Holleran JD, Liu W, et al. Internal architecture of the thoracic pedicle. An anatomic study. *Spine*. 1996;21(3):264–270.

Kretzler RM, Chaput C, Sciubba DM, et al. A computed tomography-based morphometric study of thoracic pedicle anatomy in a random United States trauma population. *J Neurosurg Spine*. 2011;14:235–243.

Kudo K, Terae S, Asano T, et al. Anterior spinal artery and artery of Adamkiewicz detected using multi-detector row CT. *Am J Neuroradiol*. 2003;24(1):13–17.

Lazorthes G, Gouaze A, Zadeh JO, et al. Arterial vascularization of the spinal cord: recent studies of the anastomotic substitution pathways. *J Neurosurg*. 1971;35:253–262.

Lee RA, van Zundert AAJ, Breedveld P, et al. The anatomy of the thoracic spinal canal investigated with magnetic resonance imaging (MRI). *Acta Anaesth Belg*. 2007;58:163–167.

Lee RA, van Zundert AJ, Botha CP, et al. The anatomy of the thoracic spinal canal in different postures. *Reg Anesth Pain Med*. 2010;35(4):364–369.

Lien SB, Lien SB, Liou NH, et al. Analysis of anatomic morphometry of the pedicles and the safe zone for through-pedicle procedures in the thoracic and lumbar spine. *Eur Spine J*. 2007;16:1215–1222.

Limthongkul W, Karaikovic EE, Savage JW, et al. Volumetric analysis of thoracic and lumbar vertebral bodies. *Spine J*. 2010;10:153–158.

Lirk P, Colvin J, Steger B, et al. Incidence of lower thoracic ligamentum flavum midline gaps. *Br J Anaesth*. 2005;94(6):852–855.

Lord MJ, Ogden JA, Ganey TM. Postnatal development of the thoracic spine. *Spine*. 1995;20(15):1692–1698.

Loughenbury PR, Wadhwani S, Soames RW. The posterior longitudinal ligament and peridural (epidural) membrane. *Clin Anat*. 2006;19:487–492.

Martirosyan NL, Feuerstein JS, Theodore N, et al. Blood supply and vascular reactivity of the spinal cord under normal and pathological conditions. *J Neurosurg Spine*. 2011;15:238–251.

Masharawi Y, Salame K. Shape variation of the neural arch in the thoracic and lumbar spine: characterization and relationship with the vertebral body shape. *Clin Anat*. 2011;24:858–867.

Masharawi Y, Salame K, Mirovsky Y, et al. Vertebral body shape variation in the thoracic and lumbar spine: characterization of its asymmetry and wedging. *Clin Anat*. 2008;21:46–54.

Masharawi YM, Peleg S, Labert HB, et al. Facet asymmetry in normal vertebral growth: characterization and etiologic theory of scoliosis. *Spine*. 2008;33(8):898–902.

Miyake H, Kiyosue H, Tanoue S, et al. Termination of the vertebral veins: evaluation by multidetector row computed tomography. *Clin Anat*. 2010;23:662–672.

Myklebust JB, Pintar F, Yoganandan N, et al. Tensile strength of spinal ligaments. *Spine*. 1988;13(5):528–531.

Nijenhuis RJ, Mull M, Wilmink JT, et al. MR angiography of the great anterior radiculomedullary artery (Adamkiewicz artery) validated by digital subtraction angiography. *Am J Neuroradiol*. 2006;27:1565–1572.

Ofiram E, Polly DW, Gilbert TJ, et al. Is it safer to place pedicle screws in the lower thoracic spine than in the upper lumbar spine? *Spine*. 2007;32(1):49–54.

Pal GP, Routal RV, Saggu SK. The orientation of the articular facets of the zygapophyseal joints at the cervical and upper thoracic region. *J Anat*. 2001;198:431–441.

Panjabi MM, Takata K, Goel V, et al. Thoracic human vertebrae: quantitative three-dimensional anatomy. *Spine*. 1991;16(8):888–901.

Panjabi MM, Oxland T, Takata K, et al. Articular facets of the human spine. *Spine*. 1993; 18:1298–1310.

Paramore CG. Dorsal arachnoid web with spinal cord compression: variant of an arachnoid cyst? Report of two cases. *J Neurosurg*. 2000;93:287–290.

Perret G, Green D, Keller J. Diagnosis and treatment of intradural arachnoid cysts of the thoracic spine. *Radiology*. 1962;79:425–429.

Petit-Lacour MC, Lasjaunias P, Iffenecker C, et al. Visibility of the central canal on MRI. *Neuroradiology*. 2000;42:756–761.

Reardon MA, Raghavan P, Carpenter-Bailey K, et al. Dorsal thoracic arachnoid web and the "scalpel sign": a distinct clinical-radiologic entity. *Am J Neuroradiol*. 2013;34(5):1104–1110.

Santillan A, Nacarino V, Greenberg E, et al. Vascular anatomy of the spinal cord. *J Neurointervent Surg*. 2012;4:67–74.

Scheuer L, Black S. *Developmental juvenile osteology*. London: Academic Press; 2000.

Scott JE, Bosworth TR, Cribb AM, Taylor JR. The chemical morphology of age-related changes in human intervertebral disc glycosaminoglycans from cervical, thoracic, and lumbar nucleus pulposus and anulus fibrosis. *J Anat*. 1994;184:73–82.

Shimizu S, Tanaka R, Kan S, et al. Origins of the segmental arteries in the aorta: an anatomic study for selective catheterization with spinal arteriography. *Am J Neuroradiol*. 2005;26:922–928.

Singer K, Edmondston S, Day R, et al. Prediction of thoracic and lumbar vertebral body compressive strength: correlations with bone mineral density and vertebral region. *Bone*. 1995;17(2):167–174.

Stringer MD, Restieaux M, Fisher AL, Crosado B. The vertebral venous plexuses: the internal veins are muscular and external veins have valves. *Clin Anat*. 2012;25:609–618.

Taylor JR, Twomey LT. Vertebral column development and its relation to adult pathology. *Aust J Physiother*. 1985;31(3):83–88.

Vandenabeele F, Creemers J, Lambrichts I. Ultrastructure of the human spinal arachnoid mater and dura mater. *J Anat*. 1996;189:417–430.

Viejo-Fuertes D, Liguoro D, Midy D, et al. Morphologic and histologic study of the ligamentum flavum in the thoraco-lumbar region. *Surg Radiol Anat*. 1998;20:171–176.

Yasui K, Hashizume Y, Yoshida M, et al. Age-related morphologic changes of the central canal of the human spinal cord. *Acta Neuropathol*. 1999;97:253–259.

Yong-Hing K, Reilly J, Kirkaldy-Willis WH. The ligamentum flavum. *Spine*. 1976; 1(4):226–234.

Yoon SP, Kim HJ, Choi YS. Anatomic variations of cervical and high thoracic ligamentum flavum. *Korean J Pain*. 2014;27(4):321–325.

Zindrick MR, Wiltse LL, Doornik A, et al. Analysis of the morphometric characteristics of the thoracic and lumbar pedicles. *Spine*. 1987;12(2):160–166.

The Lumbar Spine

*T*he lumbar spine is the most intensively investigated of the spinal regions, owing to the ubiquity of low back pain in adults. It is typically composed of five mobile vertebrae. The mobility of the lumbar segments stands in stark contrast to the restricted mobility of the thoracic segments above and immobility of the sacral segments below. No other region of the spine possesses the remarkable combination of strength, stability, multidirectional mobility, and flexibility of the lumbar spine.

4

DEVELOPMENTAL ANATOMY OF THE LUMBAR SPINE

Similar to the cervical and thoracic spine, lumbar segments are formed from a centrum and neural arches on both sides of the midline. The centra begin to ossify prior to the neural arches. Ossification proceeds from L1 to L5 and all lumbar segments are visible by the fourth fetal month (Figures 4.1a–c). At birth, three ossification centers are observed. The neurocentral synchondroses are located between the centra and neural arches. The posterior or intraneural synchondroses are located between the dorsal tips of the neural arches. The posterior synchondroses of L1–L4 fuse at about one year of age. The range of posterior synchondroseal fusion at L5 is more variable, and may take place up to 5 years of age. Nonfusion of the laminae of the lower lumbar segments is common, particularly at L5 (Figures 4.2a–d). There is 75% closure of the lumbar neurocentral synchondroses by four years of age and complete closure by 10 years of age. The typical appearance of the lumbar primary ossification centers at various ages is summarized in Figures 4.3a–p.

There are seven secondary ossification centers found within each lumbar segment, including ring apophyses along the superior and inferior margins of the vertebral body, two mammillary processes, the tips of the transverse processes, and the tip of the spinous process. The sequence of secondary ossification center closure generally starts with the mammillary processes, followed by the transverse processes, spinous processes, and ring apophyses. Complete fusion of the secondary ossification centers is usually attained by the middle of the third decade.

During the embryonic period (9–16 weeks gestation), the vertebral column elongates more rapidly than the spinal cord. This results in a change in the position of the distal spinal cord relative to that of the most caudad segments of the vertebral canal, commonly referred to as "ascent"of the cord tip. This results in a discrepancy between the sites the lumbar nerve roots exit from the spinal cord (*segmental level*) and where they exit the spinal canal into the vertebral neural foramina (*vertebral level*). For example, the L3 nerve roots exit through the L3–L4 intervertebral foramina, but because of the more rostral termination of the spinal cord, the L3 nerve roots arise from the spinal cord at the T10–T11 vertebral level.

The lumbar lordosis is a *secondary* spinal curve. The *primary* curve of the spine in utero in the first few months of life is apex posterior (kyphotic) until the secondary lordosis of the cervical spine develops when infants begin to raise their heads. The lumbar lordosis starts to form in conjunction with upright posture and progresses until 14 to 16 years of age.

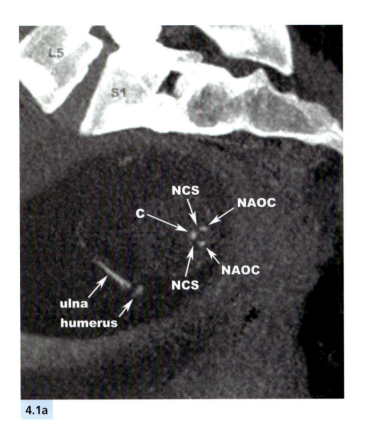

4.1a

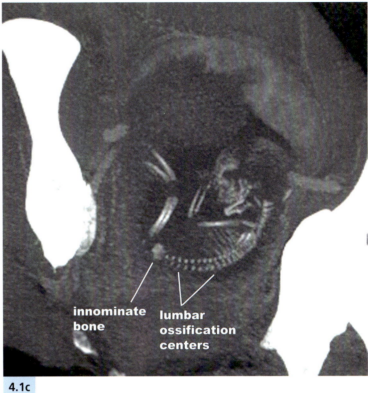

4.1c

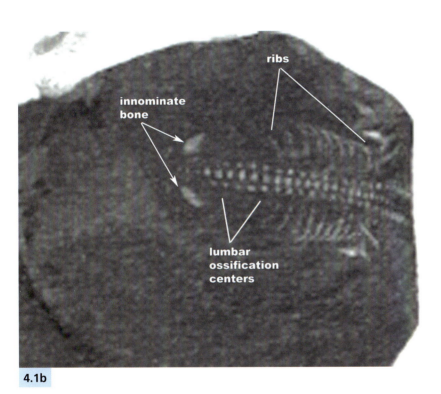

4.1b

FIGURES 4.1a–c CT performed on a female involved in a level I trauma demonstrating the fetal ossification centers at four months gestation. The primary ossification centers of the lumbar segments include a centrum (C) and two neural arches. The neurocentral synchondroses (NCS) are located between the C and the neural arch ossification centers (NAOC). The images are oriented in the (a) axial, (b) coronal, and (c) sagittal planes with respect to the fetus.

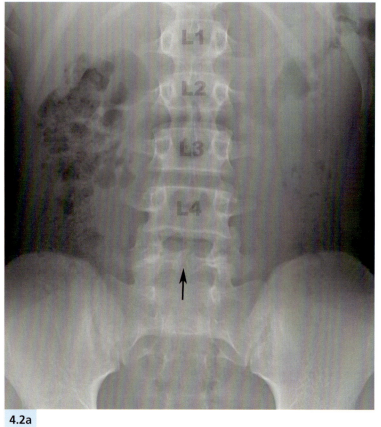

4.2a

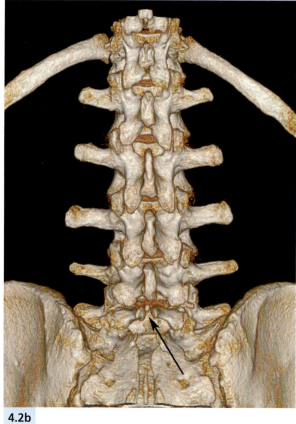

4.2b

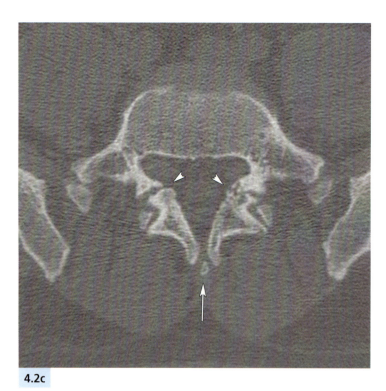

4.2c

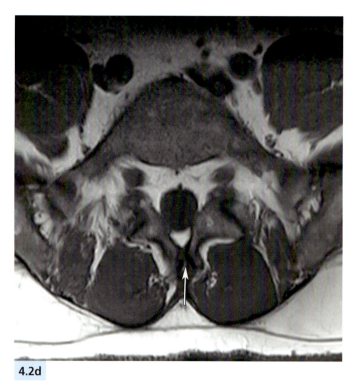

4.2d

FIGURES 4.2a–d   Spina bifida occulta at L5 demonstrated with (a) plain films, (b) surface reformatted CT from a posterior projection, (c) axial CT, and (d) axial T1-weighted TSE MR image. The arrowheads identify coexisting bilateral L5 pars interarticularis (PI) defects.

newborn

6 months

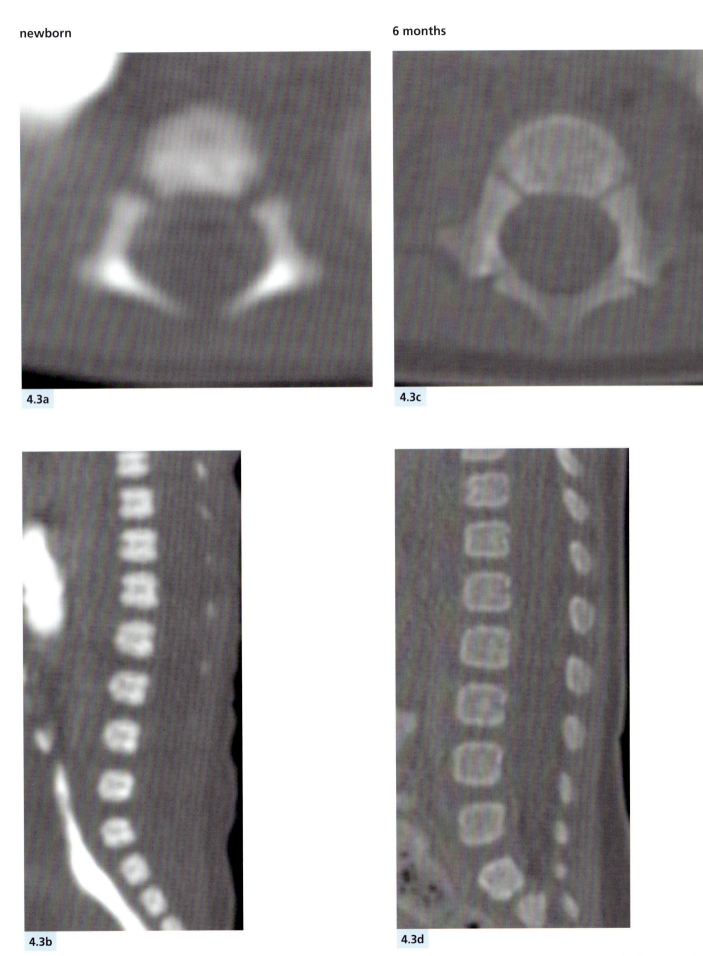

4.3a

4.3c

4.3b

4.3d

FIGURES 4.3a–p The appearance of the lumbar primary ossification centers at various ages: (a,b)—newborn, (c,d)—6 months, (e,f)—12 months, (g,h)—2 years, (i,j)—3 years, (k,l)—5 years, (m,n)—10 years, (o,p)—18 years.

(continued)

12 months

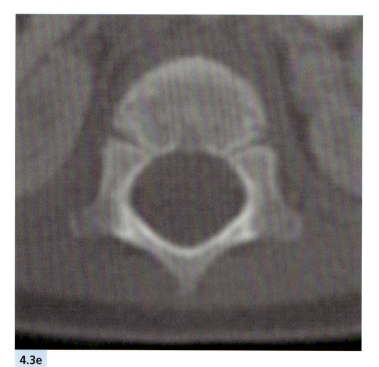

4.3e

2 years

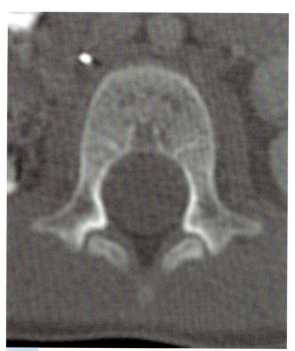

4.3g

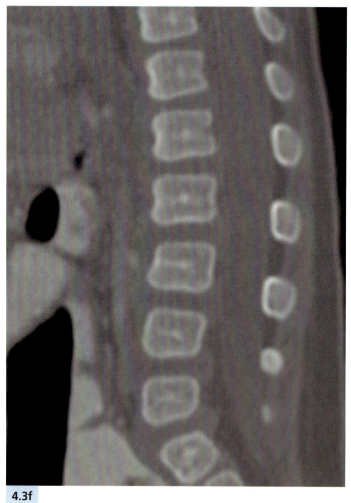

4.3f

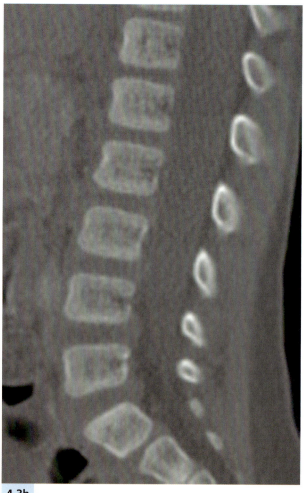

4.3h

FIGURES 4.3e–h

(*continued*)

3 years

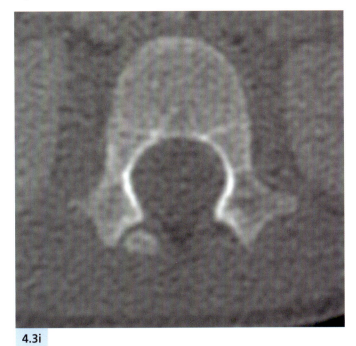

4.3i

5 years

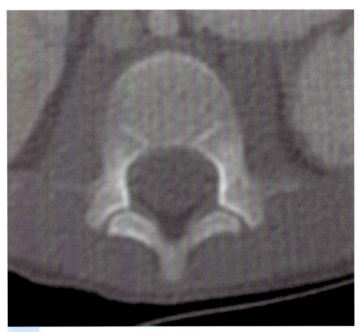

4.3k

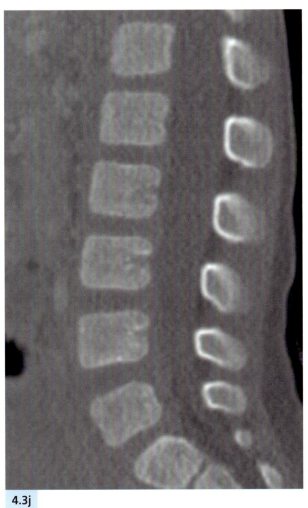

4.3j

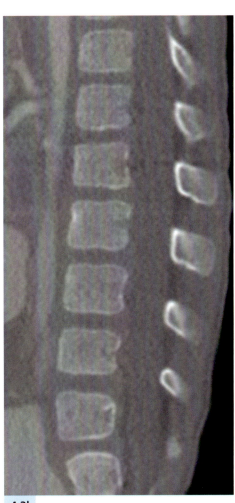

4.3l

FIGURES 4.3i–l

(continued)

10 years

18 years

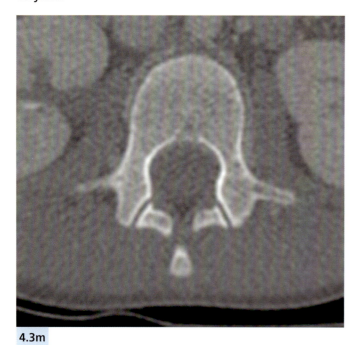

4.3m

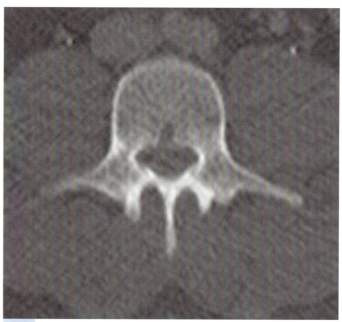

4.3o

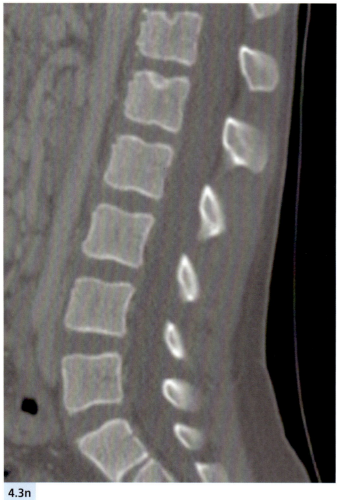

4.3n

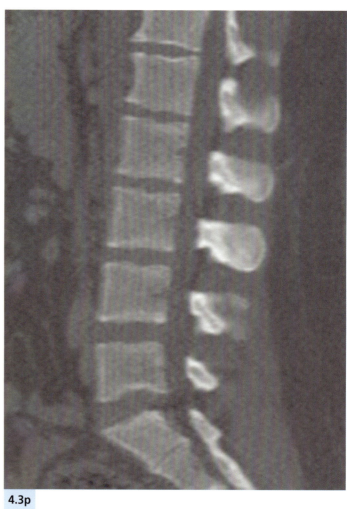

4.3p

FIGURES 4.3m–p

MULTIMODALITY ATLAS IMAGES OF THE LUMBAR SPINE

The primary modalities used to image the lumbar spine are plain films, computed tomography (CT), and magnetic resonance imaging (MRI). The basic anatomy of the lumbar segments is presented in **Figures 4.4a–y** in order to provide a foundation for the more detailed anatomic descriptions to follow.

■ PLAIN FILMS (FIGURES 4.4a–4.4c)

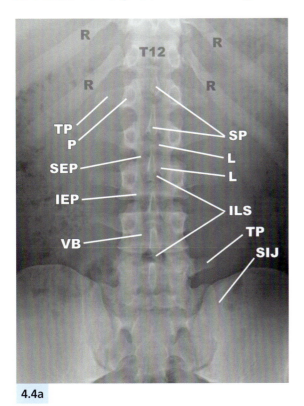

4.4a

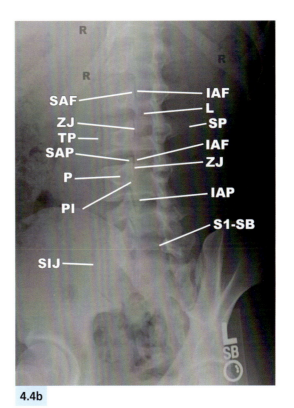

4.4b

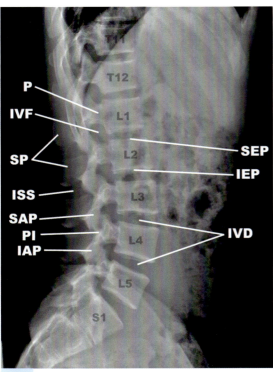

4.4c

FIGURES 4.4a–y   Multimodal image gallery demonstrating the anatomy of the lumbar spine on plain films (a–c), CT (d–q), and MR (r–y).

KEY			
IAF	inferior articular facet	**R**	rib
IAP	inferior articular process	**S1-SB**	spina bifida at S1
IEP	inferior endplate	**SAF**	superior articular facet
ILS	interlaminar space	**SAP**	superior articular process
ISS	interspinous space	**SEP**	superior endplate
IVD	intervertebral disc	**SIJ**	sacroiliac joint
IVF	intervertebral foramen	**SP**	spinous process
L	lamina	**TP**	transverse process
P	pedicle	**VB**	vertebral body
PI	pars interarticularis	**ZJ**	zygapophyseal joint

(continued)

■ CT (FIGURES 4.4d–4.4q)

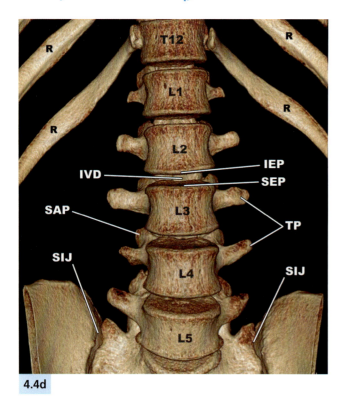

4.4d

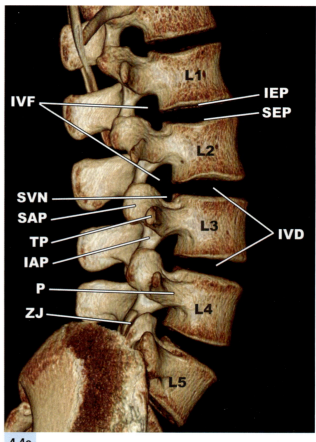

4.4e

FIGURES 4.4d–f

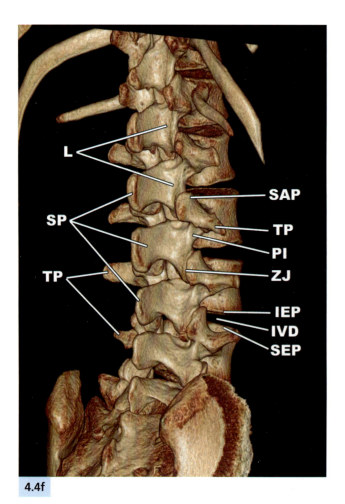

4.4f

KEY			
IAP	inferior articular process	SAP	superior articular process
IEP	inferior endplate	SEP	superior endplate
IVD	intervertebral disc	SIJ	sacroiliac joint
IVF	intervertebral foramen	SP	spinous process
L	lamina	SVN	superior vertebral notch
P	pedicle	TP	transverse process
PI	pars interarticularis	ZJ	zygapophyseal joint
R	rib		

(continued)

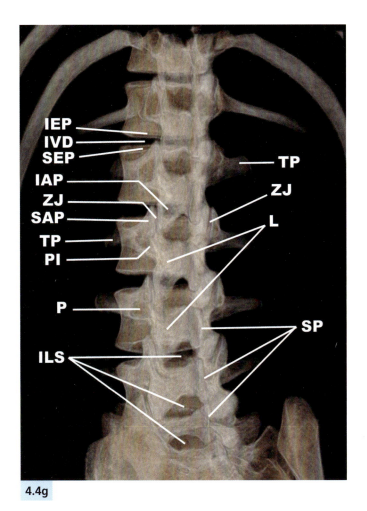

4.4g

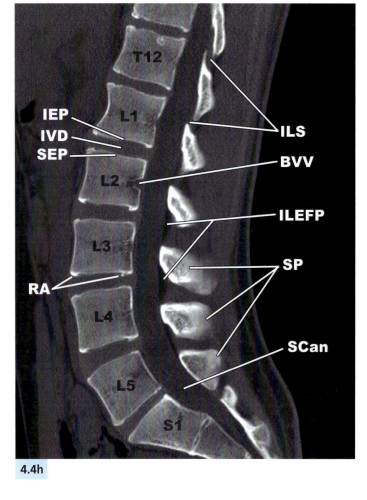

4.4h

FIGURES 4.4g–i

KEY			
BVV	basivertebral vein	**P**	pedicle
DRG	dorsal root ganglion	**PI**	pars interarticularis
IAF	inferior articular facet	**RA**	ring apophyses
IAP	inferior articular process	**SAF**	superior articular facet
IEP	inferior endplate	**SAP**	superior articular process
ILEFP	interlaminar epidural fat pad	**SCan**	spinal canal
		SEP	superior endplate
ILS	interlaminar space	**SP**	spinous process
IVD	intervertebral disc	**SVN**	superior vertebral notch
IVF	intervertebral foramen	**TP**	transverse process
IVN	inferior vertebral notch	**ZJ**	zygapophyseal joint
L	lamina		

4.4i

(*continued*)

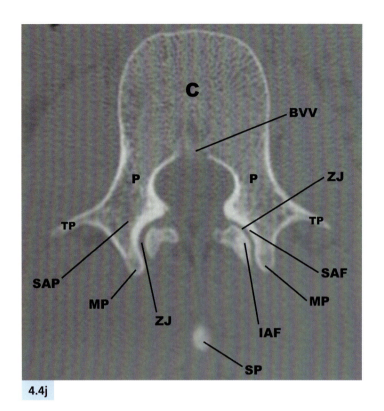

4.4j

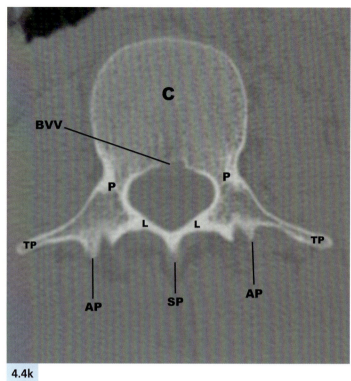

4.4k

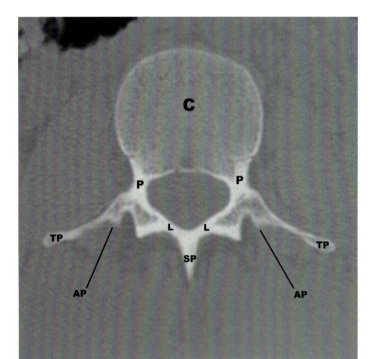

4.4l

FIGURES 4.4j–l

KEY			
AP	accessory process	SAF	superior articular facet
BVV	basivertebral vein	SAP	superior articular
C	centrum		process
IAF	inferior articular facet	SP	spinous process
L	lamina	TP	transverse process
MP	mammillary process	ZJ	zygapophyseal joint
P	pedicle		

(*continued*)

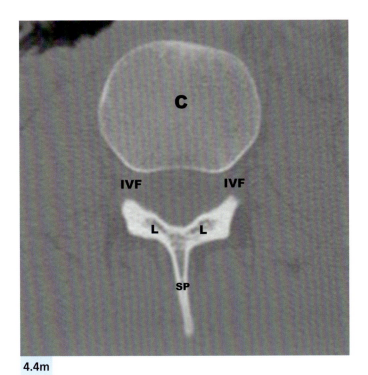

4.4m

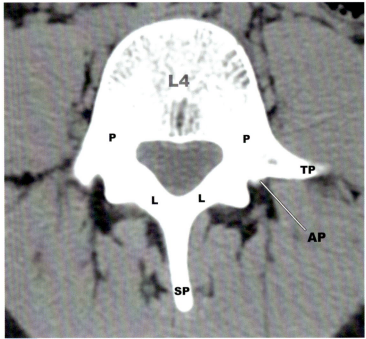

4.4n

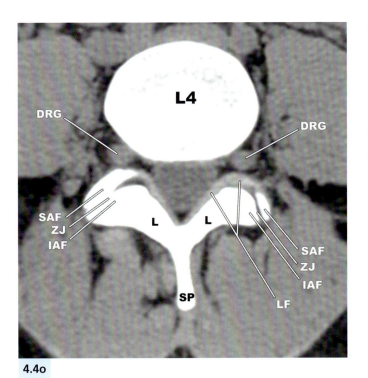

4.4o

FIGURES 4.4m–o

KEY			
AP	accessory process	LF	ligamentum flavum
C	centrum	P	pedicle
DRG	dorsal root ganglion	SAF	superior articular facet
IAF	inferior articular facet	SP	spinous process
IVF	intervertebral foramen	TP	transverse process
L	lamina	ZJ	zygapophyseal joint

(continued)

FIGURES 4.4p,q

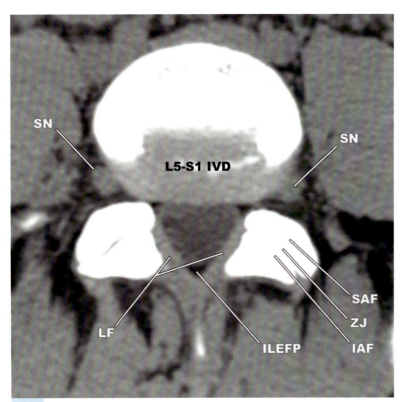

4.4p

KEY			
IAF	inferior articular facet	P	pedicle
ILEFP	interlaminar epidural fat pad	SAF	superior articular facet
ILL	iliolumbar ligament	SN	spinal nerve
IVD	intervertebral disc	SP	spinous process
L	lamina	TP	transverse process
LF	ligamentum flavum	ZJ	zygapophyseal joint

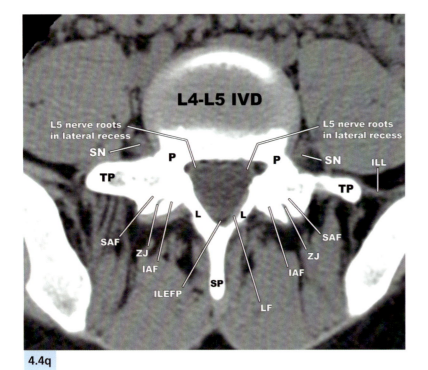

4.4q

(*continued*)

■ MR (FIGURES 4.4r–4.4y)

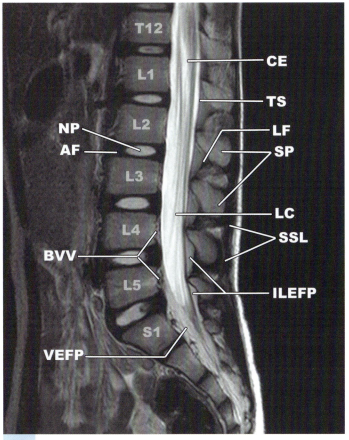

4.4r

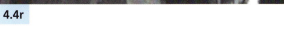

4.4s

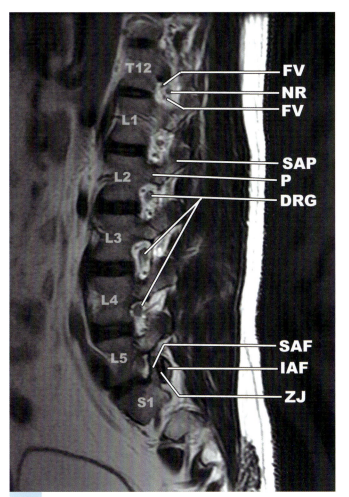

4.4t

FIGURES 4.4r–t

KEY			
AF	annulus fibrosis	LF	ligamentum flavum
ALL	anterior longitudinal ligament	NP	nucleus pulposis
		NR	nerve root
BVV	basivertebral vein	P	pedicle
CE	cauda equina	SAF	superior articular facet
DRG	dorsal root ganglion	SAP	superior articular process
FV	foraminal vein		
IAF	inferior articular facet	SP	spinous process
ILEFP	interlaminar epidural fat pad	SSL	supraspinous ligament
		TS	thecal sac
IVD	intervertebral disc	VEFP	ventral epidural fat pad
LC	lumbar cistern	ZJ	zygapophyseal joint

(continued)

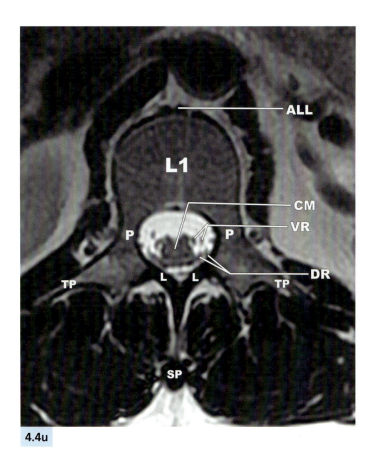

4.4u

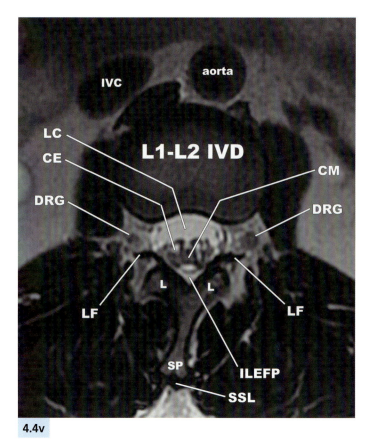

4.4v

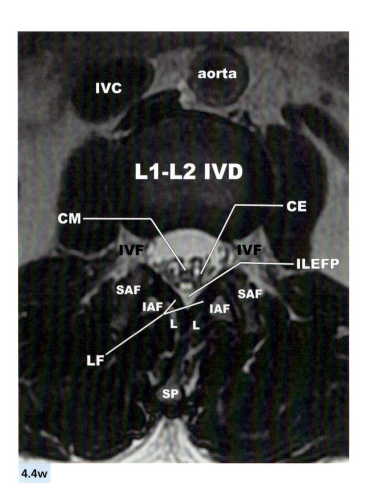

4.4w

FIGURES 4.4u–w

KEY			
ALL	anterior longitudinal ligament	**IVF**	intervertebral foramen
CE	cauda equina	**L**	lamina
CM	conus medullaris	**LC**	lumbar cistern
DR	dorsal root	**LF**	ligamentum flavum
DRG	dorsal root ganglion	**P**	pedicle
IAF	inferior articular facet	**SAF**	superior articular facet
ILEFP	interlaminar epidural fat pad	**SP**	spinous process
		SSL	supraspinous ligament
IVC	inferior vena cava	**TP**	transverse process
IVD	intervertebral disc	**VR**	ventral root

(continued)

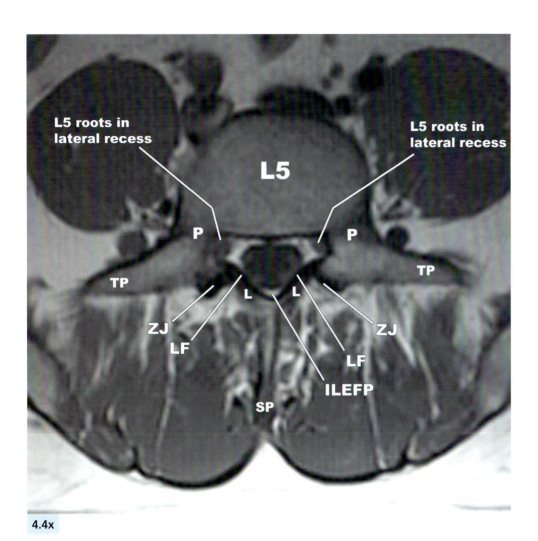

4.4x

KEY

ALL	anterior longitudinal ligament
DRG	dorsal root ganglion
IAF	inferior articular facet
ILEFP	interlaminar epidural fat pad
L	lamina
LF	ligamentum flavum
MVL	meningovertebral ligament
P	pedicle
SAF	superior articular facet
SP	spinous process
TP	transverse process
ZJ	zygapophyseal joint

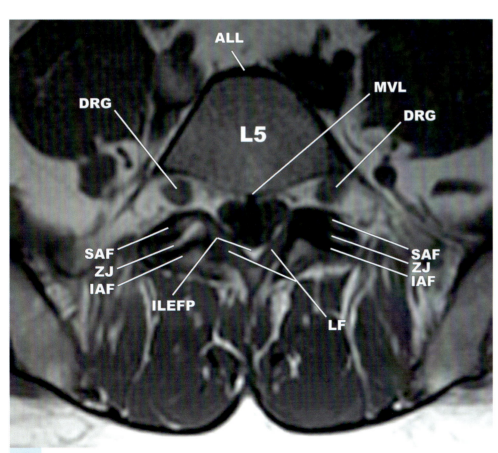

4.4y

OSTEOLOGY OF THE LUMBAR SEGMENTS

The lumbar lordosis is more pronounced than the cervical lordosis and results from a combination of vertebral body and intervertebral disc wedging. The vertebral body wedging at L4 and L5 is the opposite of that seen in the thoracic segments, with greater height anteriorly than posteriorly. The lumbar vertebral bodies are greater in size in the transverse dimension than the anterior to posterior dimension. In the axial plane, the L1–L4 vertebral bodies have a dorsal concavity that produces a kidney shape (**Figure 4.5**). The L5 vertebral body has a convex dorsal margin, forming an ellipse (Figure 4.4y). The bone mineral content, trabecular density, volume, and compressive strength of the lumbar vertebral bodies increase L1–L3 and decrease slightly L4–L5. The strength and stiffness of the posterolateral aspect of the L3–L5 vertebral endplates is greater than the central aspects of the vertebral endplates.

The lumbar pedicles are shorter than the thoracic pedicles. They are larger in height than width. The width of the lumbar pedicles increases L1–L5 (**Figure 4.6**). They arise more inferiorly from the vertebral body than the thoracic pedicles, forming shallow superior vertebral notches. The inferior vertebral notches, formed by upward concavity along the inferior margin of the pedicles, are comparatively deep. The L1 pedicles are smaller in caliber than the T10–T12 pedicles. They are angled anteromedial to posterolateral in the transverse plane. This angle increases from L1 to L5. In the sagittal plane, the lumbar pedicles are angled slightly anterosuperior to posteroinferior. The lumbar pedicle is commonly accessed for percutaneous vertebral biopsies (**Figure 4.7a**), vertebral augmentation (**Figures 4.7b–d**), and occasionally disc aspiration/biopsy.

The transverse processes of the lumbar segments are flat and primarily oriented in the coronal plane, with slight posterolateral angulation. They increase in length L1–L3 and

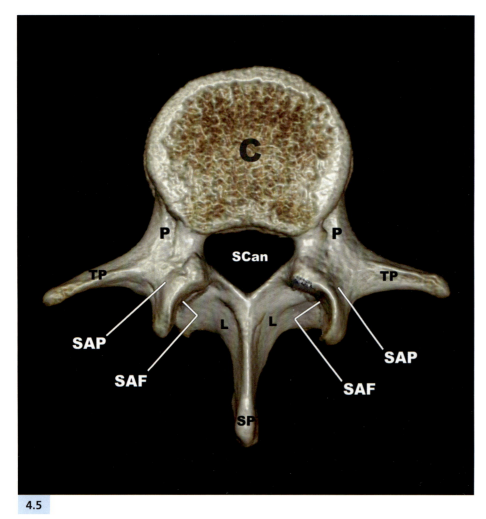

4.5

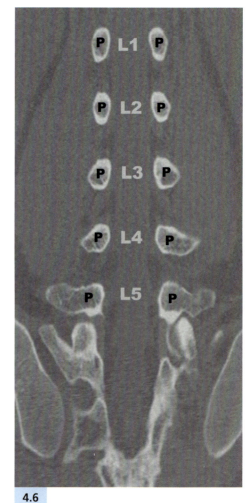

4.6

FIGURE 4.5 Surface rendered CT image from a superior projection demonstrating the shape of the L1-L4 vertebral bodies. The transverse dimension is greater than the anterior to posterior dimension and the posterior wall of the centrum (C) is concave. L—lamina, P—pedicle, SAF—superior articular facet, SAP—superior articular process, SCan —spinal canal, SP—spinous process, TP—transverse process.

FIGURE 4.6 Coronal curved reformatted CT image demonstrating the ovoid shape of the lumbar pedicles (P), which increase in size and are progressively posterolaterally oriented from L1-L5.

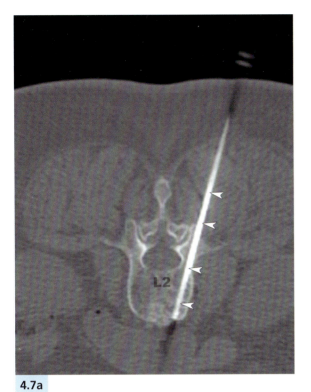

4.7a

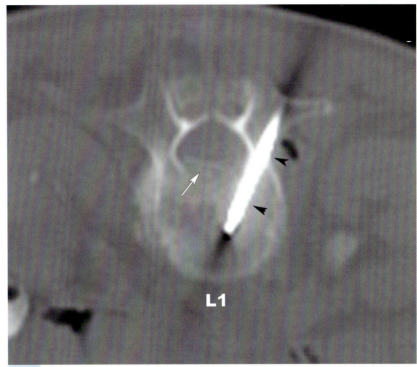

4.7b

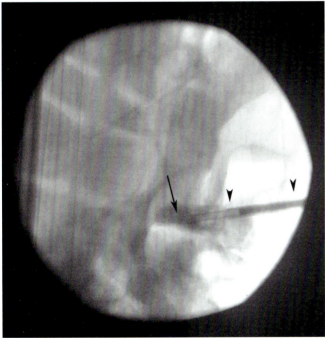

4.7c

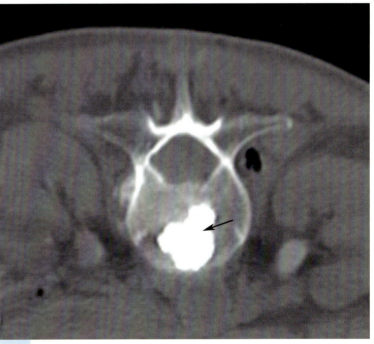

4.7d

FIGURES 4.7a–d   (a) Axial image from a CT-guided biopsy. The needle (arrowheads) traverses the left pedicle en route to the lytic lesion within the vertebral body (VB). (b) CT-guided left-sided transpedicular needle (arrowheads) approach to the L1 VB for kyphoplasty of a compression fracture that has retropulsed fragments (white arrow). (c) Lateral fluoroscopic image demonstrating positioning of the needle (arrowheads) within the pedicle and injection of methyl methacrylate cement into a previously formed cavity (arrow). (d) Axial CT fluoroscopic image shows good distribution of cement within the central and anterior aspect of the L1 VB (arrow).

decreases L4–L5. The L5 transverse processes are thicker (AP) and broader (craniad to caudad) than the L1–L4 transverse processes. The lumbar transverse processes arise at the pedicle-lamina junction just posterior to the intervertebral foramina and anterior to the articular processes. There are small posteriorly projecting osseous protuberances located at the junction of the transverse processes and lamina along their posteroinferior margin, called *accessory processes* (**Figure 4.8**). They represent the sites of attachment of the longissimus thoracis and intertransversarii lumborum muscles and are not found outside of the lumbar segments.

The laminae of the lumbar segments are broad, flat, and vertically-oriented. In the sagittal plane, they are angled slightly anterosuperior to posteroinferior. The superior margins of the lumbar laminae have a downward concavity. The inferior margins of the lumbar laminae have an upward concavity. This results in round to ovoid lumbar interlaminar spaces (**Figure 4.9**). The height of the lumbar laminae is less than that of the lower thoracic lamina. Laminar height in the lumbar spine increases slightly L1–L3 and then decreases L4–L5. As a result, the L1–L2 to L3–L4 interlaminar spaces are similar in size. The L4–L5 and L5–S1 interlaminar spaces are large (Figure 4.9). The width of the lumbar laminae increases L1–L5.

The short segment of bone that occupies the space between the superior and inferior articular processes is called the pars interarticularis. The trabecular pattern within the L4 and L5 pedicles suggests additional stress on the pars interarticularis at these levels. Further, the cortical bone of the laminae is thickest in the region of the pars interarticularis. Despite this reinforcement, fractures (defects) of the pars interarticularis are common. Defects in the pars interarticularis are most common at L5 (85%–95%), with L4 (5%–15%) the next most affected level. On lumbar plain x-rays, the pars interarticularis is easily identified as the "neck"of the Scottie dog (Figures 4.4b, 4.4f, 4.4g). The pars defect is visible on plain x-ray as a "broken neck"of the Scottie dog (**Figure 4.10a**) or a discontinuity of the pars interarticularis on parasagittal CT (**Figure 4.10b**) or MR (**Figure 4.10c**) images.

The superior and inferior articular processes of the lumbar spine arise from the superior and inferior margins of the par interarticularis, respectively. The superior articular processes are vertically oriented and their facets face posteromedially. The inferior articular processes are also vertically oriented and their facets face anterolaterally. The superior articular facets have a concave curvature and are positioned more anteriorly. The inferior articular facets have a convex curvature and are located more posteriorly (**Figures 4.11**, 4.4g, 4.4i, 4.4j, 4.5). The zygapophyseal joints are discussed in the following.

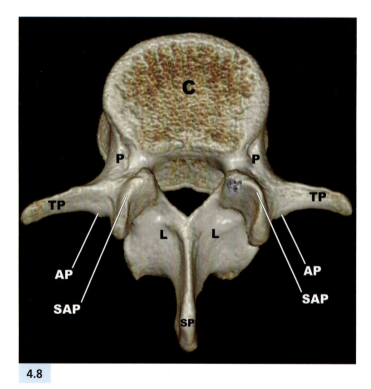

4.8

FIGURE 4.8 Surface rendered reformatted CT image showing the accessory processes (AP) positioned at the junction of the transverse processes (TP) and lamina (L) along the posteroinferior margin. C—centrum, P—pedicle, SAP—superior articular process, SP—spinous process, TP—transverse process.

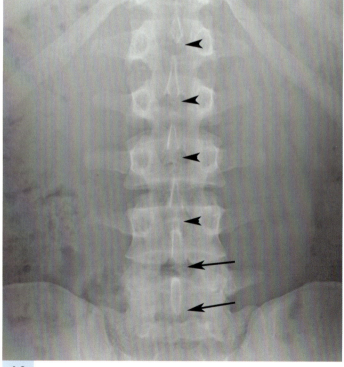

4.9

FIGURE 4.9 Frontal projection plain film of the lumbar spine demonstrating the round to ovoid configuration of the lumbar interlaminar spaces (ILS) (black arrowheads). The L4-L5 and L5-S1 ILSs (black arrows) are larger than the L1-L2, L2-L3, and L3-L4 ILSs.

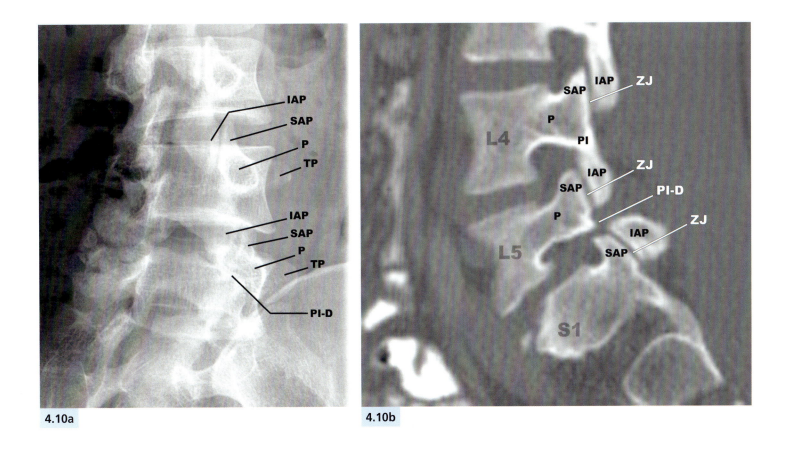

4.10a

4.10b

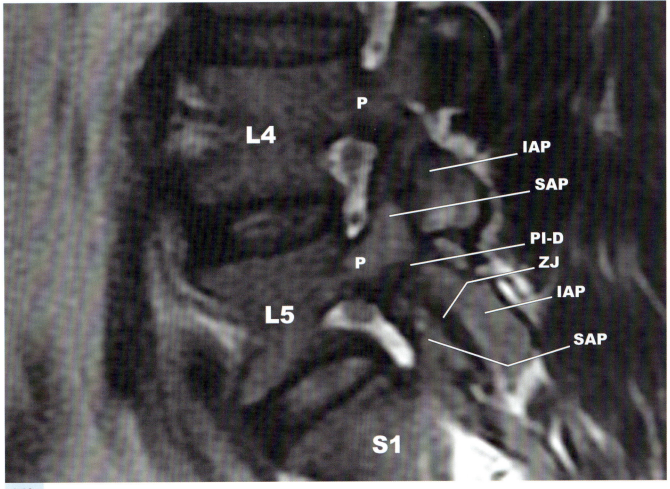

4.10c

FIGURES 4.10a–c   Pars interticularis defects (PI-D) at L5 displayed on (a) plain films, (b) CT, and (c) MR. IAP—inferior articular process, P—pedicle, PI—pars interarticularis, SAP—superior articular process, TP—transverse process, ZJ—zygapophyseal joint

The *mamillary processes* are bony projections that arise from the superior articular processes and project posteriorly. The multifidi lumborum muscles attach to the mamillary processes. There is a shallow depression located between the accessory and mamillary processes, the *mamillo-accessory notch* (**Figure 4.12**), that is bridged by the mamillo-accessory ligament (MAL). The MAL calcifies approximately 10% of the time and may form a discreet foramen. The medial branches of the dorsal rami are housed within the mamillo-accessory notches. This notch is a target in CT-guided percutaneous medial branch denervation procedures.

The spinous processes of the lumbar segments are broad, flat, rectangular, and project in a straight line posteriorly. The lumbar spinous processes decrease in size in the AP and craniocaudal dimensions L1–L4. The L5 spinous process is typically significantly smaller, projects slightly inferiorly and often has an apex posterior triangular configuration. The lumbar spinous processes may undergo elongation and progressive squaring with age.

A wide range of spinal canal configurations have been reported, the details of which are beyond the scope of this text. Generally speaking, the upper lumbar spinal canal is round to ovoid and the lower spinal canal is trefoil to triangular in shape. The spinal canal normally measures greater than 13 mm AP in the mid-sagittal plane (area 1.45 cm²). Lumbar spinal canal dimensions vary in accordance with multiple factors that include height, ethnicity, and dynamic factors. Greater overall body height is correlated with larger mid-sagittal spinal canal diameters. Smaller canal diameters have been reported in Asian and Egyptian populations relative to European and African populations.

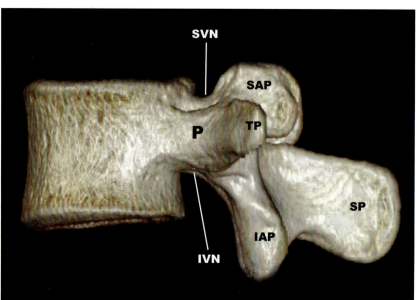

FIGURE 4.11 Surface rendered reformatted CT image from a lateral projection shows the vertical orientation of the superior articular processes (SAP) and inferior articular processes (IAP). The SAP arise more anteriorly than the inferior articular processes. IAP—inferior articular process, IVN—inferior vertebral notch, P—pedicle, SAP—superior articular process, SP—spinous process, SVN—superior vertebral notch, TP—transverse process.

4.11

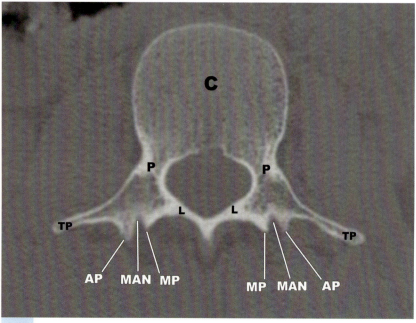

FIGURE 4.12 Axial CT image demonstrating the shallow groove located between the accessory (AP) and mamillary processes (MP), the mamillo-accessory notch (MAN). The medial branch of the dorsal ramus is reliably located within the mamillo-accessory notch, which can be utilized as a target in CT-guided percutaneous denervation procedures. C—centrum, L—lamina, P—pedicle, TP—transverse process.

4.12

THE ZYGAPOPHYSEAL JOINTS

The superior and inferior articular processes of the lumbar segments arise from the pars interarticularis of the lamina. The superior articular facets arise on the dorsal surfaces of the superior articular processes and face posteromedially. The inferior articular facets arise on the ventral surfaces of the inferior articular processes and face anterolaterally (Figures 4.4f, 4.4g, 4.4i, 4.4j, 4.5, 4.11). The facet surfaces are lined by a thin layer of smooth articular cartilage, are surrounded by a fibrous capsule, and are lubricated by synovial fluid. There are prominent fibrofatty pads along the superior and inferior recesses of the zygapophyseal joint capsules. The articular surfaces are variably curved. The lumbar zygapophyseal joints are oriented posterolaterally. This degree of posterolateral angulation increases from L1–L2 to L4–L5. The L5–S1 zygapophyseal joints are generally smaller, flatter, and more variable in orientation than the other lumbar levels. The zygapophyseal joints may display mixed orientations, with one of the joints more coronally-oriented and the other more sagittally oriented, termed *facet tropism* (**Figure 4.13**). Facet tropism may also refer to differential size of the facets and is often a precursor to facet degeneration.

The zygapophyseal joints allow a wide range of motion in the lumbar segments, including flexion (60 degrees), extension (25 degrees), and lateral flexion (25 degrees). However, the configuration of the zygapophyseal joints significantly limits rotational motion of the lumbar segments.

Percutaneous access to the zygapophyseal joint capsules for diagnostic or therapeutic injections is most commonly performed with CT or fluoroscopic guidance. Depending on the level of the zygapophyseal joint, the joint is accessed from variable posterolateral obliquities (**Figures 4.14a, 4.14b**).

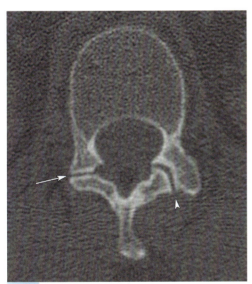

FIGURE 4.13   Facet tropism. The left zygapophyseal joint (ZJ) is oriented posterolaterally (arrowhead) and the right ZJ is coronally-oriented (arrow).

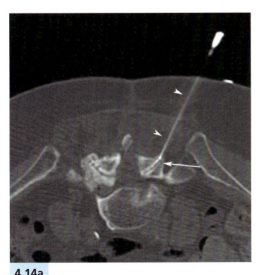

4.14a   4.14b

FIGURES 4.14a,b   CT-guided facet injections. (a) Left and (b) right zygapophyseal joint (arrows) steroid injections displaying the typical posterolateral approach of the needles (arrowheads).

LUMBOSACRAL TRANSITIONAL ANATOMY

Lumbosacral transitional vertebrae (LSTV) are anatomic normal variants that are common in the general population. There is a wide range of prevalence estimates, ranging from 4% to 35.9%, that are derived from varying sample sizes and populations. The most commonly encountered LSTV is an L5 segment that is partially or completely incorporated into the sacrum, called *sacralization*. When the S1 segment displays lumbar-type features, it is referred to as *lumbarization*. However, a wide range of anomalies are observed at the lumbosacral transition.

A useful classification system for LSTV has been published by Castellvi, et al (1984). Type I LSTV are dysplastic transverse processes, triangular in shape, and measuring at least 19 mm in width. In type II, there is an enlarged transverse process that forms a diarthrodial joint with the adjacent sacral ala. Type III LSTV displays solid bony fusion of the transverse process and sacral ala, instead of a diarthrodial joint. Type IV LSTV show a mixture of type II and type III features. The modifiers "a"or "b"are added to indicate unilaterality or bilaterality, respectively. The Castellvi classification is summarized in **Table 4.1** and examples of the subtypes are displayed in **Figures 4.15a–e**.

The Castellvi system is based upon visualizing the osseous anatomy of the lumbosacral junction, which is optimally evaluated with plain films or CT. The identification of LSTV is generally more difficult with MR. O'Driscoll, et al (1996) addressed this issue by developing a system designed to identify LSTV on MR based on S1–S2 disc morphology. Disc material is absent in type I. In type II, there is rudimentary disc material that does not extend the AP

TABLE 4.1   Castellvi Lumbosacral Transitional Vertebra Classification System

TYPE	FEATURES
I	Dysplastic, triangular transverse process (> 19 mm in width)
II	Large transverse process that follows the contour of the sacral ala; forms an apparent diarthrodial joint between the transverse process and sacrum
III	Large transverse process that fuses with the sacrum
IV	Type II on one side and type III on the other

a—unilateral, b—bilateral

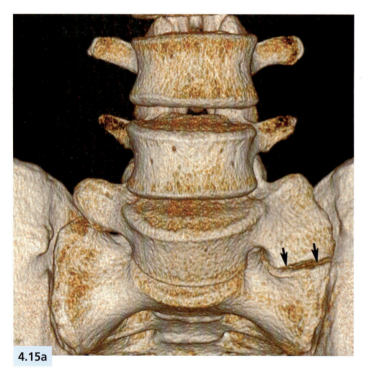

4.15a

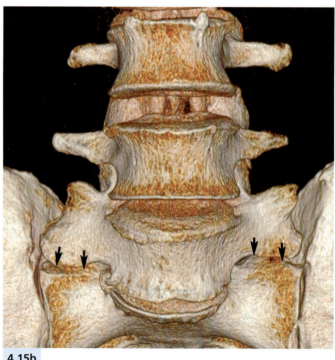

4.15b

FIGURES 4.15a–e   The Castellvi classification of lumbosacral transitional vertebrae. Surface rendered reformatted CT images from a frontal projection demonstrating: (a) left-sided diarthrodial joint (arrows) or type IIa, (b) bilateral diarthrodial joints (arrows) or type IIb, (c) fusion of the left transverse process (TP) to the sacrum (arrows) or type IIIa, (d) bilateral fusion of the TPs to the sacrum (arrows) or type IIIb, and (e) type II morphology on the right (arrowheads), and type III morphology on the left (arrows) or type IV.

(continued)

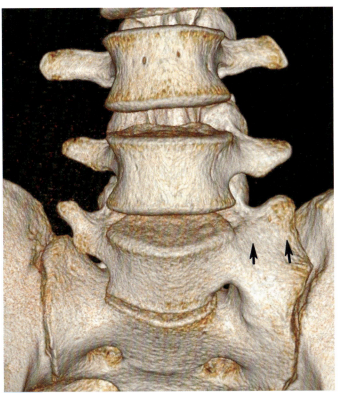

4.15c

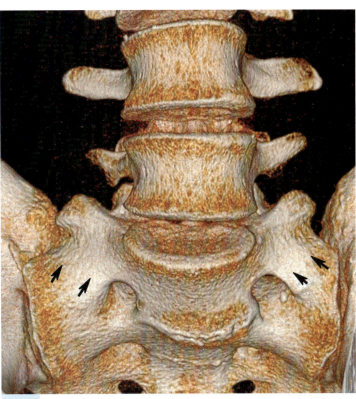

4.15d

FIGURES 4.15c–e

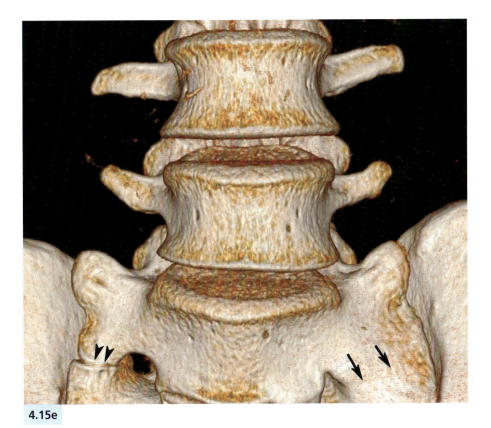

4.15e

length of the sacrum. The type III disc extends the entire AP length of the sacrum. Type IV discs are similar in morphology to type III discs, with squaring of what is presumed to be the S1 segment. Type I is not associated with LSTV. Type II is rarely associated with LSTV. Type III may or may not be associated with LSTV. Type IV morphology is correlated with the presence of Castellvi III and IV transitional anatomy. The O'Driscoll method is demonstrated in **Figures 4.16a–d**.

Accurate numbering of the lumbosacral segments is important in order prevent wrong level surgical or interventional procedures. Traditional methods of lumbar segmental numbering, such as counting down from the last set of ribs, are prone to error. A large number of anatomic landmarks have been tested in order to identify a structure that allows for accurate segmental numbering, without success. The only techniques that are nearly foolproof are the use of "counting" sagittal MR sequences that image from C2 to the sacrum (**Figure 4.17**), whole spine CT, and whole spine plain films.

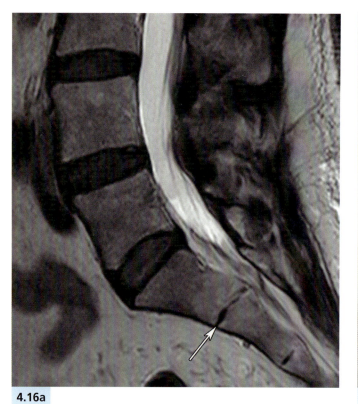

4.16a

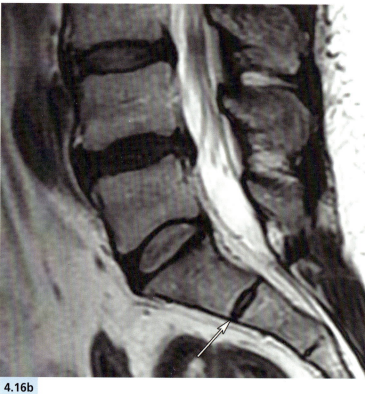

4.16b

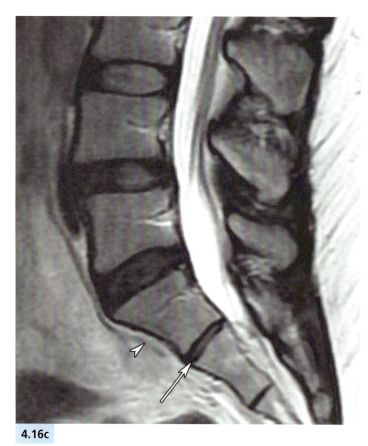

4.16c

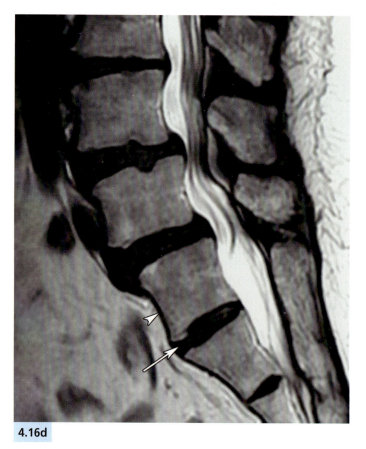

4.16d

FIGURES 4.16a–d   O'Driscoll disc classification system. (a) Disc material is absent (arrow). (b) Disc material (arrow) is present, but does not extend the entire length of the sacrum. (c) Disc material extends the entire length of the sacrum in the AP dimension. The vertebral body (VB) above (arrowhead) tapers from craniad to caudad. (d) Disc material (arrow) extends the entire length of the sacrum in the AP dimension and the VB above (arrowhead) maintains a squared appearance (arrowhead).

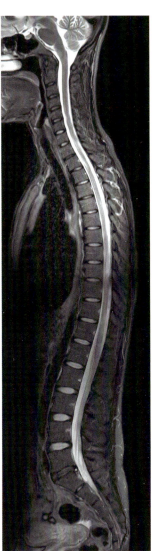

4.17

FIGURE 4.17 Large field of view short-TI inversion recovery (STIR) image of the whole spine in the sagittal plane obtained for the purpose of accurate vertebral numbering.

THE LATERAL RECESSES AND INTERVERTEBRAL FORAMINA

The lateral recesses and neural foramina form a canal through which the nerve roots and spinal nerves exit the spinal canal and vertebral column. The *lateral* or *subarticular recess* is bounded by the thecal sac medially, the pedicle laterally, the dorsolateral margin of the vertebral body and disc anteriorly, and superior articular process posteriorly (Figures 4.4q, 4.4x). The narrowest part of the lateral recess is located at the superior margin of the corresponding pedicle, due to the slight anterior angulation of the superior articular process. The "height" of the lateral recess is measured from the anterior margin of the superior articular process to the posterolateral margin of the vertebral body, at the superior margin of the pedicle. A height of 5 mm or greater is normal. The L5 lateral recesses shorter (AP) and wider (transverse) than any other spinal level.

Immediately superior to their exit into the intervertebral foramina, transiting lumbar nerve roots within their dural sleeves are laterally located within the spinal canal within the lateral recess. Degenerative hypertrophy of the superior articular process can result in lateral recess stenosis and nerve root impingement. If radicular symptoms are present, they will generally be localized to the dermatome one level below the level of lateral recess abnormality. For example, lateral recess stenosis at L4–L5 typically produces an L5 radiculopathy.

The intervertebral (neural) foramina of the lumbar spine transmit the L1–L5 spinal nerves within their dural sheaths, the dorsal root ganglia, the radicular (or radiculomedullary) arteries, intervertebral veins, the sinuvertebral nerve, and lymphatic vessels. Also contained within the intervertebral foramina is epidural fat and ligaments (discussed in the following). The size of the lumbar intervertebral foramina slightly decreases L1–L5 in the craniocaudad dimension (Figure 4.4t). The L5–S1 intervertebral foramina are smaller in size than the other lumbar foramina and have a different shape, appearing as an up-side-down egg. The L1–L2 to L4–L5 intervertebral foramina have a keyhole shape when viewed in the sagittal plane, with a rounded superior component and a vertically-oriented ovoid inferior component (Figures 4.4c, 4.4e, 4.4i, 4.4t).

The superior component of the intervertebral foramen is relatively immobile and is bounded by the inferior vertebral notch of the pedicle rostrally, the posterior margin of the vertebral body ventrally, and the anterior margin of the inferior articular process dorsally. The inferior component of the intervertebral foramen is mobile and its margins are formed by the superior vertebral notch of the pedicle caudally, the posterior margin of the intervertebral disc ventrally, and anterior margin of the superior articular process dorsally (Figure 4.4i). In extension, the dimensions of the intervertebral foramina all decrease, particularly the craniocaudad dimension. In flexion, the dimensions of the foramina are maximal.

The exiting spinal nerves within their dural sleeves are positioned just inferior to the pedicles within the lumbar intervertebral foramina. This is an important anatomic relationship to consider when performing spine interventions, in order to prevent spinal nerve injury. The pedicle is used as an anatomic reference point for the performance of selective nerve root blocks and transforaminal epidural steroid injections under fluoroscopic guidance. On posterolateral oblique fluoroscopic images, the "eye" of the Scottie dog corresponds to the pedicle viewed en face (**Figures 4.18a, 4.18b**).

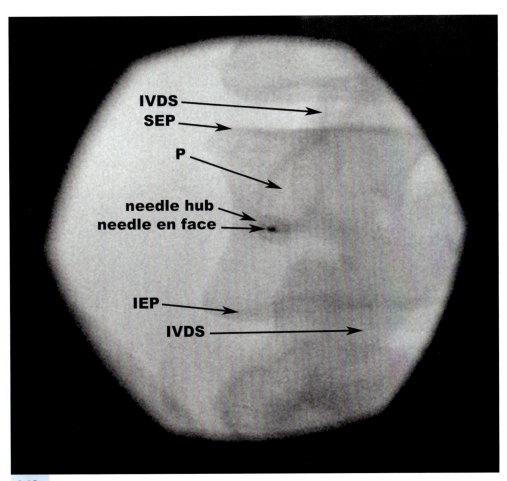

4.18a

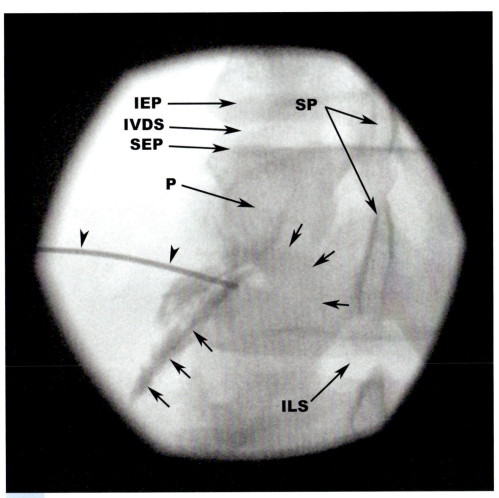

4.18b

FIGURES 4.18a,b Fluoroscopically guided selective nerve root block. (a) Posterolateral oblique fluoroscopic image demonstrates the needle on target with the 6 o'clock position of the pedicle (P). The needle was then advanced to the spinal nerve (SN), where contrast was injected. (b) AP projection fluoroscopic image showing the needle (arrowheads) positioned under the pedicle (P). Contrast outlines the exiting SN and refluxes into the dorsal epidural space (arrows). IEP—inferior endplate, ILS—interlaminar space, IVDS—intervertebral disc space, SEP—superior endplate, SP—spinous process.

THE INTERVERTEBRAL DISCS OF THE LUMBAR SPINE

Intervertebral disc and vertebral shape are the primary determinants of the lumbar lordosis. The lumbar intervertebral discs are taller anteriorly than posteriorly, particularly at L4–L5 and L5–S1 (Figures 4.4r, 4.4s). The lumbar discs are the tallest of the spinal column and increase in cross sectional area L1–L2 to L4–L5. The L5–S1 disc is shorter than the rest of the lumbar discs. The weight-bearing capacity of the lumbar intervertebral discs is greater than that of the cervical and thoracic discs. This is likely related to a preferential accumulation of degenerative changes within the lumbar intervertebral discs that has been documented in a variety of age groups. The proportion of the L5–S1 disc composed of nucleus pulposis is higher than any other intervertebral disc and its rate of degeneration is more rapid.

The appearance of the intervertebral discs varies with age on T2-weighted MR images. The nucleus pulposis and inner annulus fibrosis display hyperintense signal while the outer annulus fibrosis displays low signal (**Figures 4.19a, 4.19b**). In the first decade, the hyperintense T2 signal of nucleus pulposis and inner annulus is well-delineated from the low signal of the thin outer annulus. As early as the third decade, a thin, transversely oriented band of low signal may be seen at the center of the nucleus pulposis on sagittal MR images that correlates with collagen deposition, referred to as the *internuclear cleft* (**Figure 4.20**). With increasing age, there is a progressive decrease in water and proteoglycan content and an increase in collagen content within the intervertebral discs that correlates with decreasing T2 signal. In the eighth and ninth decades, the fibrous content of the intervertebral discs is marked, correlating with diffusely decreased signal on T2 and reduced delineation of the nucleus pulposis and annulus fibrosis.

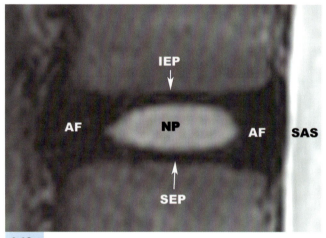

4.19a

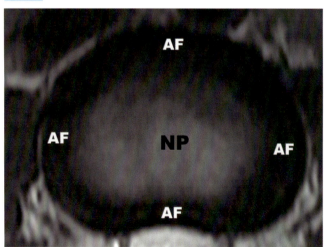

4.19b

FIGURES 4.19a,b Lumbar intervertebral disc (IVD). (a) Sagittal and (b) axial T2-weighted TSE images demonstrate the hypointense outer annulus fibrosis (AF) and hyperintense nucleus pulposis (NP). The inner AF is hyperintense on T2-weighted images and is indistinguishable from the nucleus pulposis. IEP—inferior endplate, SAS—subarachnoid space, SEP—superior endplate.

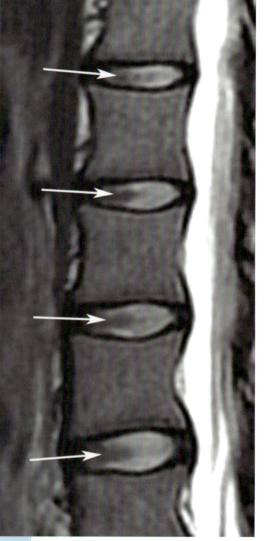

4.20

FIGURE 4.20 Sagittal T2-weighted TSE image demonstrating thin hypointense lines (internuclear clefts) bisecting the nucleus pulposis (NP) at multiple levels (arrows).

LIGAMENTOUS ANATOMY OF THE LUMBAR SPINE

The major ligaments of the lumbar spine include the anterior longitudinal ligament, posterior longitudinal ligament, ligamenta flava, interspinous ligaments, and supraspinous ligament.

The *anterior longitudinal ligament* (ALL) is a multilayered structure that measures greater in transverse dimension in the lumbar segments. The greatest average tensile strength of the ALL is observed in the lumbar region. A feature that is unique to the lumbar ALL is an increase in width at the level of the intervertebral discs and decreased width of the intervening space. The width of the ALL at the disc level gradually increases L1–L5. The anterior to posterior thickness of the ALL is greatest at the vertebral body levels and thinnest at the intervertebral disc levels. The ALL is firmly adherent to the anterior superior and inferior endplates, infrequently adherent to the intervertebral discs, and variably adherent to the central portion of the vertebral bodies. The lumbar ALL is shown in Figures 4.4s, 4.4u, 4.4y.

The *posterior longitudinal ligament* (PLL) extends along the dorsal margins of the lumbar vertebral bodies to the sacrum. The PLL contains two layers, superficial and deep. The superficial layer forms a ligamentous band that extends multiple levels. The deep fibers are shorter and extend along the margin of the dorsal annulus. The central band of the PLL decreases in size L1–L5. The PLL maintains firm attachments to the superior and inferior endplates in the lumbar spine. There are also firm attachments lateral to the central band at the level of the intervertebral discs. The PLL doesn't attach to the central aspect of the vertebral bodies or the central aspect of the intervertebral discs. The greatest average tensile strength of the PLL is found in the lumbar region. The imaging features of the lumbar PLL are shown in **Figure 4.21**.

The *ligamenta flava* are found throughout the lumbar segments (**Figures 4.22a, 4.22b**, 4.4o, 4.4p, and 4.4v). The anterior to posterior thickness of the ligamenta flava is greatest in the lumbar spine, particularly at L4–L5. The medial aspects of the ligamenta flava are thicker than the lateral components that form the anterior capsules of the zygapophyseal joints. The ligamenta flava of the lumbar spine are contiguous at the midline. However, small discontinuities are found at the medial margins of the ligamenta flava that transmit bridging veins connecting the posterior internal and external vertebral venous plexuses, like that seen in the cervical and thoracic segments. Spinal canal diameter decreases with axial loading, largely due to bulging of the ligamenta flava, with a lesser contribution from bulging of the intervertebral discs. A reduction in mid-sagittal spinal canal diameter is known to occur in extension, also largely due to bulging of the ligamenta flava.

The *interspinous ligaments* extend from the inferior margins of the spinous processes above to the superior margins of the spinous processes below in the sagittal plane and from the root to the apex of the spinous processes in the transverse plane. They are composed of three different components. The anterior component is paired, attaches to the ligamenta flava on both sides of the midline, and has elastic properties similar to the ligamenta flava. The fibers of the middle component have an S-shape and project from the anterior superior margin of the spinous process below to the posterior inferior margin of the spinous process above. The posterior component is comprised of fiber bundles that attach to the posterior superior margin of the spinous process and extend superiorly to blend with the supraspinous ligament. This component may properly be considered part of the supraspinous ligament. The main function of the interspinous ligaments is restriction of acute flexion.

The *supraspinous ligament* of the lumbar spine is well-formed in the upper lumbar segments, but rarely extends caudal to L4. Below L4, it is composed of the intermingled fibers of the thoracolumbar fascia and the aponeuroses of the longissimus and multifidus muscles. There are legitimate arguments against the presence of a supraspinous "ligament" in the lumbar spine that are beyond the scope of this text. The imaging features of the supraspinous ligament are shown in Figures 4.4r, 4.4s, and 4.4v.

The *iliolumbar ligaments* (ILL) typically project from the transverse processes of L5 to the sacrum and iliac crests (Figure 4.4q). However, the ILL can also arise from L4 or S1. Its attachments are variable in the setting of lumbosacral transitional anatomy. The functions of the ILL likely include stabilization of the lumbosacral junction and protection of the L5–S1 intervertebral disc from excess wear and tear.

The denticulate ligaments are found within the lumbar segments superior to the conus medullaris and are absent at the levels of the cauda equina (caudal to T12–L1 or L1–L2). The lumbar intertransverse ligaments are typically poorly visualized on conventional imaging examinations and are not discussed here. The meningovertebral ligaments are discussed in the context of the epidural space.

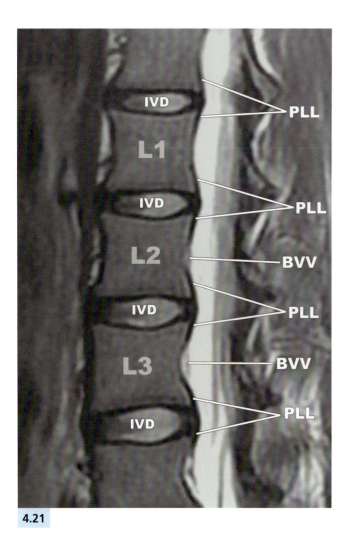

FIGURE 4.21   Sagittal T2-weighted TSE image showing the hypointense posterior longitudinal ligament (PLL) as thickening over the dorsal margins of the vertebral bodies at the superior and inferior endplates, with thinning/absence over the basivertebral veins (BVV). IVD—intervertebral disc.

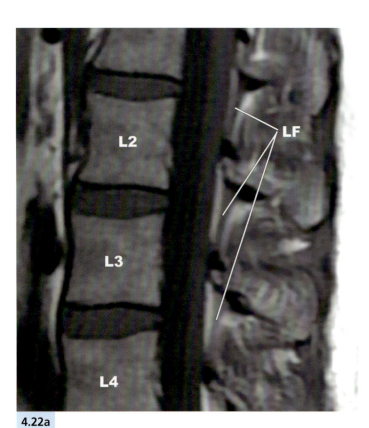

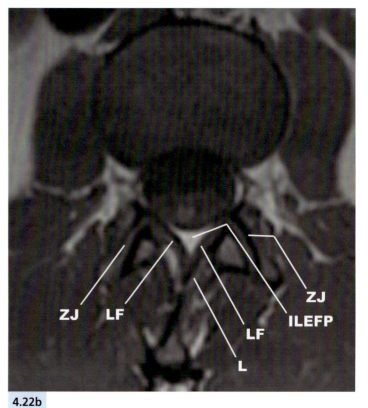

FIGURES 4.22a,b   The ligamenta flava (LF) appear as hypointense bands on (a) sagittal and (b) axial T1-weighted images. The ligamenta flava are positioned just dorsolateral to the triangular interlaminar epidural fat pad (ILEFP) and anteromedial to the lamina (L). ZJ—zygapophyseal joint.

ARTERIAL ANATOMY OF THE LUMBAR SPINE

The segmental branches supplying the lumbar segments arise from the longitudinal arteries of the lumbar spine, which include the aorta, median sacral artery, and occasionally the iliolumbar arteries (**Figure 4.23a**). The L1–L4 segmental branches are large in caliber and arise from the dorsal margin of the aorta. The L5 segmental branches are smaller in caliber, arise from the dorsal margin of the median sacral artery or iliolumbar arteries, and are variably present (**Figure 4.23b**). The lumbar segmental arteries generally arise from separate ostia on both sides of the midline, arising from a common origin approximately 10% of the time. In the upper lumbar spine, the segmental arteries take a slight superior course from their ostia to the vertebral level they supply. At L3 and L4, the ostia of the segmental arteries arise at the center of their corresponding vertebral bodies. The lumbar segmental branches course posteriorly along the lateral margins of the vertebral bodies under tendinous arches forming the origins of the psoas muscles and subsequently give off anterior (ventral) and posterior (dorsal) rami (**Figures 4.23c**).

The anterior rami ultimately supply the abdominal wall. The posterior rami give off spinal arterial and muscular arterial branches. The muscular branches supply the paraspinal muscles and posterior elements. The spinal branches course through the intervertebral foramina and give off anterior and posterior radicular arteries. The radicular arteries may supply the nerve roots, dura mater, spinal ganglia, spinal cord, or combinations of the above. In the lumbar spine, one or two radicular arteries contribute to the anterior spinal artery. The posterior radicular arteries are smaller in size and greater in number. The radicular arteries can become anterior or posterior radiculomedullary arteries, or both. There is a tendency for the anterior radiculomedullary arteries to arise on the left side in the lumbar spine, as is the case in the thoracic spine.

The great radicular artery of Adamkiewicz travels with the L1 or L2 nerve roots in approximately 10% of the population. The artery of Adamkiewicz typically originates on the left when it arises in the lumbar segments. In approximately 15% of the population, there is a high origin of the Adamkiewicz artery (T5–T8). In these cases, an anterior radiculomedullary artery arising from the lumbar segments is present; called the *artery of the conus medullaris*. The artery of Adamkiewicz is discussed in greater detail in Chapter 3.

At the level of the conus medullaris, the anterior and posterior spinal arteries form a dense anastomotic network that has the appearance of a basket. The artery of the filum terminale arises from this anastomotic basket and courses along the ventral aspect of the filum. The portion of the vasa corona located along the dorsal cord surface at the level of the lumbar enlargement is more prominent than the adjacent thoracic segments, a pattern that is also observed at the cervical enlargement. The rich arterial supply to the distal cord and conus is reflected in the central arteries, which are increased in number, larger in caliber, display greater overlap, and project deeper into the central spinal cord than the cervical and thoracic regions. The capillary beds within the distal cord and conus are more extensive than the mid-thoracic spinal cord.

The cauda equina has a dual arterial supply. The ventral roots are supplied proximally by the vasa corona and radicular branches from the anterior vasa corona (*ventral proximal radicular arteries*). They are supplied distally by radicular branches (*distal radicular branches*). The dorsal roots are supplied proximally by the vasa corona and radicular branches of the posterior spinal arteries (*dorsal proximal radicular arteries*). They are supplied distally by radicular branches (*distal radicular branches*). The dorsal distal radicular arteries form a dense plexus around the dorsal root ganglia. The proximal and distal radicular branches anastomose at the proximal one-third of the length of the lumbar roots. Special adaptations to a mobile environment with the lumbosacral roots include numerous arteriovenous anastomoses and arterial coiling. The arterial pedicles provide approximately one-third of the nutrients required by the lumbosacral nerve roots. The remaining two-thirds is supplied directly through the CSF.

The blood supply to the lumbar vertebral bodies is complex. The lumbar segmental arteries give off 10 to 20 *primary periosteal arteries* that supply the anterolateral walls of the vertebral bodies superiorly and inferiorly. An arcade of arteries arising from posterior rami of the lumbar segmental arteries supply the posterior vertebral bodies. Periosteal branches from the anterior and posterior systems form the *metaphyseal anastomosis* which supplies the upper and lower portions of the vertebral bodies. The metaphyseal anastomosis gives off small caliber penetrating arteries called *metaphyseal arteries*, which supply wedge shaped territories that point centrally. Penetrating branches of the lumbar segmental arteries called *equatorial arteries* penetrate along the anterolateral margin of the vertebral body and supply the central aspect of the vertebral body. Perforating branches called *nutrient arteries* enter the posterior wall of the vertebral bodies and supply the central aspect of the vertebral body. These two systems anastomose in the neural foramina.

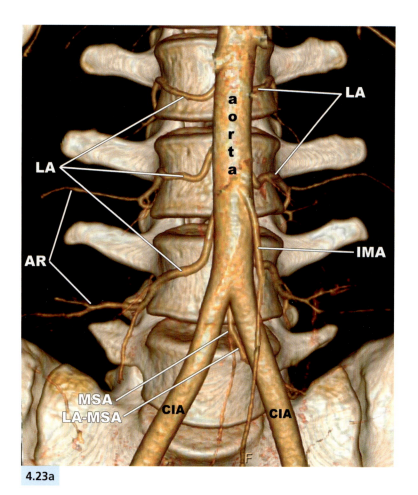

4.23a

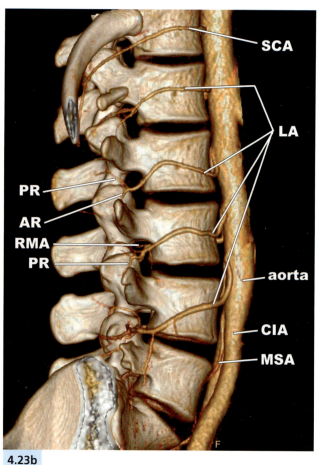

4.23b

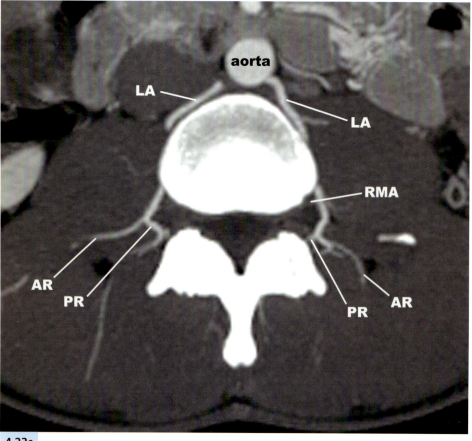

4.23c

FIGURES 4.23a–c 3D surface reformatted images in the (a) frontal and (b) lateral projections showing the main longitudinal arteries of the lumbar spine, the aorta and the median sacral artery (MSA). The L1-L4 lumbar arteries (LA) arise from the posterior midline of the aorta and course along the lateral margins of the vertebral bodies. The left L5 lumbar artery (LA-MSA) arises from the median sacral artery. (c) Axial maximum intensity projection CT angiographic image showing the lumbar arteries arising from the dorsal margin of the aorta and giving off anterior (AR) and posterior rami (PR). A small caliber radiculomedullary artery (RMA) arises directly from the left lumbar artery. CIA—common iliac artery, IMA—inferior mesenteric artery, SCA—subcostal artery.

VENOUS ANATOMY OF THE LUMBAR SPINE

The venous drainage of the subaxial lumbar spine, distal cord, and conus is carried out through a densely interconnected venous network that has intrinsic, extrinsic, and extradural divisions that are similar in many respects to the subaxial cervical and thoracic spinal levels (**Figures 4.24a–d**). However, the system of venous drainage within the lumbar spine has several specialized features that reflect to the unique neural anatomy at these levels.

The anterior and posterior radiculomedullary veins drain the spinal cord and spinal nerve roots and function to connect the extrinsic and extradural systems. The *great anterior radiculomedullary vein* (GARV) is the largest vein draining the anterior cord in the thoracolumbar region. The GARV typically originates T11–L3 and has a morphology that is similar to the artery of Adamkiewicz (**Figure 4.25**). The two vessels can be differentiated by their location (GARV is usually lower), morphology (GARV is usually serpentine), length (GARV has a longer intradural course), and caliber (GARV has larger diameter). The two vessels are best differentiated when temporal information is available, such as the information provided by conventional angiography, time resolved MR angiography, or CT angiography. The radiculomedullary veins and anterior and posterior external vertebral venous plexuses drain into the intervertebral veins.

The caliber of the anterior median spinal vein is greatest in the lumbar segments. It travels with the anterior spinal artery to the conus and usually continues as the *vein of the filum terminale*. The anterior medial spinal vein and vein of the filum terminale are usually well-visualized on post contrast T1-weighted MR images (**Figures 4.24e,f**). The venous drainage of the cauda equina, like the arterial supply, has proximal and distal components. The *distal radicular veins* drain into the lumbar veins at the level the corresponding nerve root exits into the neural foramen. The *proximal radicular veins* drain into the venous component of the vasa corona and subsequently into the anterior and posterior longitudinal veins of the spinal cord.

The venous drainage of the vertebral bodies parallels that of the arterial supply. The *subchondral post-capillary venous network* is a group of small caliber veins that are oriented parallel to the vertebral endplates that drain the capillaries of the subchondral bone. Vertical veins drain the subchondral post-capillary venous network into a larger venous system that is also oriented parallel to the vertebral endplate, called the *horizontal subarticular collecting vein system*. This system is radially arranged and drains centrally into the *vertical veins of the vertebral body* which subsequently drain into the basivertebral veins. The basivertebral veins drain through a defect in the central and posterior vertebral body into the anterior internal vertebral venous plexus (Figures 4.24a, 4.24b, 4.24d–f). The periphery of the vertebral body drains directly into the anterior internal or external vertebral venous plexus.

The anterior and posterior internal and external venous plexuses ultimately drain into the lumbar segmental veins. The lumbar segmental veins drain into the inferior vena cava and the left common iliac vein (Figures 4.24b–f).

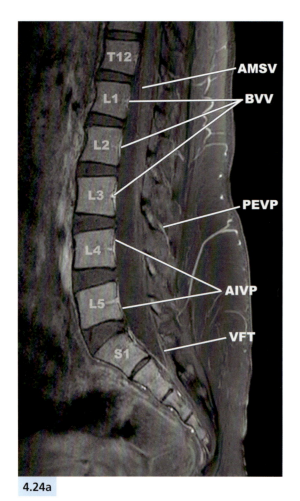

4.24a

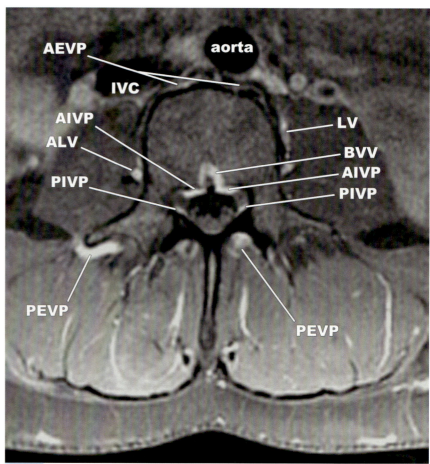

4.24b

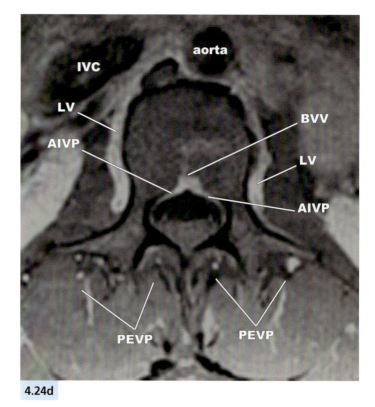

4.24c

4.24d

FIGURES 4.24a–f Post contrast T1-weighted images demonstrating the vertebral venous system. The anterior median spinal vein (AMSV) typically transitions into the vein of the filum terminale (VFT). AEVP—anterior external vertebral venous plexus, AIVP—anterior internal vertebral venous plexus, ALV—ascending lumbar vein, BVV—basivertebral vein, DRG—dorsal root ganglion, IVC—inferior vena cava, IVV—intervertebral vein, LV—lumbar vein, PEVP—posterior external vertebral venous plexus, PIVP—posterior internal vertebral venous plexus, PMSV—posterior median spinal vein.

(continued)

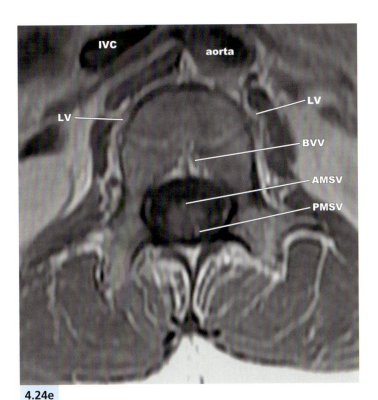

4.24e

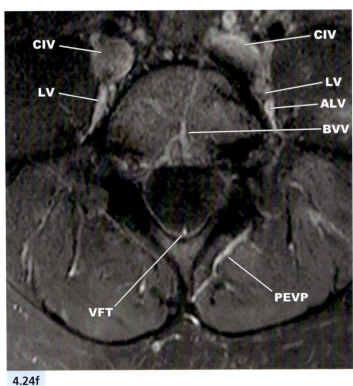

4.24f

FIGURES 4.24e,f (*Continued*) ALV—ascending lumbar vein, AMSV—anterior median spinal vein, BVV—basivertebral vein, CIV— common iliac vein, IVC—inferior vena cava, LV—lumbar vein, PEVP—posterior external vertebral venous plexus, PMSV— posterior median spinal vein, VFT—vein of the filum terminale.

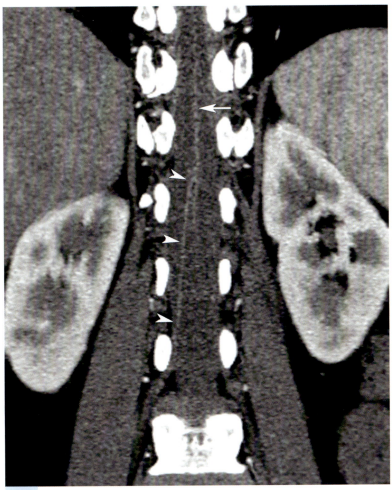

4.25

FIGURE 4.25 The great anterior radiculomedullary vein (GARV) and anterior median spinal vein (white arrow) are displayed in a coronal reformatted CT angiographic image. Although similar in appearance to the artery of Adamkiewicz, the GARV (arrowheads) is tortuous, arises from lower segments (L1 in this patient), is larger in caliber, and has a longer intradural course.

MENINGES AND SPACES OF THE LUMBAR SPINE

The basic features of the meninges (pia, arachnoid, dura) and spaces (subpial, "subdural", subarachnoid, epidural) of the lumbar spine are similar to those of the cervical and thoracic spine. However, there are notable differences that will be discussed in this section.

The pia mater of the distal cord and conus medullaris is tightly adherent to the cord parenchyma, like the pia of the cervical and thoracic spinal cord. The pia extends caudal to the conus tip adherent to a filamentous bluish structure made up of glial and ependymal cells called the *filum terminale*. The filum terminale has two components, the *filum terminale internum* and the *filum terminale externum*. The filum terminale internum extends from the conus medullaris to the fundus of the thecal sac at the S2 level. The filum exits the thecal sac and carries with it arachnoid and dura mater, forming the filum terminale externum or *coccygeal ligament* as it courses along the dorsum of the coccyx.

The subarachnoid spaces of the lumbar spine differ from the cervical and lumbar regions. The distal spinal cord, conus, and cauda equina are more posteriorly located within the thecal sac. As a result, the ventral subarachnoid space is more prominent than the dorsal subarachnoid space at the level of the distal cord and conus medullaris. The lateral subarachnoid spaces T9–L1 are relatively more restricted due to the lumbar enlargement (discussed in the following). Caudal to the conus medullaris, the primary occupants of the subarachnoid space are the roots of the cauda equina which results in a large subarachnoid space that is called the *lumbar cistern*. The lumbar cistern is accessed via the interlaminar spaces between L2–L3 and L5–S1. Using traditional surface anatomic landmarks (iliac crests), the lumbar cistern is typically accessed at L4–L5 from a midline approach. Using fluoroscopy, the lumbar cistern is typically accessed at L2–L3 or L3–L4 (**Figures 4.26a, 4.26b**). The relatively scant innervation of the dorsal thecal sac by the sinuvertebral nerves is an additional anatomic feature that makes CSF sampling within the lumbar cistern optimal.

As stated previously, the ventral and dorsal roots converge at the lateral margin of the thecal sac and exit the spinal canal through dural sleeves. The length of the dural sleeves is very short L1 and L2, due to the fact that these nerve roots exit into the intervertebral foramina near directly laterally. The dural sleeves are progressively longer L3–L5 and their obliquity, in degrees from the mid-sagittal plane, progressively decreases. That is, the lower lumbar nerve roots are progressively angled inferiorly (**Figures 4.27a–c**).

A number of dural sleeve variants have been described in the lumbar segments. The most commonly identified variant on imaging examinations is two adjacent nerve roots sharing a common dural sleeve, referred to as *conjoined nerve roots*. Conjoined nerve roots are most commonly observed on imaging studies at L5–S1. Conjoined nerve roots are discussed in more detail in Chapter 5. Other dural sleeve variants include intraforaminal communicating branches and the presence of two spinal nerves with their own dural sleeves exiting the same intervertebral foramen. Dural root sleeve variants are frequently unrecognized on imaging studies and may raise the level of difficulty of surgical procedures. The last two dural sleeve variants are generally not well demonstrated on imaging examinations.

The dorsal epidural fat pads in the lumbar spine are more prominent than the thoracic fat pads. The lumbar dorsal epidural fat pads have the shape of an isosceles triangle in the transverse plane, with the vertex oriented posteriorly and a base that abuts the dorsal margin of the thecal sac and may assume the shape of the thecal sac or display an anterior convexity. In the sagittal plane, the dorsal epidural fat pads have a flat anterior margin that forms to the thecal sac and a rounded posterior margin that forms to the ligamenta flava (Figures 4.4o, 4.4p, 4.4q, 4.4s, 4.4x, 4.4y). It is common to see a thin ventral epidural fat pad at L5 that is continuous with the lateral fat pads that project into the intervertebral foramina (Figures 4.4x, 4.4y).

The microscopic features and structure of the lumbar dorsal epidural fat pad differ from that of subcutaneous fat. The dorsal epidural fat pads of the lumbar spine consist of homogeneous adipocytes, sparse connective tissue, and "slits" that seem to confer sliding motion capabilities. Patients with congenital generalized lipodystrophy retain epidural fat stores. Further, a clear relationship between various metabolic conditions that increase central and truncal fat stores and epidural lipomatosis has not been made. Together, these findings imply that epidural fat has mechanical functions and limited or no metabolic function.

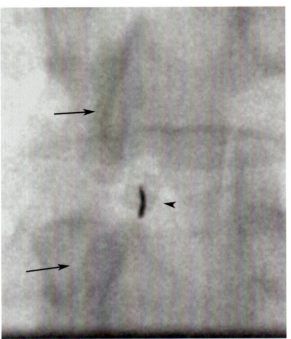

4.26a

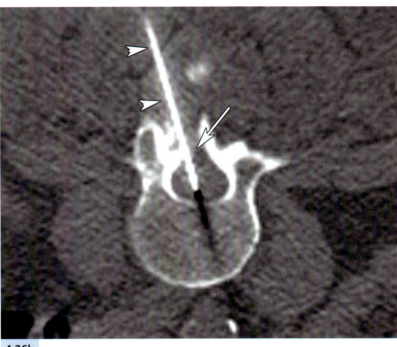

4.26b

FIGURES 4.26a,b   Image guided access to the lumbar cistern (LC). (a) Fluoroscopically-guided interlaminar approach to the subarachnoid space. The oblique approach is used in order to avoid contact with the spinous processes (arrows). The needle is viewed en face (arrowhead). (b) The interlaminar spaces (ILS) are typically well visualized with CT. The needle (arrowheads) can be seen traversing the ILS (arrow).

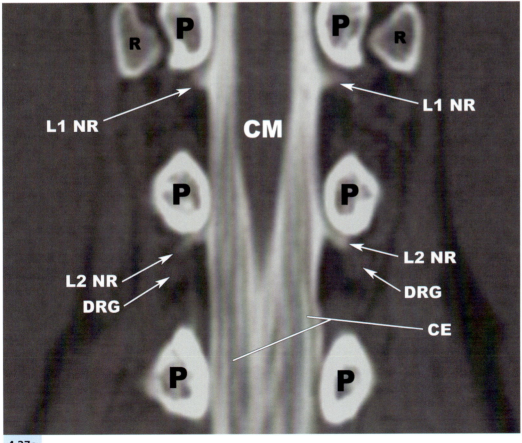

4.27a

FIGURES 4.27a–c   (a) Curved reformatted images from a CT myelogram showing the near lateral orientation of the L1 (L1 NR) and L2 nerve roots (L2 NR) as they pass through the dural sleeves. The roots of the cauda equina (CE) have a regular arrangement within the lumbar cistern (LC). Note the position of the exiting nerve roots under the pedicle (P). The L1 segment in this patient had hypoplastic ribs (R). (b) Curved reformatted CT image from a CT myelogram and (c) coronal volumetric isotropic TSE acquisition (VISTA) MR image showing the increasingly vertical orientation of the dural sleeves (arrows in b, arrowheads in c) from craniad to caudad in the lumbar spine. CM—conus medullaris, DRG—dorsal root ganglia.

(continued)

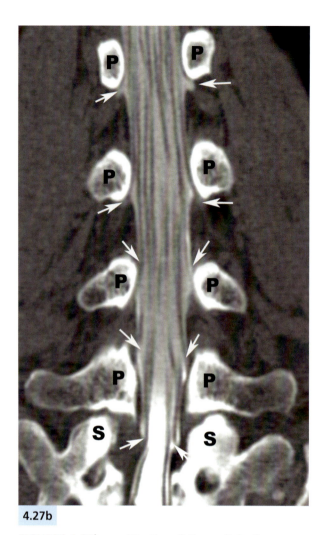

4.27b

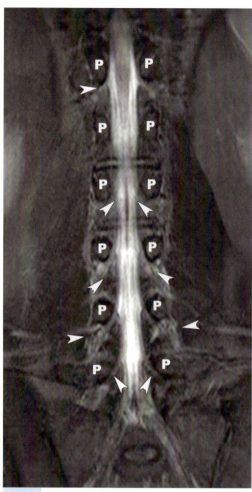

4.27c

FIGURES 4.27b,c (*Continued*) P—pedicle, S—sacrum.

Therapeutic lumbar epidural injections are performed via two primary approaches, interlaminar and transforaminal. The *interlaminar epidural injection* is generally performed from a posterolateral oblique approach, similar to the approach for fluoroscopically guided access to the lumbar cistern. There are several different techniques that are used, many of which take advantage of the negative pressure within the lumbar epidural space that produces a *loss of resistance* to light forward pressure on the plunger of the syringe when the epidural space is encountered by the needle tip. An epidurogram can be obtained simultaneous to the sensation of a loss of resistance, if contrast is hooked up to the needle hub during needle advancement into the epidural space. The *selective nerve root block* and *transforaminal epidural steroid injection* are both performed from a posterolateral oblique approach, with transforaminal epidural access performed from a slightly more lateral approach. On fluoroscopy, the target is the 6 o'clock position under the Scotty dog eye. All three techniques are typically performed with fluoroscopic or CT guidance, although other imaging modalities have been employed. Examples of these techniques are shown in **Figures 4.28a, 4.28b**, 4.18a, 4.18b.

The thecal sac has relatively more connective tissue attachments to the bony spinal canal in the lumbar spine than the cervical and thoracic spine. These connective tissue attachments have been given a variety of names, but will be referred to in this text as the meningovertebral ligaments. These fibroelastic bands attach the outer margin of the dural sac to the periosteum of the bony canal elements. They are present early in development (11 weeks gestation) and are variable in number, position, and morphology. The meningovertebral ligaments frequently compartmentalize the epidural space, and may explain a variety of thecal sac configurations. This compartmentalization may result in barriers to the spread of Medications administered to the epidural space or result in suboptimal epidural catheter placement. Meningovertebral ligaments within the ventral epidural space at the midline attach to the posterior longitudinal ligament and may act as a barrier that prevents extension of extruded disc material across the midline. Lateral meningovertebral ligaments project into the lateral recesses and neural foramina. Failure to recognize the meningovertebral ligaments during surgical interventions may lead to inadvertent CSF leaks or epidural hemorrhage.

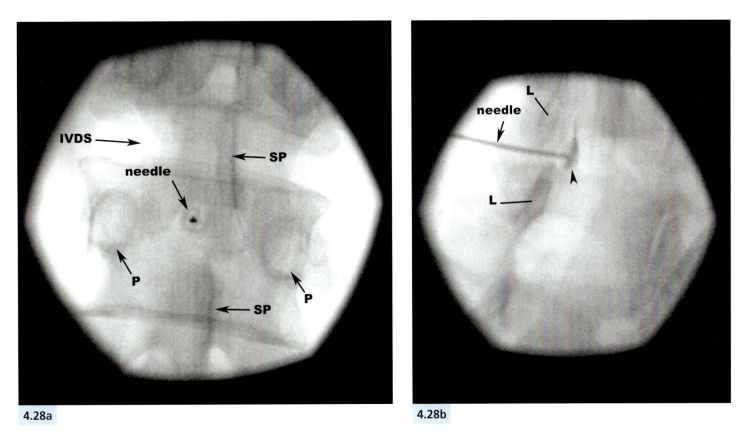

4.28a

4.28b

FIGURES 4.28a,b   (a) Posterior oblique approach fluoroscopically guided interlaminar epidural steroid injection. The needle is advanced to the edge of the upper lamina and the c-arm is rotated to a (b) lateral oblique orientation. The needle is deflected under the upper lamina (L) and advanced to the epidural space. A loss of resistance is experienced and iodinated contrast is simultaneously injected to confirm needle position (black arrowhead). A steroid admixture is subsequently injected. IVDS—intervertebral disc space, P—pedicle, SP—spinous process.

NEURAL ANATOMY OF THE LUMBAR SPINE

There is a mild increase in the transverse diameter of the spinal cord T9–L1 that is referred to as the *lumbar enlargement*. This enlargement is typically not perceptible on axial or sagittal image series and is best demonstrated in the coronal plane (Figure 4.27a). The lumbar enlargement corresponds to an increase in gray matter associated with the lumbar and sacral plexuses (L1–S4 spinal nerves). The lumbar, sacral, and coccygeal segmental levels of the cord are positioned from T10 to L1.

The distal-most aspect of the spinal cord tapers to a point, called the *conus medullaris* (Figures 4.4u–w, 4.27a). The position of the conus medullaris is usually L1–L2, varying in a normal distribution (range T12–L3). If the conus medullaris is positioned below L3, it is generally agreed to be abnormal. A conus position at L3 is indeterminate and may require additional evaluation for cord tethering. The tip of the conus is most commonly centrally located (50%), but can also be dorsally (30%), or ventrally deviated (14%).

The *ventriculus terminalis* is a normal ependyma-lined cavity within the conus that is contiguous with the central canal of the spinal cord. The ventriculus terminalis is generally not visible on conventional imaging studies. Occasionally, there is focal, smooth dilatation of the ventriculus terminalis that can be visualized on imaging studies (**Figure 4.29**). It is considered a benign finding if the patient is asymptomatic, the conus is normally positioned, the surrounding cord is normal, and the fluid contained within follows CSF on all pulse sequences.

The cauda equina is comprised of the L2–L5 and S1–S5 nerve roots. The L2–S5 nerve roots are regularly arranged in layers within invaginations of the arachnoid mater. The nerve roots that will exit through the more rostral vertebrae are positioned ventrolaterally. The nerve roots that will successively exit from the more caudal vertebrae are positioned in sequential order from ventrolaterally to dorsomedially. The lumbar nerve roots increase in caliber and length L1–L5. The lumbar dorsal root ganglia increase in size L1–L5 and are nearly always positioned within the neural foramina (**Figure 4.30**).

The S2–S5 roots maintain a dorsomedial position within the lumbar cistern from L2–L3 to L4–L5. At the L5–S1 level, the S1 roots are engaged to exit along the ventrolateral aspect of the lumbar cistern. The S2–S4 roots are arranged in order from ventrolateral to dorsomedial. The motor roots of each segment are located ventromedial to the sensory roots and are smaller in caliber than the sensory roots (**Figure 4.31**). The S1 nerve roots are shorter in length than the L4 and L5 nerve roots due to the fact that the S1 dorsal root ganglia are usually located within the spinal canal.

There is a progressive decrease in the size of the dorsal root entry zones (*linea radocularis dorsalis*) from craniad to caudad S1–S5. This corresponds to a gradual decrease in the number of rootlets contributing to the dorsal roots. Typically, one to two rootlets contribute to the ventral roots S1–S4. The S5 ventral roots are variably present. There is a progressive decrease in the caliber and cross sectional area of the ventral and dorsal nerve roots S1–S5. The dorsal roots are larger in caliber and cross sectional area than the ventral roots.

It is common (20%) to encounter small caliber rootlets connecting the roots of adjacent segments along their intradural course. These small caliber anastomoses are commonly encountered and can be simple rami or more complex configurations. These intersegmental anastomoses are more commonly observed in the dorsal roots. Anastomoses between ventral and dorsal roots are uncommon, if they occur at all.

The filum terminale internum extends from the conus tip to the fundus of the thecal sac (Figure 4.31). It progressively decreases in diameter from the level of the conus tip to the distal thecal sac. The filum terminale internum should generally not exceed 2 mm in diameter. Occasionally, fibrolipoma of the filum terminale internum is visualized on axial or sagittal MR images as linear T1 hyperintense signal (**Figures 4.32a, 4.32b**). This falls on the mild end of the spectrum of premature disjunction abnormalities and is typically clinically benign.

Ultrasound of the lumbar spine is possible in infants prior to ossification of the posterior elements. The quality of spinal ultrasound decreases progressively after 3 to 4 months of age and is generally not possible after 6 months of age due to ossification of the posterior elements. The spinal cord is hypoechoic and has a hyperechoic periphery. The walls of the central canal of the spinal cord are also hyperechoic, termed the *central echo complex*. The spinal cord is normally located one-third to one-half of the distance from the posterior spinal line to the spinolaminar line. The CSF within the subarachnoid space is hypoechoic to anechoic. The roots of the cauda equina and filum terminale are also hyperechoic and display normal phasicity during the cardiac cycle, which can be viewed in real-time ultrasound cine loops. On axial ultrasound imaging, the denticulate ligaments are visualized as thin, hyperechoic structures projecting laterally from the cord to the dura. The ultrasound features of the lumbar spine on ultrasound are displayed in **Figures 4.33a, 4.33b**.

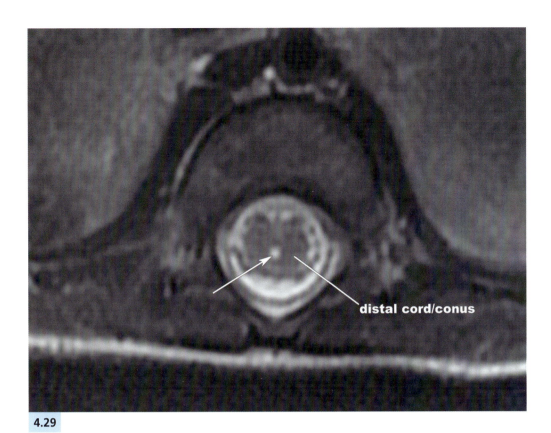

4.29

FIGURE 4.29 The ventriculus terminalis is visualized on axial T2-weighted TSE images as smooth enlargement of the central canal of the spinal cord (arrow).

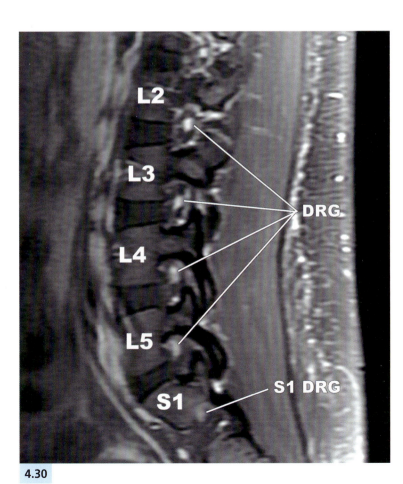

4.30

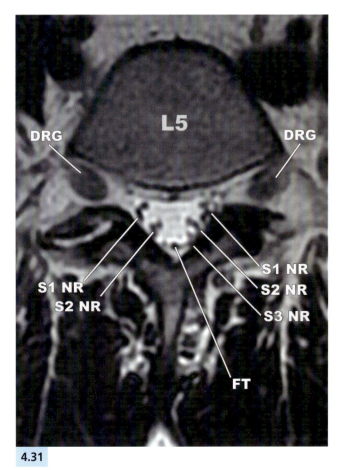

4.31

FIGURE 4.30 Parasagittal fat saturated post contrast T1-weighted image showing the increase in the size of the lumbar dorsal root ganglia (DRG) L1-L5 and location within the neural foramina. The S1 dorsal root ganglion (S1 DRG) is located within the spinal canal.

FIGURE 4.31 Axial T2-weighted TSE image showing the orderly arrangement of the S1-S3 cauda equina (CE) roots (S1 NR to S3 NR). DRG—dorsal root ganglia, FT—filum terminale, NR—nerve roots.

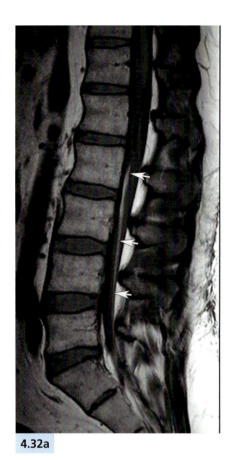

4.32a

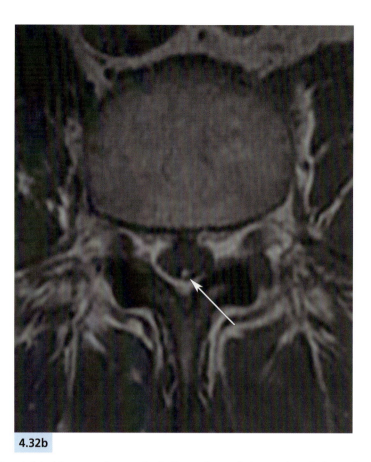

4.32b

FIGURES 4.32a,b (a) Sagittal and (b) axial T1-weighted images demonstrate linear hyperintense signal along the course of the filum terminale (arrows), consistent with fibrolipoma of the filum terminale.

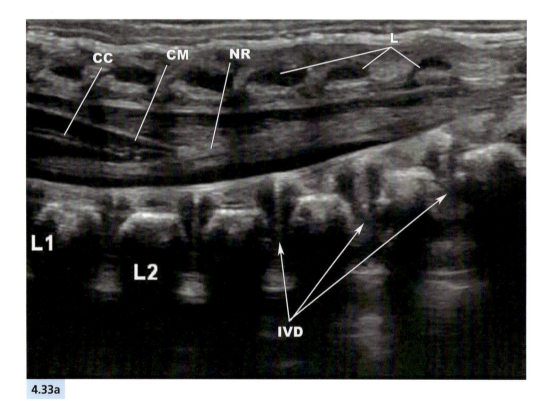

4.33a

FIGURES 4.33a,b (a) Sagittal and (b) axial ultrasound image of the lumbar spine at the level of the conus medullaris (CM). The spinal cord on ultrasound appears as an ovoid hypoechoic structure with a central echogenic complex that represents the central canal (CC) of the spinal cord. The CM is surrounded by echogenic nerve roots (NR). The nonossified spinous process (SP) is hypoechoic and allows a window into the spinal canal. The lamina (L) are ossified and create shadowing along the lateral margins of the spinal canal. The vertebral body (VB) or centrum (C) is hyperechoic and located ventral to the spinal canal. IVD—intervertebral disc.

(continued)

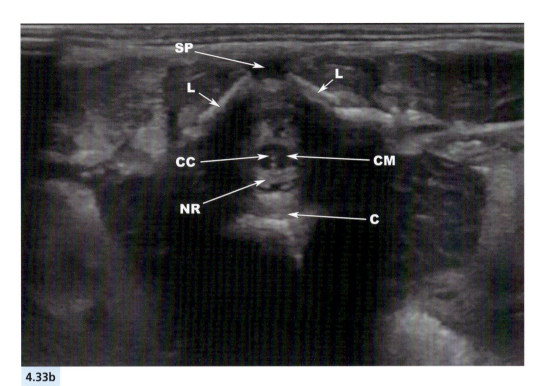

4.33b

FIGURE 4.33b   (*continued*) C—centrum, CC—central canal, CM—conus medullaris, L—lamina, NR—nerve root, SP—spinous process.

GALLERY OF ANATOMIC VARIANTS AND VARIOUS CONGENITAL ANOMALIES

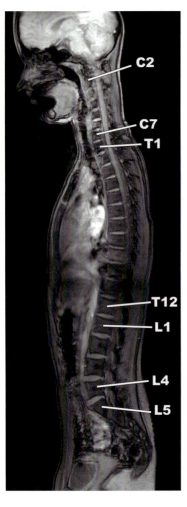

IMAGE 1   Large field of view gradient echo image obtained for counting vertebrae shows a patient with 7 cervical, 12 thoracic, and 4 mobile presacral segments. The L5 vertebra is incorporated into the sacrum ("sacralized").

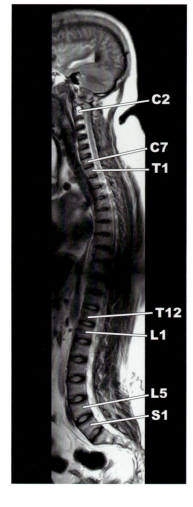

IMAGE 2   Large field of view T2-weighted image of the whole spine demonstrates 7 cervical, 12 thoracic, and 6 mobile presacral segments. The S1 segment is not incorporated into the sacrum ("lumbarized").

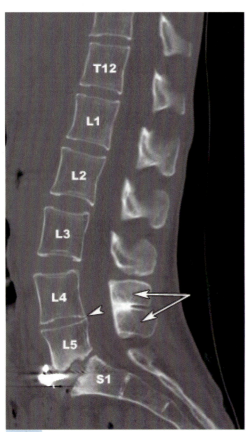

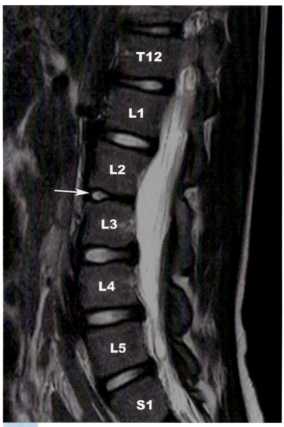

IMAGES 3a,b
(a) Sagittal reformatted CT image demonstrating partial fusion of the L4 and L5 vertebral bodies (arrowhead) and spinous processes (arrows). (b) Sagittal T2-weighted TSE image displaying partial fusion of the L2 and L3 vertebral bodies and a rudimentary L2-L3 intervertebral disc (arrow).

3a

3b

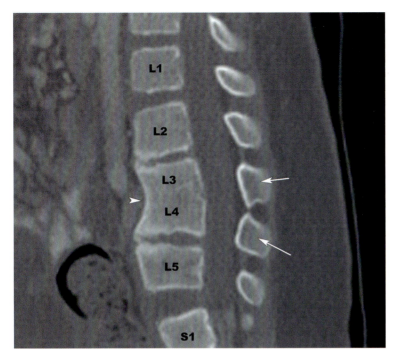

IMAGE 4   Sagittal reformatted CT image shows complete fusion of the L3 and L4 vertebral bodies (arrowhead). The fusion block is slightly angled, resulting in angulation of the L3 and L4 spinous processes (arrows).

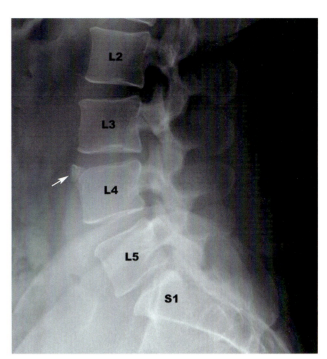

IMAGE 5   Lateral plain film of the lumbar spine displays a limbus vertebra at the L4 anterior superior endplate (arrow). The limbus vertebra is thought to result from herniation of intervertebral disc (IVD) between the centrum (C) and ring apophysis, with resultant nonfusion.

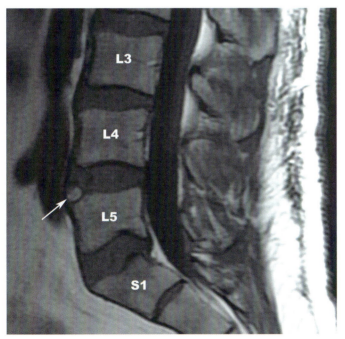

IMAGE 6   Sagittal T1-weighted TSE image demonstrating a limbus vertebra along the anterior superior endplate of L5 (arrow).

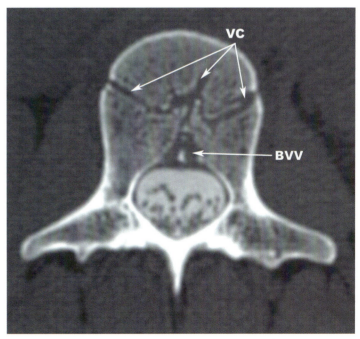

IMAGE 7   Axial image from a CT myelogram shows large venous channels (VC) draining to the basivertebral vein (BVV). Venous channels may mimic fractures in certain situations.

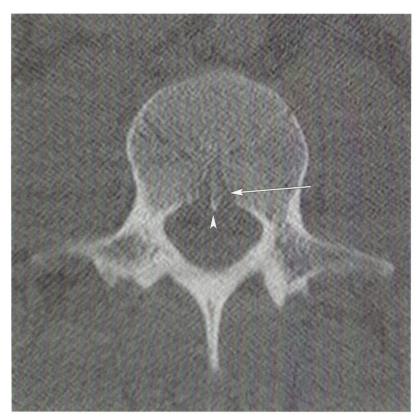

IMAGE 8 Axial CT image showing a bony spur (arrowhead) projecting dorsally from the basivertebral vein (arrow).

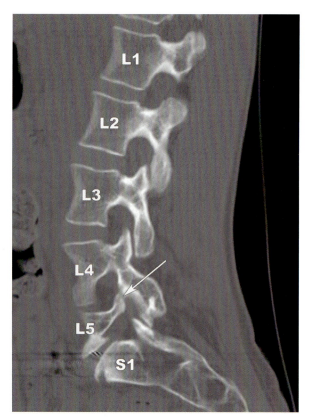

IMAGE 9 Sagittal reformatted CT image displaying a hypoplastic, nonfused L5 pedicle (arrow).

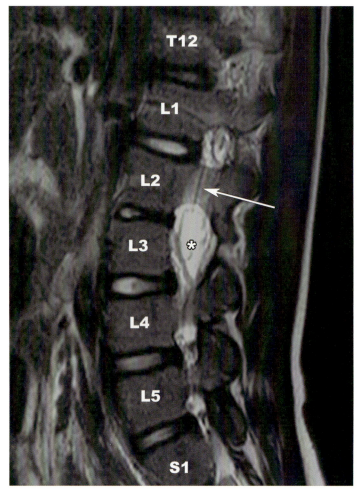

IMAGE 10 Sagittal T2-weighted TSE image shows absence of the L3 pedicle (asterisk) and broadening of the L2 pedicle (arrow).

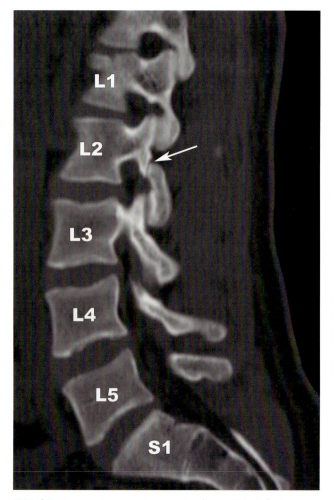

IMAGE 11 An L2 pars interarticularis (PI) defect (arrow) is displayed on a sagittal reformatted CT image.

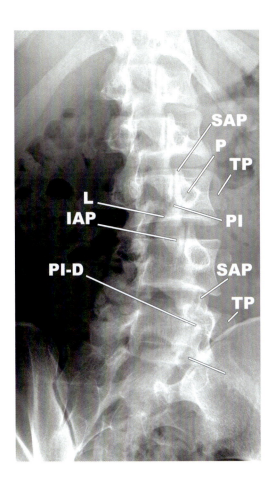

IMAGE 12   Posterolateral oblique plain film of the lumbar spine demonstrates an L5 pars interarticularis defect (PI-D). The pedicle (P) forms the "eye" of the Scotty dog, the superior articular process (SAP) the "ear", the transverse process (TP) the nose, the pars interarticularis (PI) the "neck", the inferior articular process (IAP) the "front paw", and the lamina (L) forms the "body".

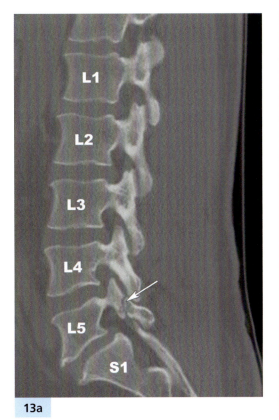

13a

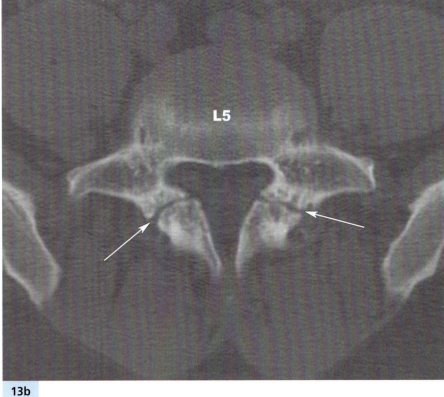

13b

IMAGES 13a,b   (a) Sagittal reformatted CT image displaying a L5 pars interarticularis (PI) defect (arrow). (b) Axial CT image showing bilateral L5 PI defects (arrows). PI defects are most commonly found at L5.

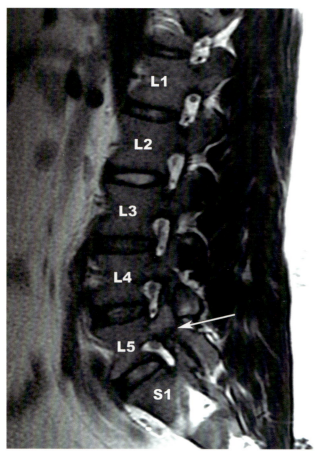

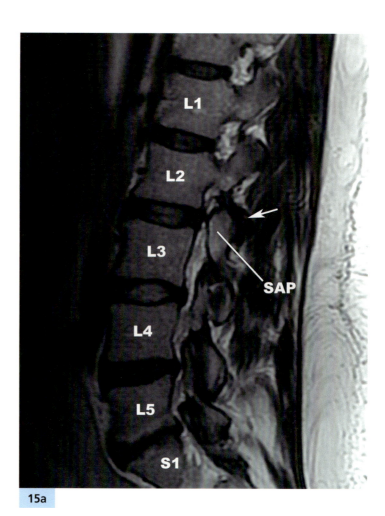

IMAGE 14 Sagittal T2-weighted TSE image showing a unilateral L5 pars interarticularis (PI) defect (arrow).

15a

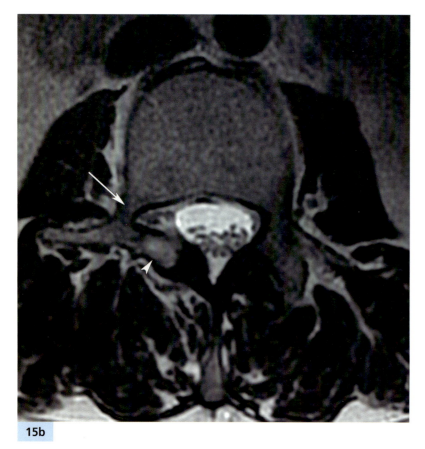

15b

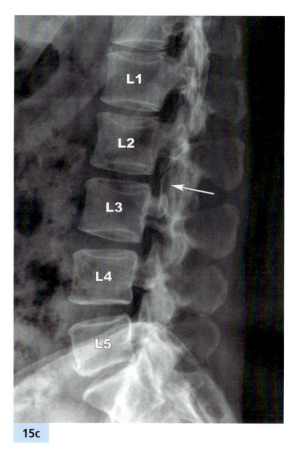

15c

IMAGES 15a–c (a) Sagittal T2-weighted TSE image demonstrating a vertically oriented, anteriorly angled L3 superior articular process (SAP). The adjacent L2-L3 zygapophyseal joint (ZJ) is degenerated out of proportion to the adjacent ZJs (arrow). (b) Axial T2-weighted image from the same patient better demonstrates the anterior displacement and rotation of the SAP (arrowhead) and an ipsilateral hypoplastic pedicle (arrow). (c) Plain film from the same patient showing the same anomalous SAP (arrow).

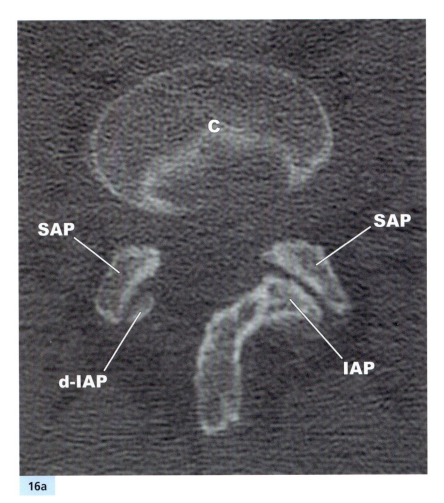

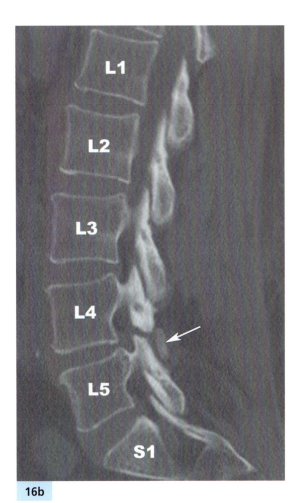

16a

16b

IMAGES 16a,b   (a) Axial CT image showing a dysplastic right lamina and right inferior articular process (d-IAP). (b) Sagittal CT image shows the dysplastic, nonfused inferior articular process (arrow). C—centrum, IAP—inferior articular process, SAP—superior articular process

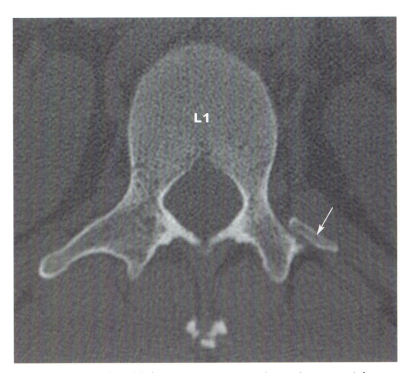

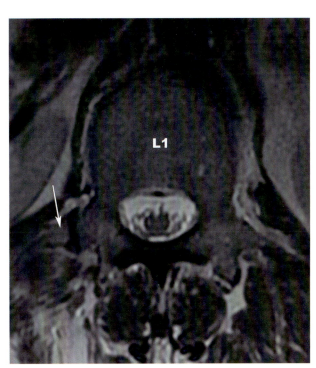

IMAGE 17   Nonfused left transverse process (arrow) on an axial CT image.

IMAGE 18   The appearance of the nonfused right transverse process (arrow) on an axial T2-weighted TSE image.

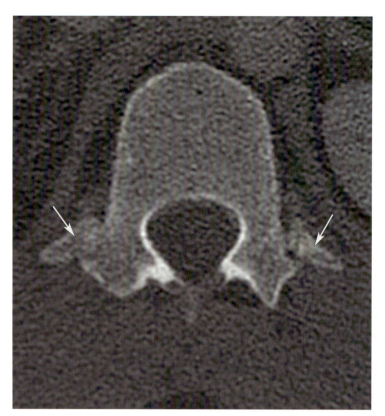

IMAGE 19   Structures that are intermediate in morphology between transverse processes and ribs at L1 (arrows).

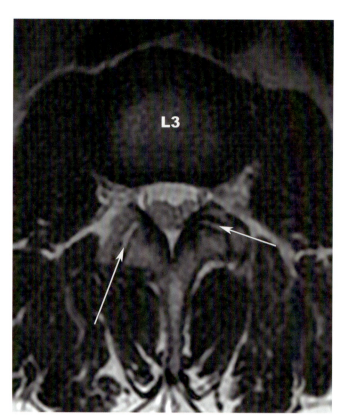

IMAGE 20   Facet tropism: The left zygapophyseal joint (short arrow) is more coronally oriented than the right zygapophyseal joint (long arrow).

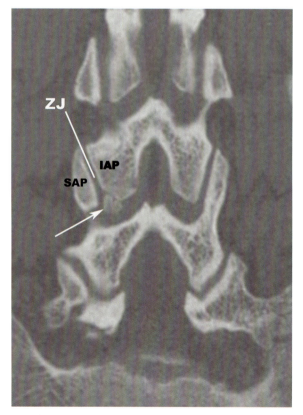

IMAGE 21   Coronal reformatted CT image displaying an ossicle (arrow) at the tip of the right L4 inferior articular process (IAP), occasionally referred to as the "Oppenheimer ossicle." SAP—superior articular process, ZJ—zygapophyseal joint.

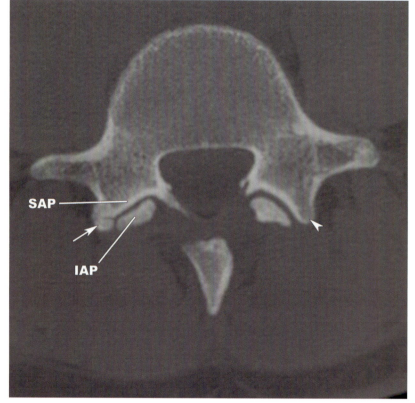

IMAGE 22   Axial CT image shows a nonfused right mammillary process (arrow). The typical appearance of the mammillary process is seen on the left (arrowhead). IAP—inferior articular process, SAP—superior articular process.

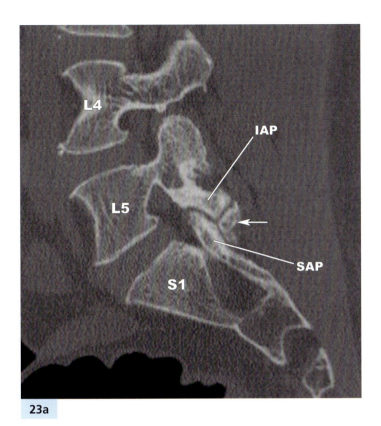

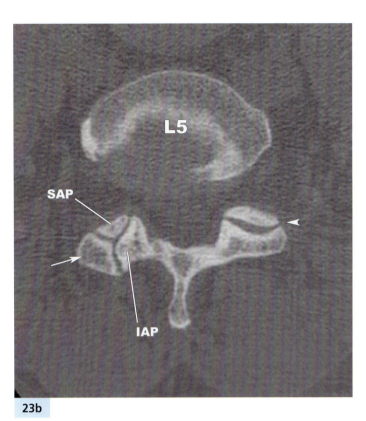

23a

23b

IMAGES 23a,b   (a) Sagittal and (b) axial CT images showing the right L5-S1 zygapophyseal joint formed by dysplastic superior (SAP) and inferior articular processes and facets (IAP). There is a triangular ossicle located along its posterolateral margin (arrow). The left zygapophyseal joint is oriented in the coronal plane (arrowhead).

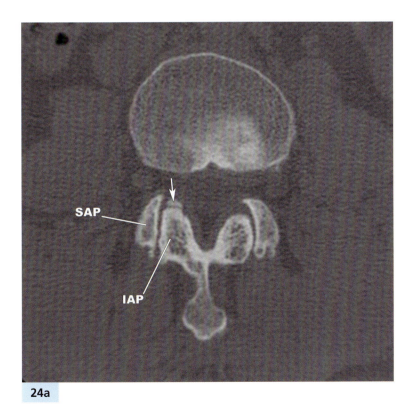

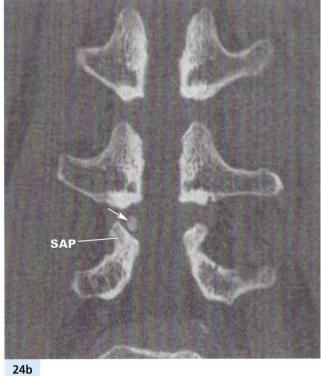

24a

24b

IMAGES 24a,b   (a) Axial and (b) coronal CT images demonstrating a small ossicle (arrow) associated with the superior articular process (SAP). IAP—inferior articular process.

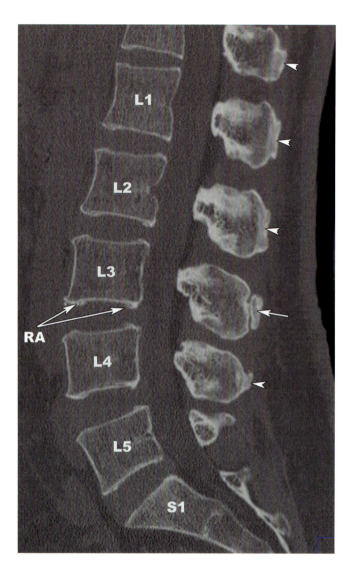

IMAGE 25   Sagittal reformatted CT image displaying partially fused (arrowheads) and nonfused (arrow) spinous process secondary ossification centers in a 45-year-old male. Partial fusion of the ring apophyses (RA) is visible at multiple levels.

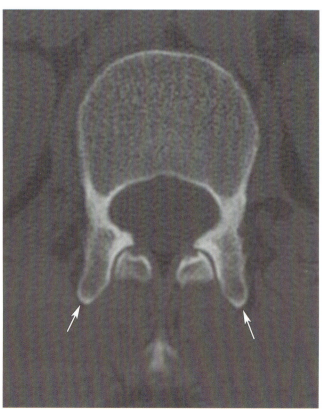

IMAGE 26   Axial CT image shows prominent, elongated mammillary processes (arrows).

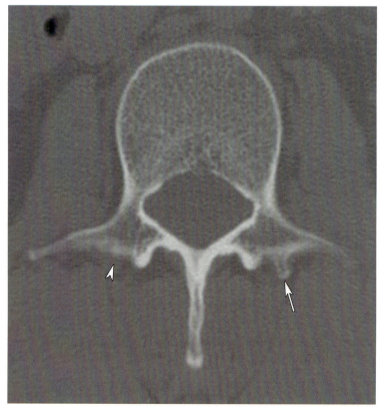

IMAGE 27   Axial CT image demonstrating an elongated accessory process on the left (arrow) and the subtle dorsal bump (arrowhead) that is the typical appearance of the accessory process.

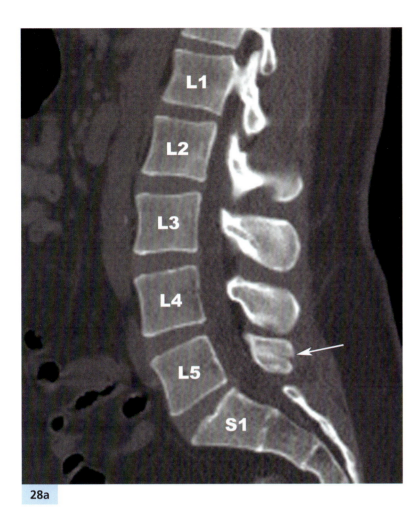

28a

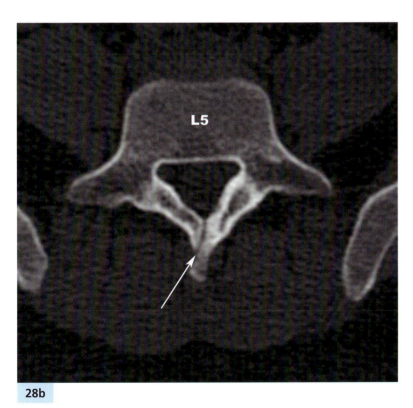

28b

IMAGES 28a,b   (a) Sagittal and (b) axial images show a bifid L5 spinous process (arrows).

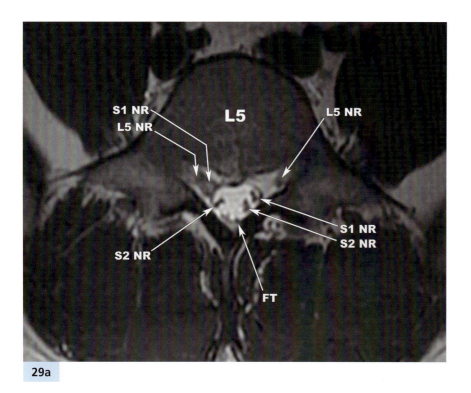

29a

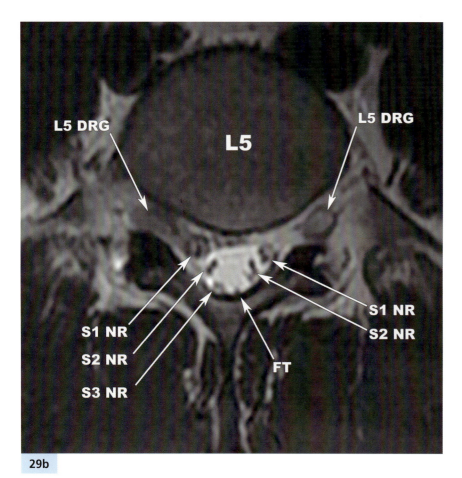

29b

IMAGES 29a,b   Consecutive (a = superior, b = inferior) T2-weighted TSE axial images demonstrating common right L5 and S1 dural sleeves, resulting in close approximation of the right L5 (L5 NR) and S1 (S1 NR) nerve roots within the subarticular recess. The typical configuration of the L5 and S1 nerve roots is present on the left. The transiting S2 nerve roots (S2 NR) and S3 nerve roots (S3 NR) are seen posteromedially. DRG—dorsal root ganglion, FT—filum terminale.

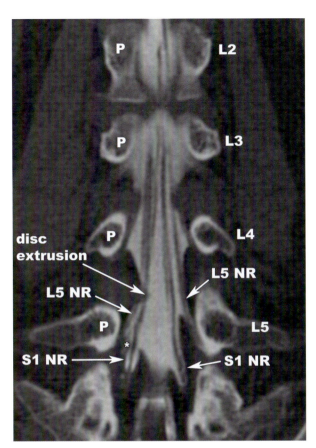

IMAGE 30 Coronal curved reformatted CT myelogram displays common right L5 and S1 dural sleeves (*) and contiguity of the L5 (L5 NR) and S1 nerve roots (S1 NR). The typical configuration is seen on the left. An extruded disc mildly deviates the right L5 and S1 nerve roots. P—pedicle.

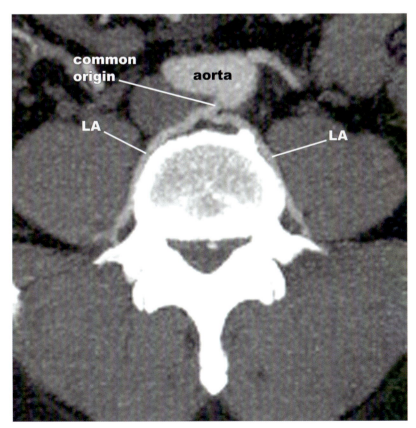

IMAGE 31 Axial maximum intensity projection image from a CT angiogram displays a common origin of the left and right lumbar arteries from the aorta, a common anatomic variant. LA—lumbar artery.

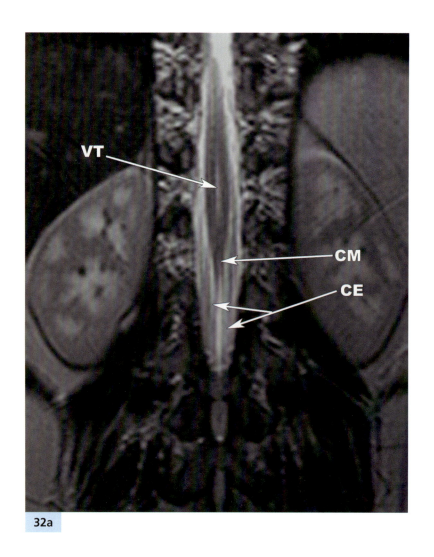

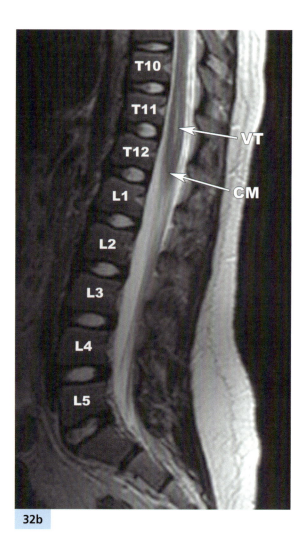

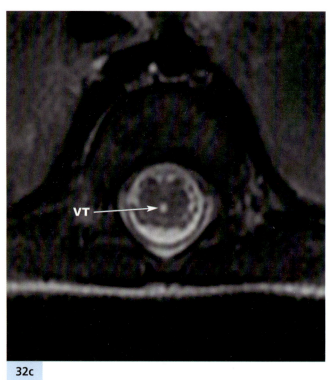

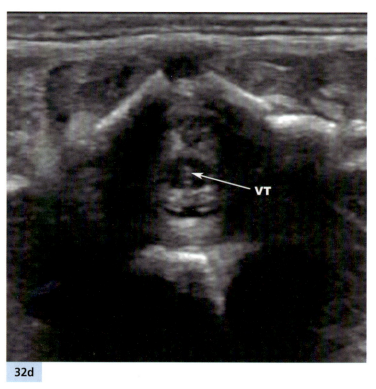

IMAGES 32a–d   Coronal (a), sagittal (b), and axial (c) T2-weighted TSE images showing smooth prominence of the central canal of the spinal cord within the distal cord and conus medullaris (CM), the typical appearance of the ventriculus terminalis (VT). (d) Axial ultrasound image showing the ventriculus terminalis. CE—cauda equine.

SUGGESTED READINGS

Abrams HL. The vertebral and azygous venous systems, and some variations in systemic venous return. *Radiology*. 1957;69:508–526.

Aihara T, Takahashi K, Ono Y, et al. Does the morphology of the iliolumbar ligament affect lumbosacral disc degeneration? *Spine*. 2002;27(14):1499–1503.

Albert M, Mulhern D, Torpey MA, et al. Age estimation using thoracic and first two lumbar vertebral ring epiphyseal union. *J Foren Sci*. 2010;55(2):287–294.

Alicioglu B, Sarac A, Tokuc B. Does abdominal obesity cause increase in the amount of epidural fat? *Eur Spine J*. 2008;17(10):1324–1328.

Alleyne CH, Cawley CM, Shengelaia GG, et al. Microsurgical anatomy of the artery of Adamkiewicz and its segmental artery. *J Neurosurg*. 1998;89:791–795.

Altinkaya N, Yildirim T, Demir S, et al. Factors associated with the thickness of the ligamentum flavum: is ligamentum flavum thickening due to hypertrophy or buckling? *Spine*. 2011;36(16):E1093–E1097.

Arai Y, Shitoto K, Takahashi M, et al. Magnetic resonance imaging observation of the conus medullaris. *Hosp for Joint Diseases*. 2001;60:10–12.

Bagnall KM, Harris PF, Jones PRM. A radiographic study of the human fetal spine 1. The development of the secondary cervical curvature. *J Anat*. 1977;123(3):777–782.

Bagnall KM, Harris PF, Jones PRM. A radiographic study of the human fetal spine 2. The sequence of development of ossification centres in the vertebral column. *J Anat*. 1977;124(3):791–802.

Bagnall KM, Harris PF, Jones PRM. A radiographic study of the human fetal spine 3. Longitudinal growth. *J Anat*. 1979;128(4):777–787.

Barson AJ. The vertebral level of termination of the spinal cord during normal and abnormal development. *J Anat*. 1970;106:489–497.

Bartynski WS, Lin L. Lumbar root compression in the lateral recess: MR imaging, conventional myelography, and CT myelography comparison with surgical confirmation. *Am J Neuroradiol*. 2003;24:348–360.

Beaujeux R, Wofram-Gabel R, Kehrli P, et al. Posterior lumbar epidural fat as a functional structure? Histologic specificities. *Spine*. 1997;22(11):1264–1269.

Beers GJ, Carter AP, McNary WF. Vertical foramina in the lumbosacral spine: CT appearance. *Am J Neuroradiol*. 1984;5:617–619.

Bertram C, Prescher A, Furderer S, et al. Attachment points of the posterior longitudinal ligament and their importance for thoracic and lumbar spine fractures. *Orthopade*. 2003;32(10):848–851.

Bley TA, Duffek CC, Francois CJ, et al. Presurgical localization of the artery of Adamkiewicz with time-resolved 3.0-T MR angiography. *Radiology*. 2010;255(3):873–881.

Bogduk N. The lumbar mamillo-accessory ligament. Its anatomical and neurosurgical significance. *Spine*. 1981;6(2):162–167.

Bogduk N. The innervation of the vertebral column. *Aust J Physio*. 1985;31(3):89–94.

Bose K, Balassubramaniam P. Nerve root canals of the lumbar spine. *Spine*. 1984;9:16–18.

Botsford DJ, Esses SI, Ogilvie-Harris DJ. In vivo diurnal variation in intervertebral disc volume and morphology. *Spine*. 1994;19(8):935–940.

Botwin KP, Gruber RD. Lumbar spinal stenosis: anatomy and pathogenesis. *Phys Med Rehabil Clin N Am*. 2003;14:1–15.

Cardoso HFV, Rios L. Age estimation from stages of epiphyseal union in the presacral vertebrae. *Am J Phys Anthrop*. 2011;144(2):238–247.

Castellvi AE, Goldstein LA, Chan DPK. Lumbosacral transitional vertebrae and their relationship with lumbar extradural defects. *Spine*. 1984;9(5):493–495.

Ciric I, Mikhael MA, Tarkington JA, et al. The lateral recess syndrome: a variant of spinal canal stenosis. *J Neurosurg*. 1980;53:433–443.

Coleman LT, Zimmerman RA, Rorke LB. Ventriculus terminalis of the conus medullaris: MR findings in children. *Am J Neuroradiol*. 1995;16:1421–1426.

Cramer, GD, Darby SA. *Clinical Anatomy of the Spine, Spinal Cord, and Ans*. 3rd ed. St. Louis, MO: Elsevier; 2014.

Cramer GD, Cantu JA, Dorsett RD, et al. Dimensions of the lumbar intervertebral foramina as determined from the sagittal plane magnetic resonance imaging scans of 95 normal subjects. *J Manipulative Physiol Ther*. 2003;26(3):160–170.

Crock HV, Yoshizawa H, Kame SK. Observations on the venous drainage of the human vertebral body. *J Bone Joint Surg*. 1973;55(3):528–533.

d'Avella, Mingrino S. Microsurgical anatomy of lumbosacral spinal roots. *J Neurosurg*. 1979;51:819–823.

De Andres J, Reina MA, Maches F, et al. Epidural fat: considerations for minimally invasive spinal injection and surgical therapies. *J Neurosurg Rev*. 2011;1(S1):45–53.

Demondion X, Vidal C, Glaude E, et al. The posterior lumbar ramus: CT-anatomic correlation and propositions of new sites of infiltration. *Am J Neuroradiol*. 2005;26:706–710.

Demondion X, Lefebvre G, Fisch O, et al. Radiographic anatomy of the intervertebral cervical and lumbar foramina (vessels and variants). *Diagn Interv Imaging*. 2012;93(9):690–697.

Dick EA, Patel K, Owens CM, et al. Spinal ultrasound in infants. *Brit J Radiol*. 2002;75:384–392.

Djindjian M. The normal vascularization of the intradural filum terminale in man. *Surg Radiol Anat.* 1998;10:201–209.

Duggal N, Lach B. Selective vulnerability of the lumbosacral spinal cord after cardiac arrest and hypotension. *Stroke.* 2002;33:116–126.

Edelson JG, Nathan H. Stages in the natural history of the vertebral end-plates. *Spine.* 1988;13(1):21–26.

El-Rakhawy M, El-Shahat AE, Labib I, et al. Lumbar vertebral canal stenosis: concept of morphometric and radiometric study of the human lumbar vertebral canal. *Anatomy.* 2010;4:51–62.

Garg A, Fleckenstein JL, Peshock RM, et al. Peculiar distribution of adipose tissue in patients with congenital generalized lipodystrophy. *J Clin Endocrinol Metab.* 1992;75(2):358–361.

Geers C, Lecouvet FE, Behets C, et al. Polygonal deformation of the dural sac in lumbar epidural lipomatosis: anatomic explanation by the presence of meningovertebral ligaments. *Am J Neuroradiol.* 2003;24:1276–1282.

Gilchrist RV, Slipman CW, Isaac Z, et al. Vascular supply to the lumbar spine: an intimate look at the lumbosacral nerve roots. *Pain Physician.* 2002;5(3):288–293.

Gouzien P, Cazalbou C, Boyer B, et al. Measurements of the normal lumbar spinal canal by computed tomography. *Surg Radiol Anat.* 1990;12(2):143–148.

Grenier N, Greselle JF, Vital JM, et al. Normal and disrupted longitudinal ligaments: correlative MR and anatomic study. *Radiology.* 1989;171(1):197–205.

Griessenauer CJ, Raborn J, Foreman P, et al. Venous drainage of the spine and spinal cord: a comprehensive review of its history, embryology, anatomy, physiology, and pathology. *Clin Anat.* 2014 doi:1002/ca.22354

Hansasuta A, Tubbs RS, Oakes WJ. Filum terminale fusion and dural sac termination: study in 27 cadavers. *Pediatr Neurosurg.* 1999;30(4):176–179.

Hansson T, Suzuki N, Hebelka H, et al. The narrowing of the lumbar spinal canal during loaded MRI: the effects of the disc and ligamentum flavum. *Eur Spine J.* 2009;18(5):679–686.

Hauck EF, Wittkowski W, Bothe HW. Intradural microanatomy of the nerve roots S1-S5 at their origin from the conus medullaris. *J Neurosurg Spine.* 2008;9:207–212.

Hasegawa T, Mikawa Y, Watanabe R, et al. Morphometric analysis of the lumbosacral nerve roots and dorsal root ganglia by magnetic resonance imaging. *Spine.* 1996;21(9):1005–1009.

Hill AR, Gibson PJ. Ultrasound determination of the normal location of the conus medullaris in neonates. *Am J Neuroradiol.* 1995;16:469–472.

Kim NH, Lee HM, Chung IH, et al. Morphometric study of the pedicles of the thoracic and lumbar vertebrae in Koreans. *Spine.* 1994;19(12):1390–1394.

Lazorthes G, Gouaze A, Zadeh JO. Arterial vascularization of the spinal cord. Recent studies of the anastomotic substitution pathways. *J Neurosurg.* 1971;35(3):253–262.

Lien SB, Liou NH, Wu SS. Analysis of anatomic morphometry of the pedicles and the safe zone for through-pedicle procedures in the thoracic and lumbar spine. *Eur Spine J.* 2007;16(8):1215–1222.

Limthongkul W, Karaikovic EE, Savage JW, et al. Volumetric analysis of thoracic and lumbar vertebral bodies. *Spine J.* 2010;10:153–158.

Mahato NK. Anatomy of lumbar interspinous ligaments: attachment, thickness, fibre orientation and biomechanical importance. *Int J Morphol.* 2013;31(1):351–355.

Mahato NK. Mamillo-accessory notch and foramen: distribution patterns and correlation with superior lumbar facet structure. *Morphologie.* 2014;98(323):176–181.

Martirosyan NL, Feuerstein JS, Theodore N, et al. Blood supply and vascular reactivity of the spinal cord under normal and pathological conditions. *J Neurosurg Spine.* 2011;15:238–251.

Masharawi Y, Salame K, Mirovsky Y, et al. Vertebral body shape variation in the thoracic and lumbar spine: characterization of its asymmetry and wedging. *Clin Anat.* 2008;21:46–54.

Masharawi YM, Peleg S, Labert HB, et al. Facet asymmetry in normal vertebral growth: characterization and etiologic theory of scoliosis. *Spine.* 2008;33(8):898–902.

Miyake H, Kiyosue H, Tanoue S, et al. Termination of the vertebral veins: evaluation by multidetector row computed tomography. *Clin Anat.* 2010;23:662–672.

Myklebust JB, Pintar F, Yoganandan N, et al. Tensile strength of spinal ligaments. *Spine.* 1988;13(5):528–531.

Nicholson AA, Roberts GM, Williams LA. The measured height of the lumbosacral disc in patients with and without transitional vertebrae. *Br J Radiol.* 1988;61(726):454–455.

O'Driscoll CM, Irwin A, Saifuddin A. Variations in morphology of the lumbosacral junction on sagittal MRI: correlation with plain radiography. *Skeletal Radiol.* 1996;25:225–230.

Ofiram E, Polly DW, Gilbert TJ, et al. Is it safer to place pedicle screws in the lower thoracic spine than in the upper lumbar spine? *Spine.* 2007;32(1):49–54.

Oh CH, Park JS, Choi WS, et al. Radiological anatomical consideration of conjoined nerve root with a case review. *Anat Cell Biol.* 2013;46:291–295.

Ohshima H, Hirano N, Osada R, et al. Morphological variation of lumbar posterior longitudinal ligament and the modality of disc herniation. *Spine.* 1993;18(16):2408–2411.

Oppenheimer, A. Supernumerary ossicle at the isthmus of the neural arch. *Radiology.* 1942; 39(1):98–100.

Oxland TR, Grant JP, Dvorak MF, et al. Effects of endplate removal on the structural properties of the lower lumbar vertebral bodies. *Spine.* 2003;28(8):771–777.

Panjabi MM, Oxland T, Takata K, et al. Articular facets of the human spine. *Spine.* 1993;18:1298–1310.

Pech P, Haughton VM. CT appearance of unfused ossicles in the lumbar spine. *Am J Neuroradiol.* 1985;6:629–631.

Pooni JS, Hukins DW, Harris PF, et al. Comparison of the structure of human intervertebral discs in the cervical, thoracic and lumbar regions of the spine. *Surg Radiol Anat.* 1986;8(3):175–182.

Ratcliffe JF. The arterial anatomy of the developing human dorsal and lumbar vertebral body. A microarteriographic study. *J Anat.* 1981;4:625–638.

Rydevik B, Holm S, Brown MD, et al. Diffusion from the cerebrospinal fluid as a nutritional pathway for spinal nerve roots. *Acta Physiol Scand.* 1990;138(2):247–248.

Saifuddin A, Burnett SJ, White J. The variation of position of the conus medullaris in an adult population. A magnetic resonance imaging study. *Spine.* 1998;23(13):1452–1456.

Santillan A, Nacarino V, Greenberg E, et al. Vascular anatomy of the spinal cord. *J Neurointervent Surg.* 2012;4:67–74.

Scheuer L, Black S. *Developmental juvenile osteology.* London: Academic Press; 2000.

Schmid MR, Stucki G, Duewell S, et al. Changes in cross-sectional measurements of the spinal canal and intervertebral foramina as a function of body position: in vivo studies on an open-configuration MR system. *Am J Roentgenol.* 1999;172(4):1095–1102.

Shimizu S, Tanaka R, Kan S, et al. Origins of the segmental arteries in the aorta: an anatomic study for selective catheterization with spinal arteriography. *Am J Neuroradiol.* 2005;26:922–928.

Scott JE, Bosworth TR, Cribb AM, Taylor JR. The chemical morphology of age-related changes in human intervertebral disc glycosaminoglycans from cervical, thoracic, and lumbar nucleus pulposus and annulus fibrosis. *J Anat.* 1994;184:73–82.

Scuderi GJ, Vaccaro AR, Brusovanik GV, et al. Conjoined lumbar nerve roots: a frequently underappreciated congenital abnormality. *J Spinal Disord Tech.* 2004;17:86–93.

Shefi S, Soudack M, Konen E, et al. Development of the lumbar lordotic curvature in children from age 2 to 20 years. *Spine.* 2013;38(10):E602–8. doi: 10.1097/BRS.0b013e31828b666b.

Song SJ, Lee JW, Choi JY, et al. Imaging features suggestive of a conjoined nerve root on routine axial MRI. *Skeletal Radiol.* 2008;37:133–138.

Scapinelli R, Stecco C, Pozzuoli A, et al. The lumbar interspinous ligaments in humans: anatomical study and review of the literature. *Cells Tissues Organs.* 2006;183(1):1–11.

Siemionow K, H A, Masuda K, et al. The effects of age, sex, ethnicity, and spinal level on the rate of intervertebral disc degeneration: a review of 1712 intervertebral discs. *Spine.* 2011;36(17):1333–1339.

Singer K, Edmondston S, Day R, et al. Prediction of thoracic and lumbar vertebral body compressive strength: correlations with bone mineral density and vertebral region. *Bone.* 1995;17(2):167–174.

Stringer MD, Restieaux M, Fisher AL, Crosado B. The vertebral venous plexuses: the internal veins are muscular and external veins have valves. *Clin Anat.* 2012;25:609–618.

Syrmou E, Tsitsopoulos PP, Marinopoulos D, et al. Spondylolysis: a review and appraisal. *Hippokratia.* 2010;14(1):17–21.

Taylor JR, Twomey LT. Vertebral column development and its relation to adult pathology. *Aust J Physiother.* 1985;31(3):83–88.

Torun F, Tuna H, Buyukmumcu M, et al. The lumbar roots and pedicles: a morphometric analysis and anatomical features. *J Clin Neuroscience.* 2008;15(8):895–899.

Vandenabeele F, Creemers J, Lambrichts I. Ultrastructure of the human spinal arachnoid mater and dura mater. *J Anat.* 1996;189:417–430.

Wagner M, Sether LA, Yu S, et al. Age changes in the lumbar intervertebral disc studied with magnetic resonance and cryomicrotomy. *Clin Anat.* 1988;1(2):92–103.

Wall EJ, Cohen MS, Massie JB, et al. Cauda equina anatomy I: intrathecal nerve root organization. *Spine.* 1990;15(12):1244–1247.

Weiler C, Schietzsch M, Kirchner T, et al. Age-related changes in human cervical, thoracal and lumbar intervertebral discs exhibit a strong intra-individual correlation. *Eur Spine.* 2012;21(6):S810–S818.

Wiltse LL, Fonseca AS, Amster J, et al. Relationship of the dura, Hofmann's ligaments, Batson's plexus, and a fibrovascular membrane lying on the posterior surface of the vertebral bodies and attaching to the deep layer of the posterior longitudinal ligament: an anatomic, radiologic, and clinical study. *Spine.* 1993;19(8):1030–1043.

Wilson DA, Prince JR. MR imaging determination of the location of the normal conus medullaris throughout childhood. *AJR.* 1989;152:1029–1032.

Yasui K, Hashizume Y, Yoshida M, et al. Age-related morphologic changes of the central canal of the human spinal cord. *Acta Neuropathol.* 1999;97:253–259.

Zhang H, Socato DJ, Nurenberg P, et al. Morphometric analysis of neurocentral synchondrosis using magnetic resonance imaging in the normal skeletally immature spine. *Spine.* 2010;35(1):76–82.

Zindrick MR, Wiltse LL, Doornik A, et al. Analysis of the morphometric characteristics of the thoracic and lumbar pedicles. *Spine.* 1987;12(2):160–166.

The Sacrum and Coccyx

5

*T*he complex structure of the sacrum reflects its multiple functions, including: allowing for bidirectional axial load shifting between the upper body and the lower extremities, formation and stabilization of the pelvic girdle, protection and transmission of the sacral spinal nerves, and serving as an origin or attachment site for several lower extremity muscles. The varied articulations of the sacrum include an amphiarthrodial (symphyseal) joint with the coccyx below, fibrous and synovial joints with the iliac bones bilaterally, discovertebral and zygapophyseal joints with the lumbar spine above.

DEVELOPMENTAL ANATOMY OF THE SACRUM AND COCCYX

The sacrum is made up of five segments that are each formed from five primary ossification centers: a centrum, two neural arches, and two costal processes located lateral to the centrum (**Figure 5.1**). Sacral secondary ossification centers include the ring apophyses, transverse processes, spinous processes, mamillary processes, anterior and posterior costal epiphyses. The sacral secondary ossification centers range in number from 35 to 37.

The presence or absence of the primary and secondary ossification centers varies according to vertebral level in the sacrum. The primary ossification centers forming the costal processes are absent at S5 and variably present at S4 (**Figure 5.2**). The secondary ossification centers of the transverse processes are variably present at S4. The secondary ossification centers of the costal epiphyses form anteriorly at S1–S4 and posteriorly S1–S2. The secondary ossification centers of the spinous processes only develop from S1 to S3. The secondary ossification centers forming the mamillary processes only develop at S1.

All primary ossification centers are present at birth and are fused by the age of 6 years, except for the laminae which fuse between 7 and 15 years of age. Nonfusion of the S1 laminae is

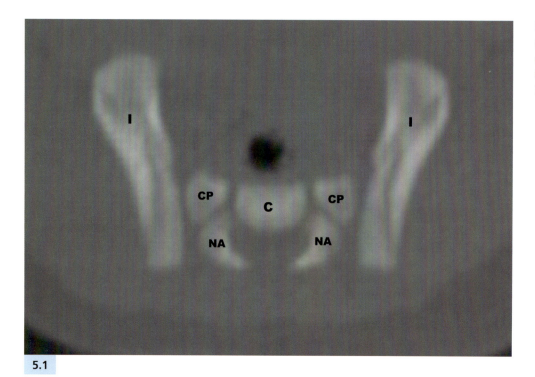

FIGURE 5.1 Axial CT image showing the sacral primary ossification centers. C—centrum, CP—costal process, I—ilium, NA—neural arch.

5.1

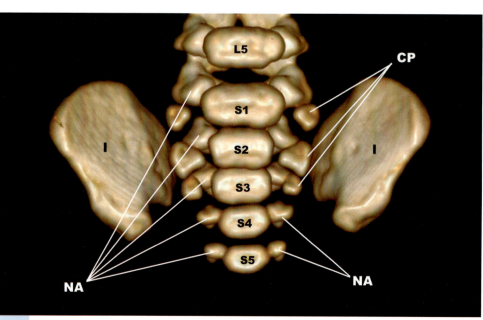

FIGURE 5.2 Surface rendered reformatted CT image demonstrating absence of the costal process (CP) ossification centers at S4 and S5 in this newborn baby. I—ilium, NA—neural arches.

5.2

a commonly observed variant (**Figure 5.3**). Fusion of the sacral vertebral bodies proceeds from caudal to rostral, beginning at age 17 to 18 years and complete by 25 years (**Figures 5.4a–c**). There is significant asymmetry in the timing of fusion of the primary and secondary ossification centers that can simulate fractures and other pathology. Complete fusion of the secondary ossification centers is not achieved until the end of the third decade.

At birth, the spine has a dorsal convex C-shape. The thoracic and sacral kyphotic curves are considered to be the primary curves of the spine. As the child assumes an upright posture, ambulates, and sleeps in the supine position, the sacral promontory rotates anteroinferiorly,

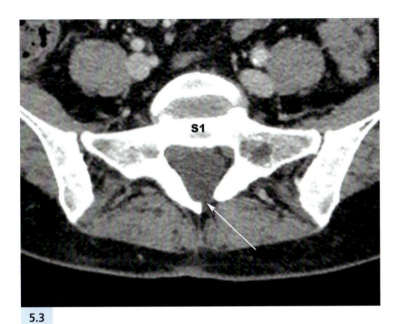

5.3

FIGURE 5.3   Axial CT image displaying nonfused S1 neural arches.

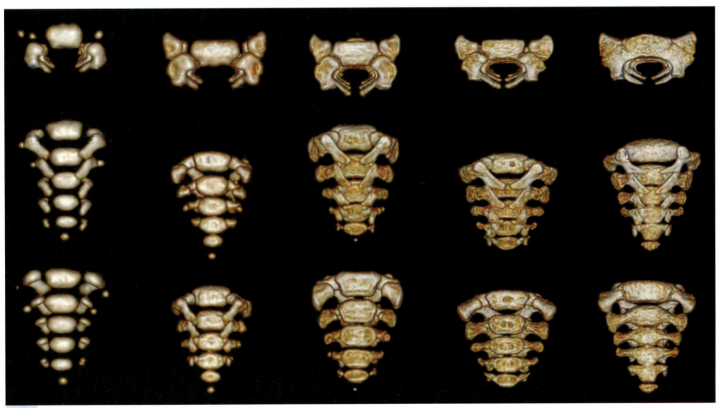

5.4a

FIGURES 5.4a–c   (a) Surface rendered reformatted CT images at various ages. The rows include axial (top), AP (middle), and posterior (bottom) projections, from left to right: newborn, 2 months, 6 months, 1 year, and 2 years. (b) Surface rendered reformatted CT images at various ages (continued). The rows include axial (top), posterior (middle), and AP (bottom) projections, from left to right: 3 years, 4 years, 5 years, 6 years, and 7 years. (c) Surface rendered reformatted CT images at various ages (continued). The rows include axial (top), posterior (middle), and AP (bottom) projections, from left to right: 8 years, 9 years, 10 years, and 11 years.

(*continued*)

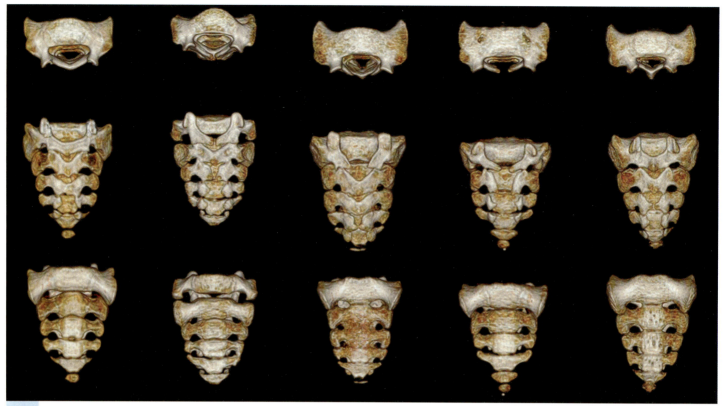

5.4b

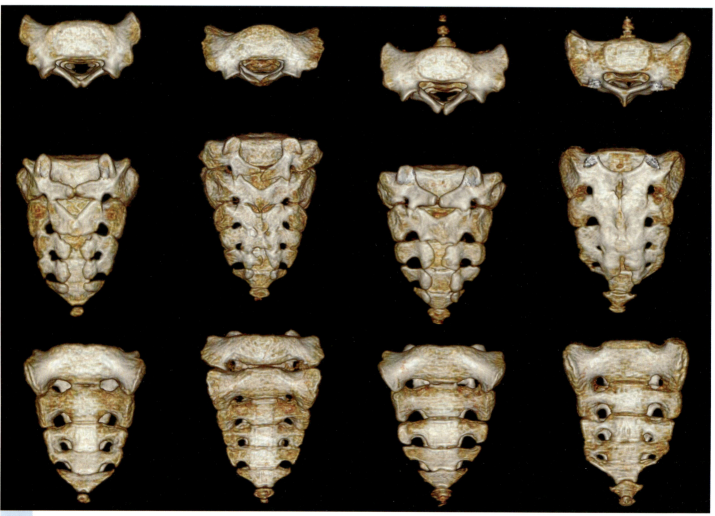

5.4c

FIGURES 5.4b,c

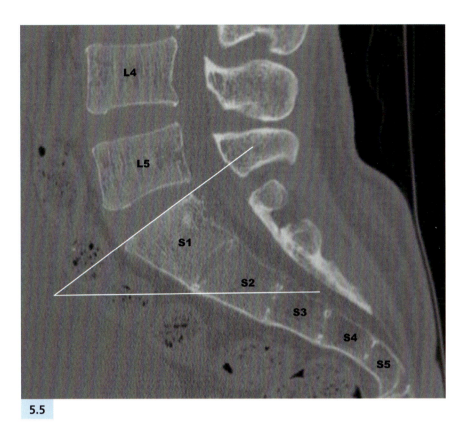

5.5

FIGURE 5.5   Ferguson's lumbosacral angle is formed by a line drawn across the superior margin of S1 and the horizontal.

the sacral kyphosis increases, and the lumbosacral angle increases to an average of 41° (standard deviation 7.68°) in adulthood. The lumbosacral angle is demonstrated in **Figure 5.5**.

The sacroiliac joints form by the 7th month of gestation. At birth the sacroiliac joints are flat and oriented to the long axis of the spine. The adult curvature of the sacroiliac joints is formed with the assumption of upright posture and ambulation.

The ossification sequence of the coccygeal segments is not completely understood. The coccygeal segments likely develop from their own primary ossification centers. However, the cornua of the Cx1 segment may arise from its own ossification center. The Cx1 ossification center is visible within the first post natal year, Cx2 between 3 and 6 years, Cx3 at 10 years, and Cx4 at puberty. The adult configuration of the coccyx takes shape in puberty.

OSTEOLOGY OF THE SACRUM

The adult sacrum is typically made up of five-fused vertebral segments that progressively decrease in size S1–S5, resulting in a triangular shape when viewed in the coronal plane (**Figure 5.6**). There are five surfaces of the sacrum, including the base, apex, dorsal, pelvic, and lateral surfaces.

The cephalad surface of the S1 segment is called the *base* of the sacrum (**Figure 5.7**). In the center of the sacral base is the ovoid articular surface upon which the L5–S1 intervertebral disc attaches. There is a bony ridge along the anterior margin of the ovoid articular surface that is called the *sacral promontory*, which marks the border of the pelvic inlet. The triangular sacral spinal canal is located immediately posterior the intervertebral articular surface that extends throughout the sacrum. The S1 superior articular processes arise along the lateral margins of the sacral canal. There are shallow notches along the lateral margins of the S1 superior articular processes that mark the position of the posterior rami of L5. The laminae and spinous process form the remainder of the sacral arch. The rudimentary spinous process forms a small, dorsally projecting ridge called the *spinous tubercle*. There are wing-like bony

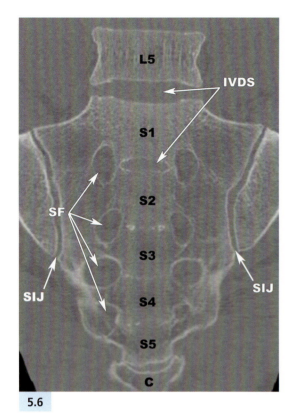

5.6

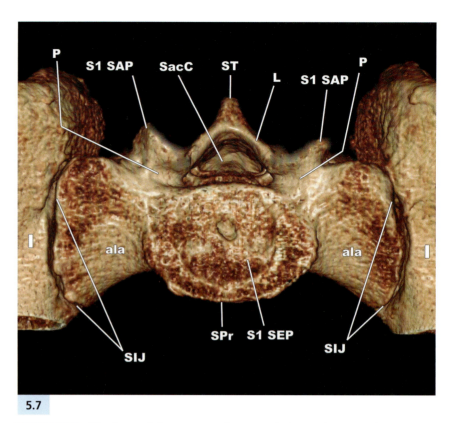

5.7

FIGURE 5.6 Curved reformat coronal CT image displaying the triangular shape of the sacrum, with the broad base superiorly and apex inferiorly. C—centrum, IVDS—intervertebral disc space, SF—sacral foramina, SIJ—sacroiliac joint.

FIGURE 5.7 The base of the sacrum. ala—sacral ala, I—ilium, L—lamina, P—pedicle, SAP—superior articular process, SacC—sacral canal, SEP—superior endplate, SIJ—sacroiliac joint, SPr—sacral promontory, ST—spinous tubercle.

projections from the S1 vertebral body on both sides that are fusion masses of the costal and transverse processes, the *sacral alae*. The medial margins of the S1 pedicles are the lateral margin of the S1 sacral foramina. The lateral margins of the S1 pedicles have not yet been defined. The large size of the S1 pedicles makes them an ideal site for pedicle screw insertion when stabilizing the lumbosacral junction from a posterior approach (**Figure 5.8**). The *apex* of the sacrum is formed by an oval facet that articulates with the coccyx.

The *dorsal surface* of the sacrum has a posterior convex curvature (**Figure 5.9**). There are three to four tubercles at the midline that represent rudimentary spinous processes, most prominent at S1. These tubercles are incorporated into an irregular ridge of bone that is called the *median sacral crest*. The laminae fuse at all levels, except S4 and S5. The nonfused laminae at S4 or S5 form a small inverted U-shaped aperture called the *sacral hiatus*. The *apex* of the sacral hiatus is located along is rostral margin. The lateral margins of the sacral hiatus are formed by the *sacral cornua*, which are the remnants of the S5 inferior articular processes that articulate with the coccyx. Variations of the sacral hiatus include closure of the sacral canal (3%), absent sacral hiatus (4%), bony septum (2%), and complete agenesis or spina bifida (1%). The sacral hiatus is a potential point of access to the sacral epidural space (see Meninges and Spaces of the Lumbar Spine section). The *intermediate sacral crest* is a small-bony ridge located just lateral to the fused laminae that represents the fused articular processes. The *posterior sacral foramina* (S1–S4) are located just lateral to the intermediate sacral crests. Lateral to the posterior sacral foramina are irregular ridges of bone formed by tubercles that arise from the fused sacral transverse processes, called the *lateral sacral crests*. The erector spinae and multifidis muscles have broad origins that include a large area spanning from the median sacral crests to the lateral sacral crests.

The *pelvic* or *ventral surface* of the sacrum is concave in the sagittal and transverse planes, forming a dorsal convex bowl (**Figure 5.10**). There are four horizontally oriented *transverse ridges* that correspond to the fused intervertebral fibrocartilages S1–S2 to S4–S5. The medial aspect of the pelvic surface is comprised of the fused S1–S5 vertebral bodies and is smooth in comparison to the dorsal surface. The sacral vertebral bodies decrease in height and width from superior to inferior, contributing to the triangular shape of the sacrum. Immediately lateral to the sacral vertebral bodies are the S1–S4 *anterior sacral foramina*. Lateral to the sacral foramina, the costal elements and transverse processes are fused into lateral masses. On plain radiographs, the

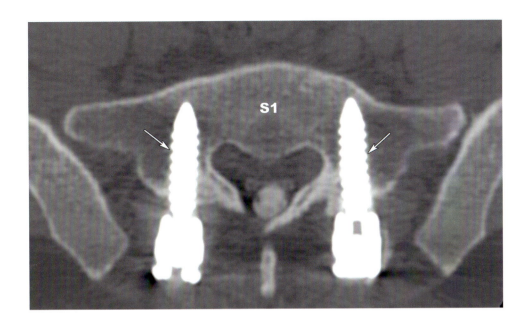

FIGURE 5.8   Axial reformatted image demonstrating large caliber bilateral S1 screws (arrows).

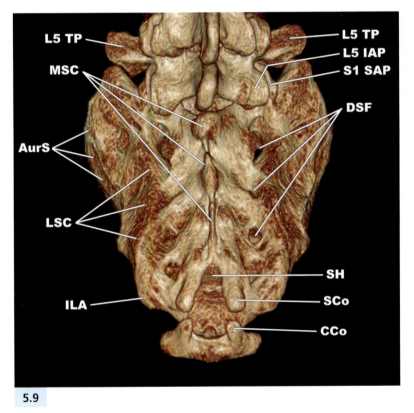

5.9

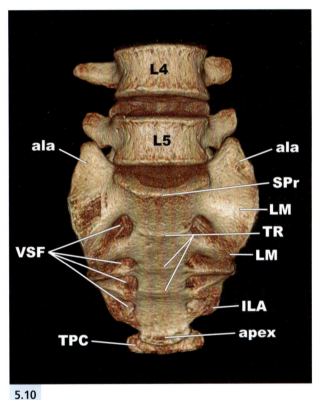

5.10

FIGURE 5.9   The dorsal surface of the sacrum. AurS—auricular surface, CCo—coccygeal cornua, DSF—dorsal sacral foramina, IAP—inferior articular process, ILA—inferolateral angle, LSC—lateral sacral crest, MSC—median sacral crest, SAP—superior articular process, SCo—sacral cornua, SH—sacral hiatus, TP—transverse process.

FIGURE 5.10   The ventral or pelvic surface of the sacrum. ala—(sacral) ala, apex—(sacral) apex, ILA—inferolateral angle, LM—lateral mass, SPr—sacral promontory, TPC—transverse process of coccyx, TR—transverse ridges, VSF—ventral sacral foramina.

inferior margins of the upper two to three costal elements form smooth *arcuate lines*, asymmetry of which can be a clue of sacral fractures or other pathology (**Figure 5.11**). The iliacus muscles attach to the S1 lateral masses. The piriformis muscles attach to the lateral masses from S1–S2 to S3–S4.

The *lateral surface* of the sacrum is C-shaped in accordance with the sacral kyphosis and tapers in the AP dimension from superior to inferior (**Figure 5.12**). There is a large, ear- or L-shaped *auricular surface* superiorly that is lined with cartilage and articulates with the ilium, forming the cartilaginous portion of the sacroiliac joint. The auricular surfaces are more posteriorly positioned in females, shifting the center of gravity posterior to the axis of support. Immediately posterior and superior to the auricular surface is an irregular, rough surface that forms an attachment site for the interosseous sacroiliac ligament and posterior sacroiliac ligament, called the *sacral tuberosity*. Inferior to the auricular surface, the lateral surface is thin and tapers progressively to the *inferior lateral angle*. The gluteus maximus and coccygeus muscles attach along the inferior lateral angles. The sacrospinous and sacrotuberous ligaments attach along the dorsal margins of the inferior lateral angles.

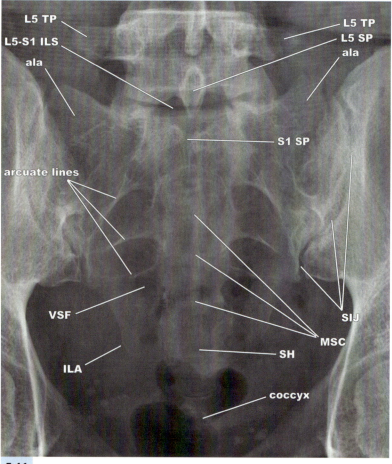

FIGURE 5.11   AP radiograph of the sacrum. The inferior margins of the upper 2–3 costal elements form the arcuate lines. ala—sacral ala, ILA—inferolateral angle, MSC—median sacral crest, SH—sacral hiatus, SIJ—sacroiliac joint, SP—spinous process, TP—transverse process, VSF—ventral sacral foramen.

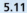

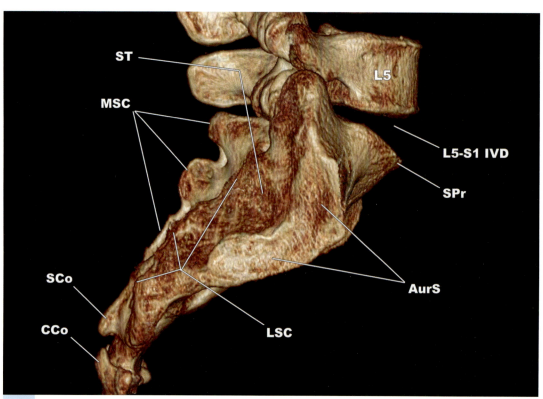

FIGURE 5.12   The lateral surface of the sacrum. AurS—auricular surface, CCo—coccygeal cornua, IVD—intervertebral disc, LSC—lateral sacral crest, MSC—median sacral crest, SCo—sacral cornua, SPr—sacral promontory, ST—sacral tuberosity.

THE SACRAL FORAMINA

The arrangement of the spinal canal and neural foramen within the sacrum is unlike that found in the rest of the spine. Outside of the sacral spine, the spinal nerves exit the neural foramina and give off anterior and posterior primary rami. Within the sacrum, there is a network of interconnected osseous channels that house the sacral nerve roots and the primary rami (**Figures 5.13a–m**).

■ AXIAL CT IMAGES FROM SUPERIOR (FIGURE 5.13a)–INFERIOR (FIGURE 5.13f)

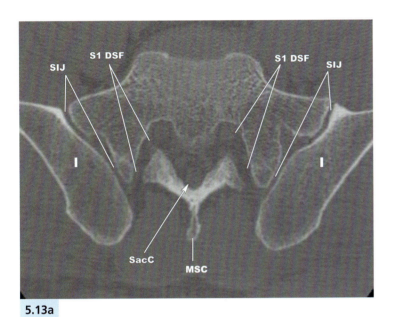

5.13a

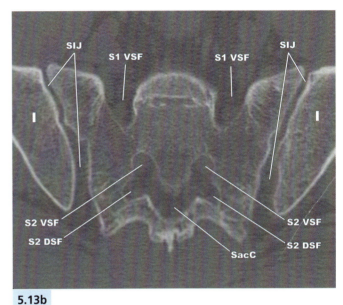

5.13b

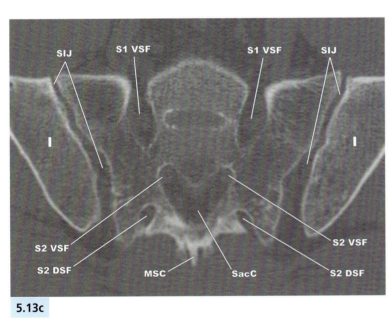

5.13c

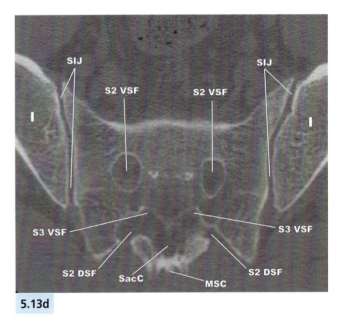

5.13d

FIGURES 5.13a–m   Axial CT images from superior (a) to inferior (f) and axial T1-weighted turbo spin echo (TSE) images angled with the long axis of the sacrum from superior (g) to inferior (m).

KEY					
DSF	dorsal sacral foramen	**MSC**	median sacral crest	**SIJ**	sacroiliac joint
I	ilium	**SacC**	sacral canal	**VSF**	ventral sacral foramen

(*continued*)

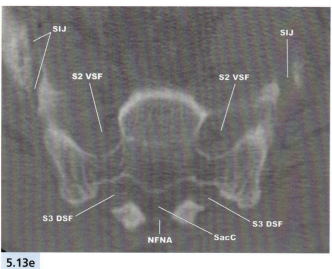

5.13e

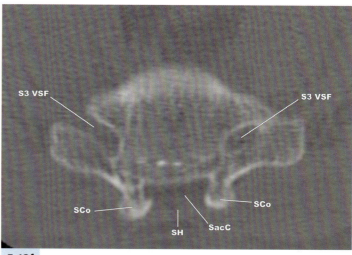

5.13f

■ AXIAL T1-WEIGHTED TSE IMAGES FROM SUPERIOR (FIGURE 5.13g)–INFERIOR (FIGURE 5.13m)

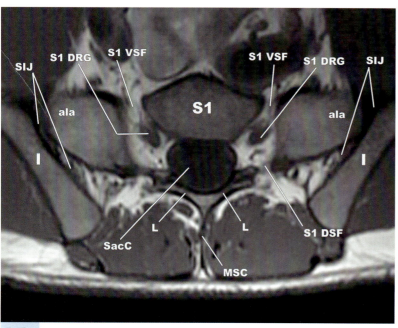

5.13g

FIGURES 5.13e–h

KEY	
ala	sacral ala
I	ilium
DRG	dorsal root ganglion
DSF	dorsal sacral foramen
L	lamina
MSC	median sacral crest
NFNA	nonfused neural arch
SacC	sacral canal
SCo	sacral cornua
SH	sacral hiatus
SIJ	sacroiliac joint
VSF	ventral sacral foramen

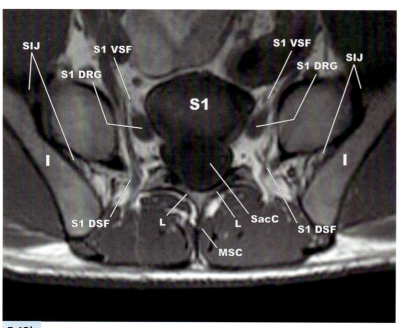

5.13h

(continued)

FIGURES 5.13i–k

KEY	
I	ilium
DRG	dorsal root ganglion
DSF	dorsal sacral foramen
L	lamina
MSC	median sacral crest
SacC	sacral canal
SIJ	sacroiliac joint
VR	ventral ramus
VSF	ventral sacral foramen

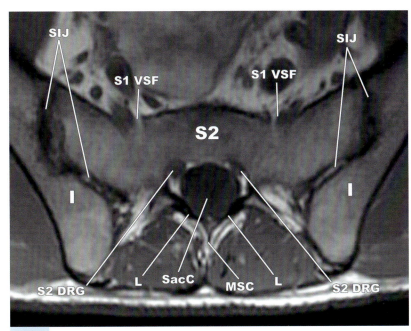

5.13i

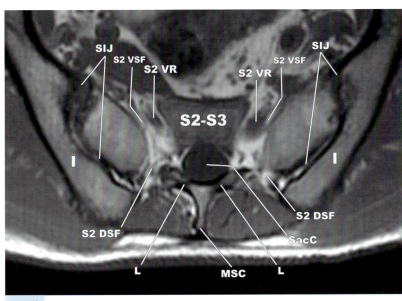

5.13j

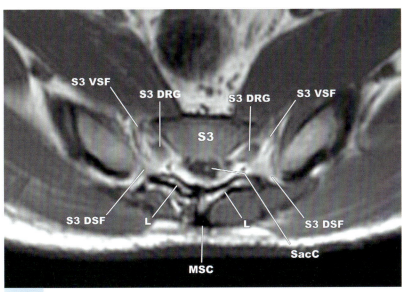

5.13k

(continued)

FIGURES 5.13l,m

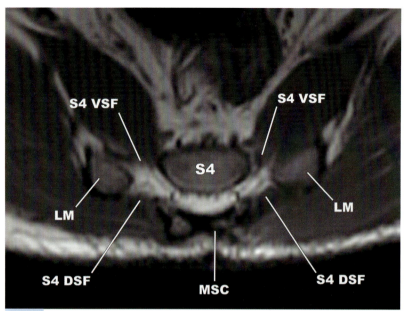

5.13l

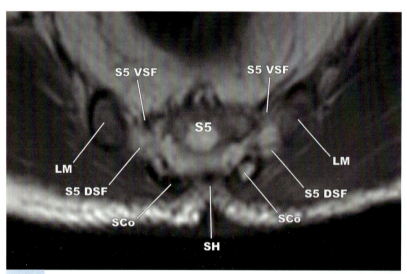

5.13m

There are typically four ventral and four dorsal sacral foramina (S1–S4). Rarely, three or five pairs of sacral foramina may be observed. The ventral foramina are funnel or trumpet shaped and transmit the ventral rami of the sacral nerves. The dorsal foramina are smaller in caliber, are more often irregular, and transmit the dorsal rami of the sacral nerves. The anterior sacral foramina are larger and more regular in shape than the posterior sacral foramina. The sacral foramina decrease in caliber from S1 to S4.

The ventral foramina are primarily vertically-oriented and course superomedial to inferolateral (**Figures 5.14a,b**). This results in an inverted Y-shaped configuration on coronal images (**Figures 5.15a,b**). The axes of the S1 and S2 dorsal foramina are oriented anteromedial to posterolateral in the transverse plane. The S3 and S4 dorsal foramina are also oriented primarily in the transverse plane, in a more anterior to posterior fashion.

The dorsal foramina of S1 are commonly accessed percutaneously when performing selective nerve root blocks. The most common imaging modalities employed are fluoroscopy and CT. Examples of fluoroscopically guided and CT-guided S1 selective nerve root injections are provided in **Figures 5.16a–c**.

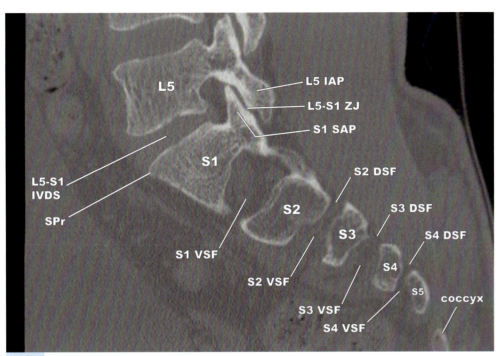

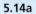
5.14a

FIGURES 5.14a,b Parasagittal (a) CT and (b) T2-weighted TSE images displaying the sacral foramina. DSF—dorsal sacral foramen, IAP—inferior articular process, IVD—intervertebral disc, IVDS—intervertebral disc space, SAP—superior articular process, SPr—sacral promontory, VSF—ventral sacral foramen, ZJ—zygapophyseal joint.

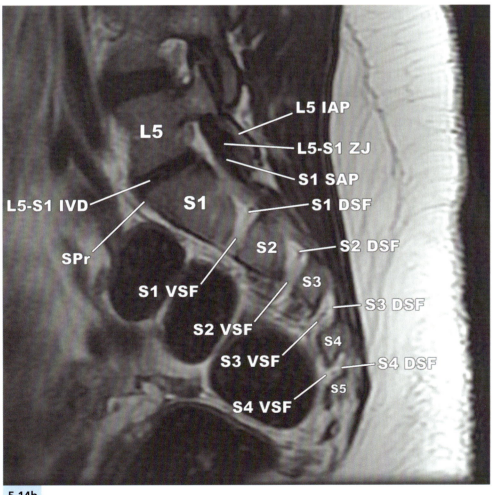
5.14b

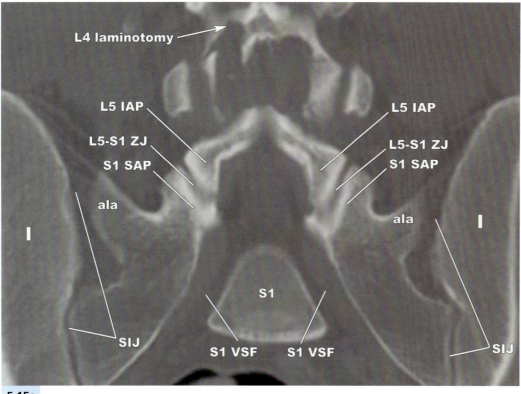

5.15a

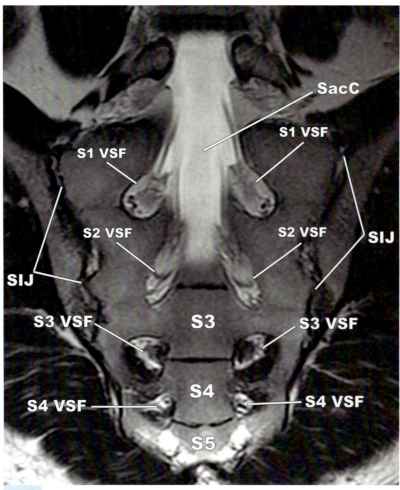

5.15b

FIGURES 5.15a,b (a) Coronal reformatted CT and (b) coronal T2-weighted TSE images showing the vertical orientation of S1 ventral foramina, forming an inverted Y-shape. A right-sided L4 laminotomy can be seen on the CT image. ala—sacral ala, I—ilium, IAP—inferior articular process, SAP—superior articular process, SacC—sacral canal, SIJ—sacroiliac joint, VSF—ventral sacral foramen, ZJ—zygapophyseal joint.

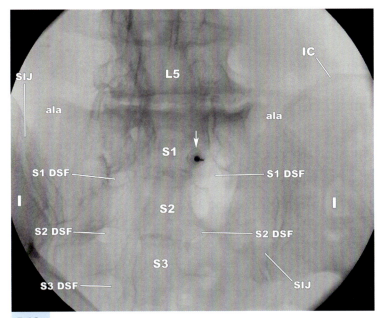

5.16a

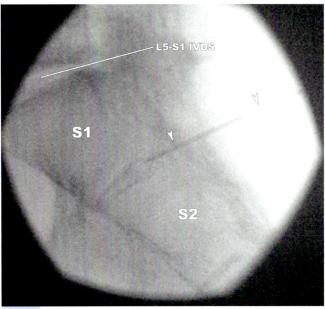

5.16b

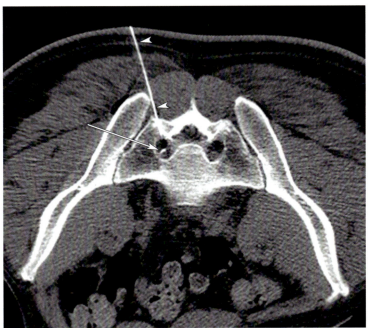

5.16c

FIGURES 5.16a–c   Image-guided S1 selective nerve root blocks. (a) Posterior oblique fluoroscopic image demonstrating the needle (arrow) aimed at the superior margin of the S1 dorsal foramen. When the needle contacts the bone along the superior rim of the S1 dorsal foramen, the C-arm is turned to a lateral position (b) and the needle (arrowheads) advanced under real time fluoroscopic guidance to the S1 nerve root. (c) CT-guided S1 selective nerve root block demonstrates the path of the needle (arrowheads) through the S1 dorsal foramen. A small amount of contrast confirms the needle position (arrow). ala—sacral ala, DSF—dorsal sacral foramen, I—ilium, IC—iliac crest, IVDS—intervertebral disc space, SIJ—sacroiliac joint.

THE L5–S1 ZYGAPOPHYSEAL JOINTS

The S1 superior articular processes project upward from the sacral base along the lateral margins of the sacral canal (Figures 5.7, 5.15a, and 5.17a–d). The superior articular facets tend to face posteriorly or posteromedially. The facet surfaces are variably curved and lined by a thin layer of smooth articular cartilage. The L5-S1 zygapophyseal joints are surrounded by a fibrous capsule and lubricated by synovial fluid. There are prominent fibrofatty pads along the superior and inferior recesses of the zygapophyseal joint capsules. The L5–S1 zygapophyseal joints are generally smaller, flatter, and more variable in orientation than the other lumbar levels. They tend to be oriented in the coronal plane, but can be oriented sagittally, or a combination of orientations.

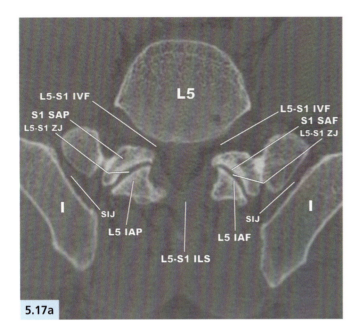

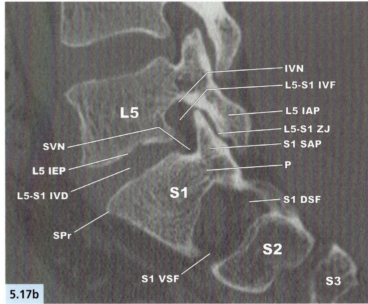

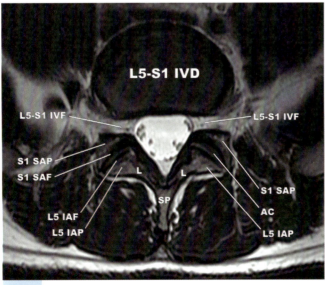

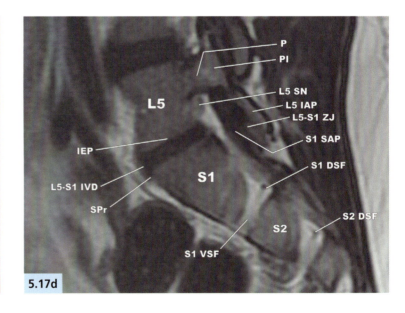

FIGURES 5.17a–d   The anatomy of the L5–S1 zygapophyseal joints displayed on (a) axial CT, (b) sagittal reformatted CT, (c) axial T2-weighted fast spin echo (FSE), and (d) sagittal T2-weighted FSE images. AC—articular cartilage, DSF—dorsal sacral foramen, I—ilium, IAF—inferior articular facet, IAP—inferior articular process, IEP—inferior endplate, ILS—interlaminar space, IVD—intervertebral disc, IVF—intervertebral foramen, IVN—inferior vertebral notch, L—lamina, P—pedicle, PI—pars interarticularis, SAF—superior articular facet, SAP—superior articular process, SIJ—sacroiliac joint, SN—spinal nerve, SP—spinous process, SPr—sacral promontory, SVN—superior vertebral notch, VSF—ventral sacral foramen, ZJ—zygapophyseal joint.

THE SACROILIAC JOINTS

The *sacroiliac joints* (SIJ) are the largest joints of the axial skeleton and are responsible for weight transfer from the upper body to the lower extremities. The SIJs have properties of synarthroses and diarthroses, allowing a small amount of motion that include gliding, nodding, tilting, translation, and rotation. There is a greater degree of SIJ motion in females and mobility is increased during pregnancy and the postpartum period.

The SIJs have cartilaginous and ligamentous portions (**Figures 5.18a–f**). The cartilaginous portions of the SIJs display features of symphyseal and diarthrodial (synovial) joints. The superior two-thirds of the cartilaginous portion of the joint are symphyseal and the inferior one-third is synovial. The SIJ capsule is thin and discontinuous posteriorly. The ligamentous portion of the SIJ is best classified as a syndesmosis and is located posterior and superior to the cartilaginous component.

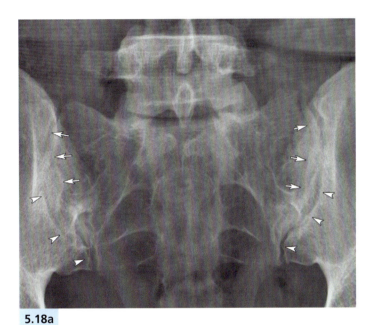

5.18a

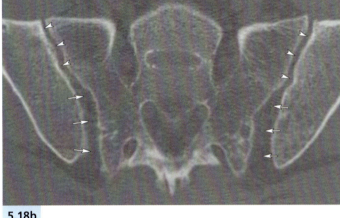

5.18b

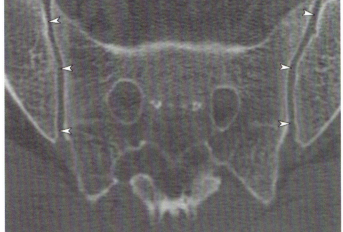

5.18c

FIGURES 5.18a–f Multimodality imaging of the sacroiliac joints. (a) AP radiographic, (b, c) axial CT, (d, e, f) axial T2-weighted TSE images demonstrating the synovial (arrowheads) and symphyseal (arrows) components of the sacroiliac joints. On AP radiographs, the synovial portion of the joints are located along the inferior 1/3–1/2 of the joint, tend to be smoother in contour, and more laterally positioned than the symphyseal portion. On MR, the short-dorsal sacroiliac ligaments are seen extending from the lateral sacral crest (LSC) to the posterior iliac crest (PIC) at S1 and S2.

(continued)

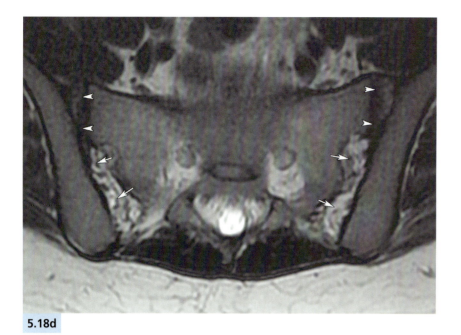

FIGURES 5.18d–f (*continued*) Multimodality imaging of the sacroiliac joints. (a) AP radiographic, (b, c) axial CT, (d, e, f) axial T2-weighted TSE images demonstrating the synovial (arrowheads) and symphyseal (arrows) components of the sacroiliac joints. On AP radiographs, the synovial portion of the joints are located along the inferior 1/3–1/2 of the joint, tend to be smoother in contour, and more laterally positioned than the symphyseal portion. On MR, the short-dorsal sacroiliac ligaments are seen extending from the lateral sacral crest (LSC) to the posterior iliac crest (PIC) at S1 and S2. LSC—lateral sacral crest, PIC—posterior iliac crest, SDSL—short dorsal sacroiliac ligament.

5.18d

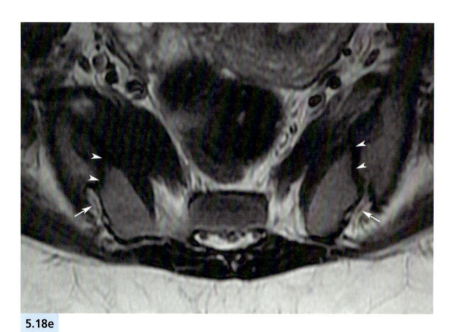

5.18e

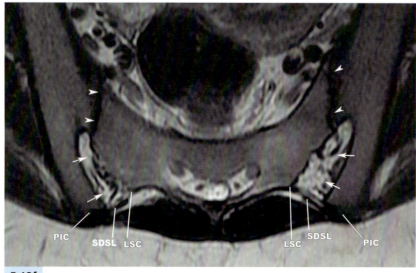

5.18f

The SIJs are primarily stabilized by several ligaments, including: the interosseous ligaments, anterior and posterior ligaments, and the accessory ligaments (iliolumbar, sacrospinous, sacrotuberous). The *interosseous sacroiliac ligaments* (ISL) connect the sacral and iliac tuberosities at the S1 and S2 levels. The ISLs have broad surfaces of bony attachment, fill the irregular spaces between the sacrum and ilia superior and posterior to the SIJ, and are the strongest SIJ supporting ligaments. The *anterior sacroiliac ligament* is made up of two thin bands located along the anterior inferior margin of the SIJ capsule. The *posterior sacroiliac ligament* has significantly greater tensile strength than the anterior sacroiliac joint and has two components, short and long. The short components are horizontally oriented and project from the iliac tuberosities to the S1–S2 transverse tubercles (Figure 5.18e). The long components are obliquely oriented and attach to the S3–S4 transverse tubercles and posterior superior iliac spines. The accessory ligaments of the SIJ are discussed in the following. Muscles that assist in SIJ stability include the gluteus maximus, biceps femoris, piriformis, and latissimus dorsi through the thoracolumbar fascia.

Therapeutic injections of the sacroiliac joints can be performed with fluoroscopic, CT, ultrasound, or MR guidance. Most commonly, fluoroscopy or CT are the modalities of choice. The posterior inferior aspect of the SIJ is targeted and contrast administered to confirm the intra-articular position of the needle (**Figure 5.19**). Extravasation of contrast injected into the SIJ capsule is commonly encountered.

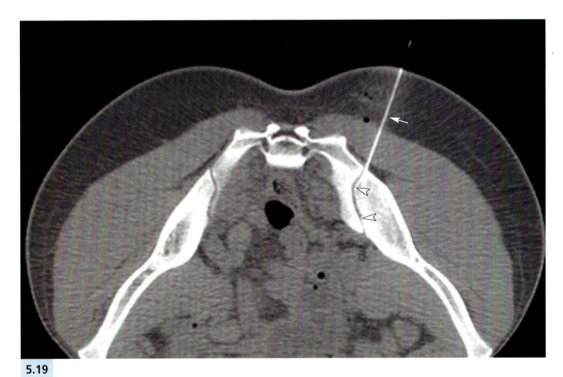

5.19

FIGURE 5.19   CT guided sacroiliac joint steroid injection. The needle (arrow) is advanced into the synovial portion of the sacroiliac joint (arrowheads) via a posterior approach.

LUMBOSACRAL TRANSITIONAL ANATOMY

Transitional anatomy at the lumbosacral junction and the related issue of segmental numbering were discussed in Chapter 4.

LIGAMENTOUS ANATOMY OF THE SACRUM

The ligamentous structures at the lumbosacral junction include the anterior and posterior longitudinal ligaments, ligamenta flava, and interspinous ligaments. The accessory ligamentous complex is comprised of the iliolumbar, sacrospinous, and sacrotuberous ligaments. The ligamentous anatomy of the sacroiliac joints was discussed previously.

The *anterior longitudinal ligament* (ALL) of the lumbar spine continues uninterrupted inferiorly to form attachments at the ventral midline the upper sacral vertebral bodies. The ALL has a broad attachment to the sacral promontory and subsequently decreases in transverse width as it courses inferiorly. The inferior continuation of the ALL is the anterior sacrococcygeal ligament. The *posterior longitudinal ligament* (PLL) is uninterrupted as it extends along the dorsal margins of the lumbar vertebral bodies to the sacrum. The PLL attaches to the dorsal midline of the sacral vertebral bodies and continues inferiorly as the posterior sacrococcygeal ligament. The *ligamenta flava* at L5–S1 are slightly thinner in the AP dimension than the adjacent L4–L5 ligamenta flava. The fibers attach to the anterior inferior margin of the L5 laminae and the posterior superior margin of the S1 laminae. The *interspinous ligament* at L5–S1 has specialized structural properties that likely act to restrict excessive acute lumbosacral flexion. The L5–S1 interspinous ligament is thicker than the other lumbar interspinous ligaments and its fibers are oriented vertically. The L5–S1 interspinous ligament is attached to the median sacral crest below and the inferior margin of the L5 spinous process above. Ligamentous anatomy at the lumbosacral junction is displayed in **Figure 5.20**.

The *iliolumbar ligaments* (ILLs) have been variously described as having two to five components and varied attachments. In general terms, the ILLs project from the L5 transverse processes to the sacrum and iliac crests. The superior bands attach to the iliac tuberosities along the superior margins of the sacroiliac joints (**Figure 5.21**). The broad inferior bands are termed the *lumbosacral ligaments* and attach to the anterosuperomedial aspects of the sacral alae. The iliolumbar ligaments primarily function to restrict multidirectional movements at the lumbosacral junction, restrict translational motion at L5–S1, protect the intervertebral disc, and assist in stabilizing the sacroiliac joints.

The *sacrospinous ligaments* extend from the lateral margin of the sacrum and coccyx to the ischial spine. They are triangular in shape, with the base at the sacrum and coccyx and the apex at the ischial spine. Rather than true ligaments, they are tendinous components of the coccygeus muscles. The sacrospinous ligaments form the posterior and inferior margins of the greater sciatic foramina. The *sacrotuberous ligaments* are classically described as attaching to the sacrum and ischial tuberosity. In point of fact, the sacrotuberous ligaments have broad attachments to the sacrum, coccyx, ischia, and ilia. The sacrotuberous and sacrospinous ligaments make up the superior and posterior margins of the lesser sciatic foramina and function to limit nutational (nodding) motion of the sacroiliac joints.

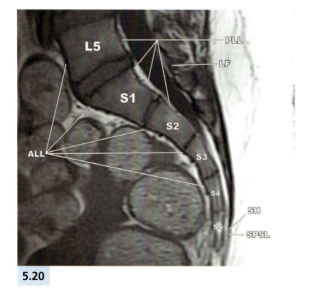

5.20

FIGURE 5.20 Sagittal T1-weighted TSE image shows the anterior longitudinal ligament (ALL), posterior longitudinal ligament (PLL), L5-S1 ligamenta flava (LF), and the superficial posterior sacrococcygeal ligament (SPSL), which covers the sacral hiatus (SH).

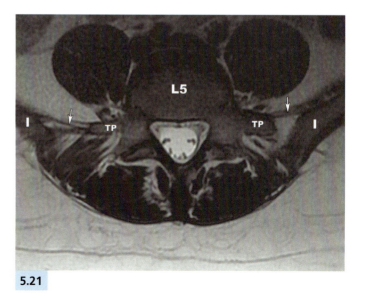

5.21

FIGURE 5.21 The iliolumbar ligaments (arrows) extend from the tips of the L5 transverse processes (TP) to the upper margins of the ilia (I).

ARTERIAL ANATOMY OF THE LUMBAR SPINE

The segmental branches supplying the sacral segments arise from the longitudinal arteries of the sacrum, which include the middle sacral and lateral sacral arteries (**Figures 5.22a,b**). The middle sacral artery typically arises from the dorsal side of the aorta, just proximal to the aortic bifurcation at the L4–L5 level, and travels along the ventral midline of the sacrum and coccyx, forming rich anastomoses with the iliolumbar and lateral sacral arteries. The lateral sacral arteries typically arise as the second branch of the internal iliac arteries. Occasionally, a lateral sacral artery may originate from the superior gluteal artery.

There are two divisions of the lateral sacral arteries, superior and inferior. The superior divisions course inferiorly and medially to anastomose with branches of the middle sacral artery. The superior divisions of the lateral sacral arteries then enter the S1 ventral foramina, where they supply the sacral nerve roots and meninges, and exit through the S1 dorsal foramina to supply the adjacent muscles and skin (**Figure 5.23**). The inferior divisions course over the

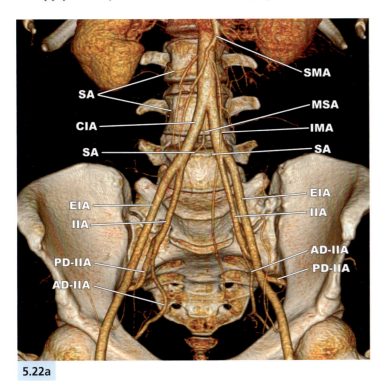

5.22a

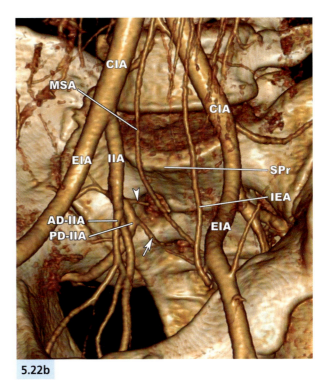

5.22b

FIGURES 5.22a,b   (a) Surface rendered CT angiogram showing the arterial supply to the sacrum. The middle sacral artery (MSA) in this individual ends in lumbar segmental arteries (SA). (b) Anterior oblique surface rendered CT angiogram shows the superior lateral sacral artery (arrowhead) and the inferior lateral sacral artery (arrow) arising from the posterior division of the internal iliac artery (PD-IIA). The superior lateral sacral artery enters the S1 ventral foramen. The inferior lateral sacral artery courses along the ventral surface of the sacrum. AD-IIA—anterior division internal iliac artery, CIA—common iliac artery, EIA—external iliac artery, IEA—inferior epigastric artery, IIA—internal iliac artery, IMA—inferior mesenteric artery, MSA—median sacral artery, PD-IIA— posterior division internal iliac artery, SA—segmental artery, SMA—superior mesenteric artery, SPr—sacral promontory.

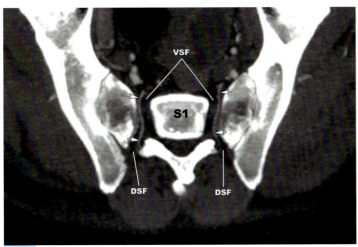

5.23

FIGURE 5.23   Axial oblique reformatted maximum intensity projection image showing the superior lateral sacral arteries (arrows) entering the S1 ventral sacral foramina (VSF), where they supply the sacral nerve roots and meninges, and exiting through the S1 dorsal sacral foramina (DSF) to supply the adjacent muscles and skin.

ventral surface of the sacrum along the medial margin of the sacral foramina. At the level of the coccyx, the inferior divisions anastomose with branches of the middle sacral artery and the contralateral lateral sacral arteries. Branches of the inferior divisions also project through the ventral and dorsal foramina to supply the sacral nerve roots, meninges, and the muscles and skin overlying the sacrum. The superior and inferior divisions of the lateral sacral arteries anastomose with the superior gluteal arteries within the soft tissues dorsal to the sacrum.

The cauda equina has a dual arterial supply. The ventral roots are supplied proximally by the vasa corona and the ventral proximal radicular arteries. They are supplied distally by the distal radicular branches. The dorsal roots are supplied proximally by the vasa corona and the dorsal proximal radicular arteries. They are supplied distally by the distal radicular branches. The proximal and distal radicular branches anastomose at the proximal one-third of the length of the sacral roots. The artery of the filum terminale arises from an anastomotic basket around the conus medullaris and courses along the ventral aspect of the filum. It travels ventral to the filum and diminishes in caliber from craniad to caudad.

VENOUS ANATOMY OF THE LUMBAR SPINE

The venous drainage of the sacrum largely parallels the arterial supply (**Figures 5.24a–e**). The *presacral venous plexus* is an extensive network of veins that is composed of longitudinal and segmental veins. The longitudinal veins of the presacral venous plexus are the *lateral sacral veins* and *middle sacral veins*. The lateral and middle sacral veins have numerous anastomoses with the horizontally oriented sacral segmental veins, called *communicating veins*. The middle sacral vein is most commonly duplicated, the communicating veins are variably present, and there may be one to two basivertebral veins. The internal iliac veins are typically single vessels (50%). Variability of the internal iliac veins includes duplication (30%) and plexiform morphology (20%).

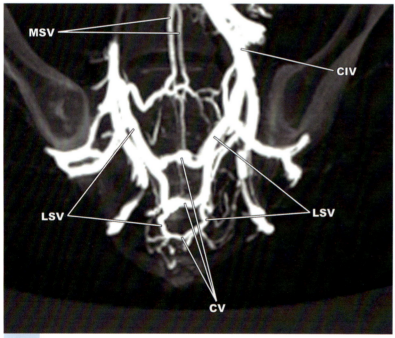

5.24a

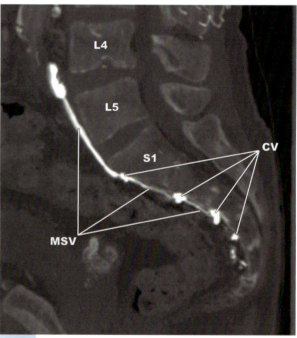

5.24b

FIGURES 5.24a–e (a) Coronal oblique reformatted maximum intensity projection image from a CT angiogram in a patient with an occluded inferior vena cava shows the presacral venous plexus. (b) Sagittal reformatted CT angiogram of the same patient with an occluded inferior vena cava demonstrating the position of the median sacral vein (MSV) and communicating veins (CV) on the pelvic surface of the sacrum. (c) Coronal reformatted image from a CT angiogram from the same patient with an occluded inferior vena cava displays the intervertebral veins (IVV) projecting through the sacral foramina. The IVV communicate freely with the lateral sacral veins and posterior external vertebral venous plexus. (d) Fat-saturated post contrast axial T1-weighted TSE image at the S1 level showing the vertebral venous plexuses. (e) Fat-saturated post contrast axial T1-weighted TSE image at the S3 level showing the intercommunication of the vertebral venous plexuses with the presacral venous plexus. CIV—common iliac vein, CV—communicating veins, LSV—lateral sacral vein, MSV—median sacral veins.

(continued)

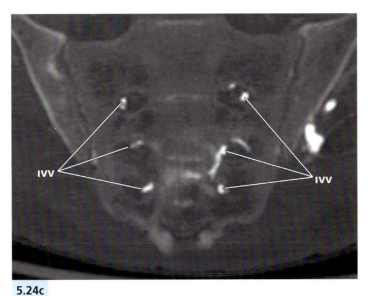

5.24c

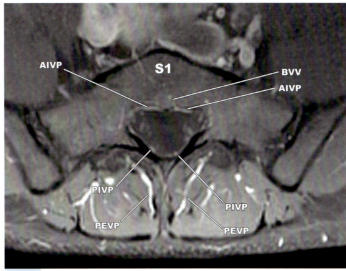

5.24d

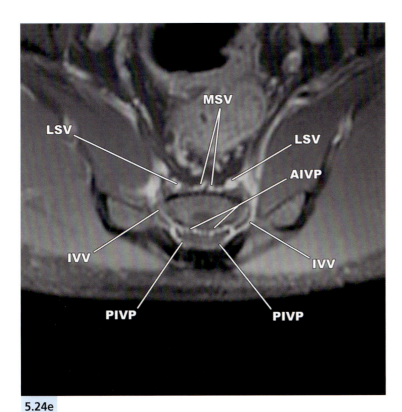

5.24e

FIGURES 5.24c–e (*continued*) AIVP—anterior internal vertebral venous plexus, BVV—basivertebral vein, IVV—intervertebral veins, LSV—lateral sacral vein, MSV—median sacral veins, PEVP—posterior external vertebral venous plexus, PIVP—posterior internal vertebral venous plexous.

The anterior and posterior internal vertebral venus plexuses continue caudally to the S4 level. The internal plexuses are significantly more prominent anteriorly and anterolaterally within the sacral canal. The internal vertebral venous plexuses communicate with the presacral vertebral venous plexus via the intervertebral and basivertebral veins. The intervertebral veins project through the sacral foramina and communicate freely with the lateral sacral veins and posterior external vertebral venous plexus. The presacral vertebral venous plexus subsequently drains to the internal iliac veins, which drain into the inferior vena cava.

MENINGES AND SPACES OF THE LUMBAR SPINE

The thecal sac typically terminates within the sacral canal. The distal thecal sac is most commonly positioned at the middle one third of S2 (**Figure 5.25**). The distal thecal sac usually tapers to a rounded point, the *fundus* of the thecal sac. However, the distal tip of the thecal sac can have a variety of configurations, from a sharp point to round. On supine MR images of the lumbar spine, this is the most posterior and inferior portion of the thecal sac. There is a grossly normal distribution thecal fundus positions, ranging from the lower one-third of L5 to the lower one-third of S3.

As stated in Chapter 4, conjoined nerve roots share a nerve root sleeve at some point along their course. Conjoined nerve roots are most commonly detected at L5–S1. The reported incidence on imaging studies is 2% to 17%, with improved detection with the use of MR. The reported incidence of conjoined nerve roots is higher on cadaveric than imaging series. MR imaging findings include: (1) asymmetric blunting of the anterolateral thecal sac ("corner sign"), (2) curvilinear extradural fat interposed between the dura and the nerve root ("fat crescent sign"), and (3) visualization of the entire spinal nerve at the disc level ("parallel sign"). The MR imaging findings associated with conjoined nerve roots are demonstrated in **Figure 5.26**.

The pia mater is tightly adherent to the filum terminale, which extends from the conus tip to the sacrum. The filum terminale internum extends from the conus medullaris to the fundus of the thecal sac at the S2 level. The filum exits the thecal sac and carries with it arachnoid and dura mater, forming the filum terminale externum or coccygeal ligament as it courses along the dorsum of the coccyx (**Figure 5.27**).

The pia mater encircling the lumbosacral nerve roots has a "gauze-like" appearance on scanning electron microscopy that allows for CSF to percolate into neural tissue. CSF is estimated to provide up to two-thirds of the nutrients to the intradural lumbosacral roots.

The sacral spinal canal is a continuation of the lumbar spinal canal that extends S1–S5 and tapers rostrally to caudally. The epidural spaces of the lumbar spine continue into the sacral

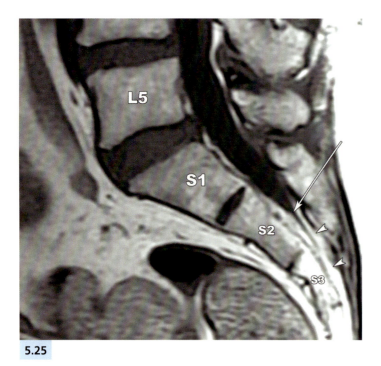

5.25

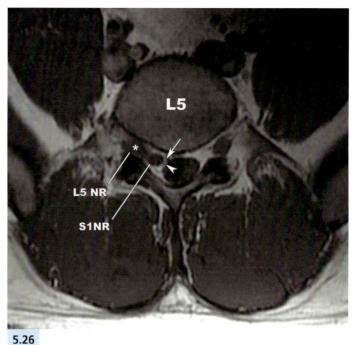

5.26

FIGURE 5.25 Sagittal T1-weighted image that shows the termination of the thecal sac at the S2 level (arrow). The fundus of the thecal sac in this case is pointed. The sacral canal caudal to the thecal sac fundus is primarily filled with fat, manifest as hyperintense signal (arrowheads).

FIGURE 5.26 The characteristic features of conjoined nerve roots on axial MR include: asymmetric contour of the ventrolateral thecal sac ("corner sign"; arrowhead), thin rim of fat between the contour deformed thecal sac and the conjoined roots ("fat crescent sign"; arrow), and the horizontal orientation of the exiting nerve root ("parallel sign"; asterisk). NR—nerve root.

spinal canal and extend to the S5 level. Because the thecal sac does not extend the length of the sacral canal, the epidural space at the levels of the thecal sac differs from the epidural space below the thecal sac termination. The varied configuration of the epidural fat pads within the upper sacral canal include thin dorsal pads, thin ventral pads, thin circumferential pads, thick ventral pads, and thick circumferential pads. Caudal to the thecal sac, the epidural space is largely composed of fat and extends to the sacral hiatus (Figure 5.25).

The position of the distal thecal sac at the S2 level and the location of the sacral hiatus at L4–L5 allow for relatively low-risk entry into the sacral spinal canal and lumbosacral epidural space. The *caudal epidural steroid injection* can be performed without or with imaging (fluoroscopic or ultrasound) guidance. Anatomic variants that may complicate this procedure include absence or high-grade stenosis of the sacral hiatus, low position of the thecal sac, and multilevel sacral spina bifida.

The density of meningovertebral ligaments anchoring the distal dural sac to the sacral canal is similar to the lower lumbar spine and greater than that seen in the cervical and thoracic regions. The meningovertebral ligaments frequently compartmentalize the epidural space, and may explain a variety of thecal sac configurations. Lateral meningovertebral ligaments project into the lateral recesses and neural foramina and anchor the dural sleeves.

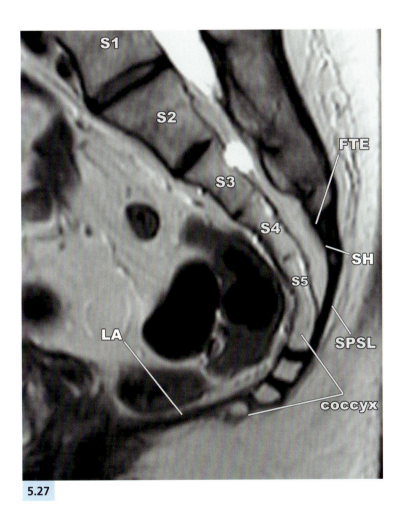

FIGURE 5.27   Sagittal T2-weighted TSE image displaying the filum terminale externum (FTE) and the superficial posterior sacrococcygeal ligament (SPSL) covering the sacral hiatus (SH). A meningeal cyst is seen at S3 within the sacral canal. LA—levator ani.

5.27

NEURAL ANATOMY OF THE LUMBAR SPINE

The cauda equina within the sacral canal is comprised of the S1–S5 nerve roots and the coccygeal nerves. There is a progressive decrease in the caliber and cross sectional area of the ventral and dorsal nerve roots S1–S5. The dorsal roots are larger in caliber and cross sectional area than the ventral roots. The S1 roots are usually shorter in length than the lower lumbar roots as a result of more proximal positioning of the dorsal root ganglia. The dorsal root ganglia decrease in length and width from S1 to S4. The S1 and S2 dorsal root ganglia are most commonly located within the sacral canal.

The S1–S5 nerve roots are arranged in layers within invaginations of the arachnoid mater. The S2–S4 roots are arranged in numerical order from ventrolateral to dorsomedial (Figures 5.28a–d). The motor roots of each segment are located ventromedial to the sensory

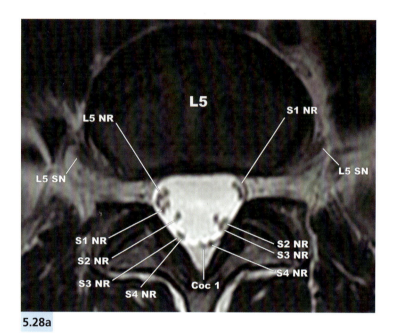

5.28a

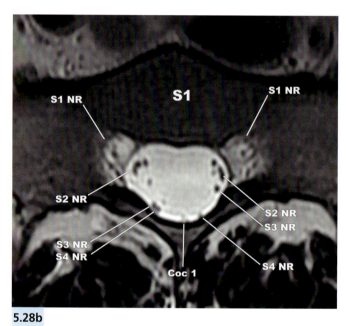

5.28b

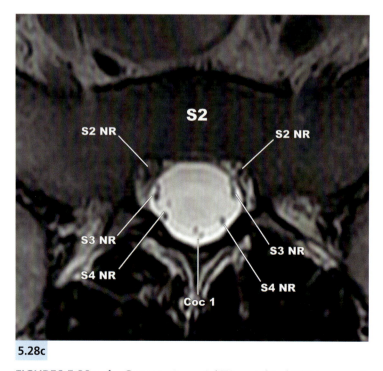

5.28c

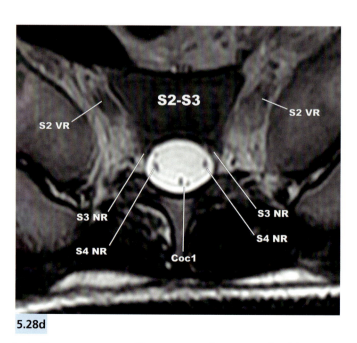

5.28d

FIGURES 5.28a–d Consecutive axial T2-weighted FSE images demonstrate the sacrococcygeal nerve roots from superior (a) to inferior (d). The reader will notice the orderly arrangement of the transiting and exiting nerve roots, the decreasing caliber of the nerve roots from S1 to S4, and the connection of small rootlets to the roots of adjacent segments along their intradural course (left S2 and S3 in image a, right S3 and S4 roots in image a, and right S3 and S4 roots in image b). Coc 1—coccygeal nerve, NR—nerve root, SN—spinal nerve, VR—ventral ramus.

roots and are smaller in caliber than the sensory roots. Intersegmental anastomoses are more commonly observed in the sacral than the lumbar nerve roots. These anastomoses are more common between the dorsal roots.

The coccygeal nerves arise from the tip of the conus medullaris, course through the posteromedial aspect of the lumbar cistern with the lower sacral nerve roots (Figures 5.28a–d), exit the sacral hiatus along with the S5 sacral nerves, and wrap around the inferior margins of the sacral cornua.

The filum terminale internum extends from the conus tip to the fundus of the thecal sac. The majority of the time, the filum fuses to the dorsal midline dura at the S1 level or below. There is a tendency of the filum to fuse at the same level as the fundus of the thecal sac. The *filum terminale externum* is the extradural continuation of the filum terminale located distal to the termination of the thecal sac within the sacral spinal canal. It attaches to the periostium of the posterior coccyx or sacrum and has been proposed to be a remnant of secondary neurulation. Fibrolipomatous infiltration of the distal aspect of the filum terminale internum is occasionally seen on axial or sagittal MR images as linear T1 hyperintense signal (**Figures 5.29a,b**). The filum terminale internum generally should not exceed 2 mm in diameter.

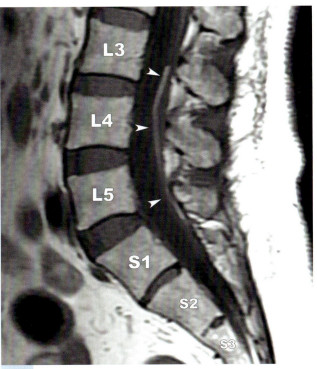

5.29a

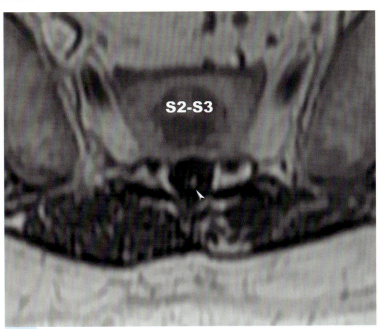

5.29b

FIGURES 5.29a,b Sagittal (a) and axial (b) T1-weighted TSE images demonstrating linear hyperintense signal following the course of the filum terminale (arrowheads) from L3 to the fundus of the thecal sac.

THE COCCYX

The coccyx typically consists of four segments (70%–80%), ranging from three to five segments. The coccygeal segments decrease in size craniad (base) to caudad (apex). The coccygeal cornua are vestigial superior articular processes that form a zygapophyseal joint with similar, inferiorly projecting sacral cornua. An S5-Coc1 fibrous disc allows a small amount of flexion and extension. However, fusion across the sacrococcygeal joint is common (57%). There is variable fusion across the intercoccygeal joints, with two (54%) and three (34%) bony segments the most common configurations. There is a range of coccygeal shapes that may be considered normal, including the presence of bony spicules, severe angulation, and subluxation (Table 5.1). The anatomy of the coccygeal segments is presented in multiple imaging modalities in Figures 5.30a–d.

The coccygeal segments serve as sites of attachment for several muscles and ligaments. The gluteus maximus attaches to the dorsolateral margins of the coccyx and levator ani muscles attach to the apex (Figure 5.27). The *anterior sacrococcygeal ligament* is the downward extension of the anterior longitudinal ligament that attaches to the anterior margin of Coc1 and Coc2. The *posterior sacrococcygeal ligament* has deep and superficial components. The deep component is the downward extension of the posterior longitudinal ligament on the ventral margin of the sacral canal that attaches to the dorsal surface of the coccyx. The superficial component covers the sacral hiatus and attaches to the dorsal coccyx (Figures 5.27 and 5.30). Additional ligaments that have attachments to the coccyx include the intracornual, lateral sacrococcygeal, and anococcygeal ligaments. The sacrotuberous and sacrospinous ligaments have extensions that attach to the posterolateral margins of the coccyx.

TABLE 5.1   Morphological Types of the Coccyx

TYPE	DEFINITION
1	Slight coccygeal curvature with apex pointing inferiorly.
2	More pronounced coccygeal curvature with apex pointing anteriorly.
3	Sharply angulated between Cx1-Cx2 or Cx2-Cx3
4	Anterior subluxation of the sacrococcygeal joint or Cx1-Cx2
5	Retroverted coccygeal apex

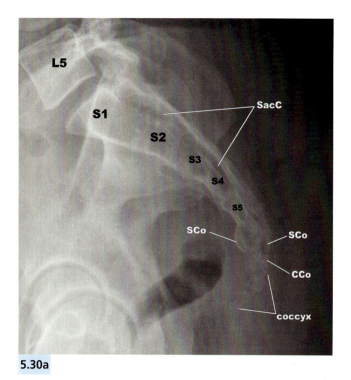

5.30a

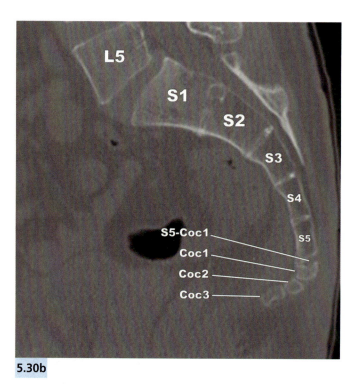

5.30b

FIGURES 5.30a–d   Anatomy of the coccyx on (a) plain radiograph, (b) sagittal reformatted CT, (c) surface reformatted CT, and (d) contrast enhanced T1-weighted FSE images. CCo—coccygeal cornua, Coc—coccygeal nerve, SacC—sacral canal, SCo—sacral cornua.

(continued)

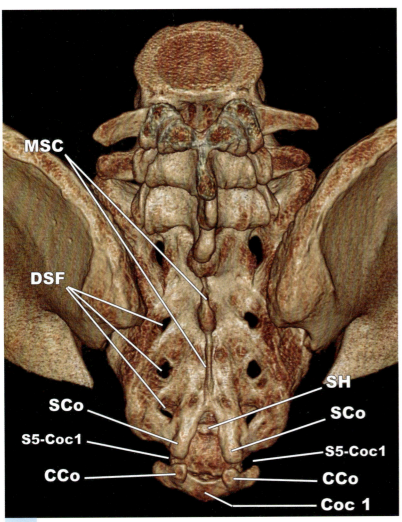

5.30c

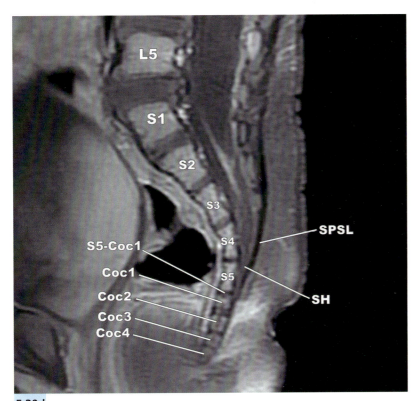

5.30d

FIGURES 5.30c,d   (*continued*) CCo—coccygeal cornua, Coc—coccygeal nerve, DSF—dorsal sacral foramina, MSC—median sacral crest, SCo—sacral cornua, SH—sacral hiatus, SPSL—superficial posterior sacrococcygeal ligament.

GALLERY OF ANATOMIC VARIANTS AND VARIOUS CONGENITAL ANOMALIES

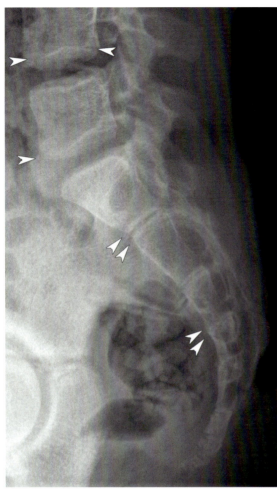

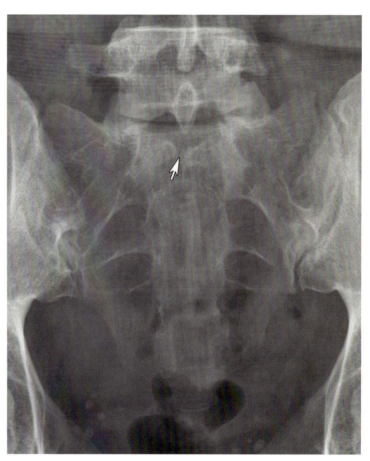

IMAGE 1   Lateral plain radiograph of the sacrum and coccyx showing the secondary ossification centers in a 13-year old (arrowheads).

IMAGE 2   AP plain radiograph showing congenital nonfusion of the S1 neural arches (arrow; spina bifida occulta).

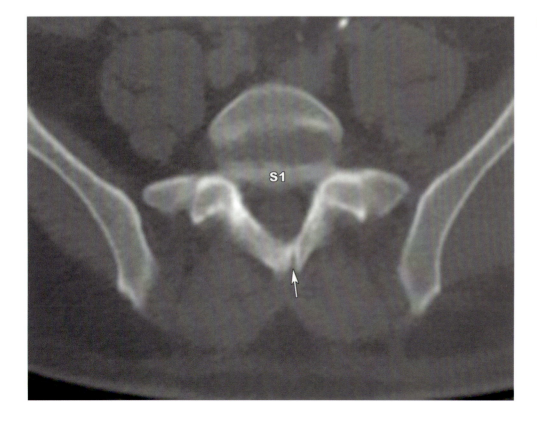

IMAGES 3   Axial CT image showing incomplete fusion of the S1 neural arches (arrow).

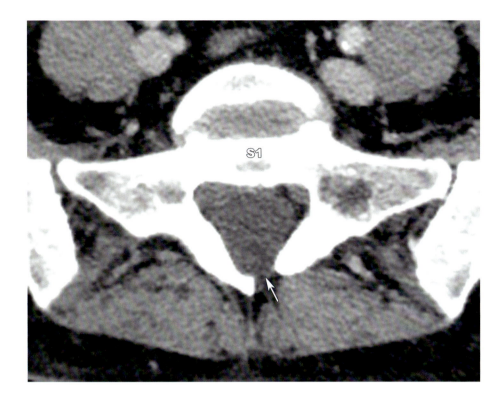

IMAGE 4   Axial CT image demonstrating nonfusion of the S1 neural arches to the left of midline (arrow).

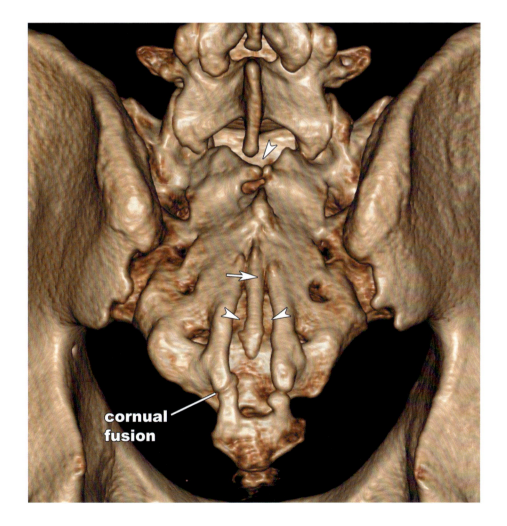

IMAGE 5   Surface reformatted image of the sacrum showing incomplete dorsal fusion (arrowheads) and a vertically oriented bony bar (arrow). Also evident is fusion across the sacral and coccygeal cornua on the patient's left side.

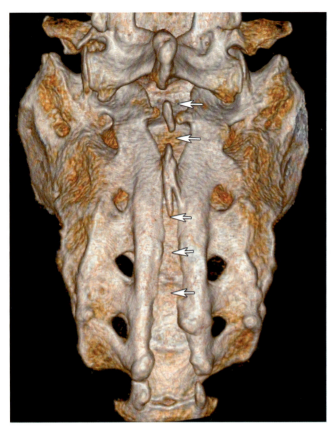

IMAGE 6 Surface reformatted image of the sacrum displaying more extensive nonfusion at S1, S2, and S3–S5 (arrows).

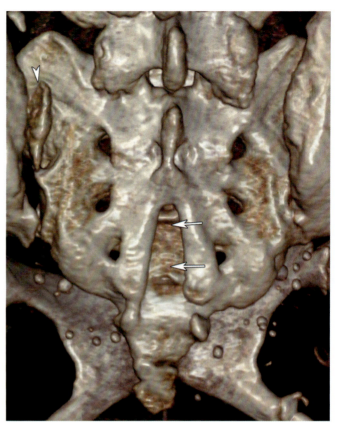

IMAGE 7 Surface reformatted image of the sacrum demonstrating neural arch nonfusion at S3 (arrows), lengthening the sacral hiatus. This patient also had a diastatic fracture of the left sacroiliac joint (arrowhead).

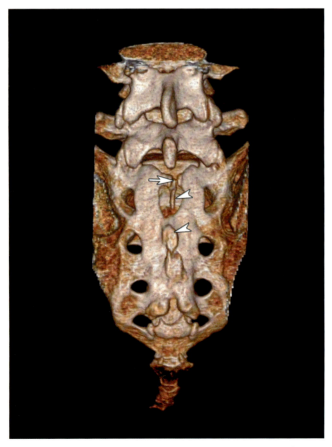

IMAGE 8 Surface rendered CT image showing nonfusion of the S1 neural elements (arrow) and rounded midline dorsal defects at S2 and S3 (arrowheads).

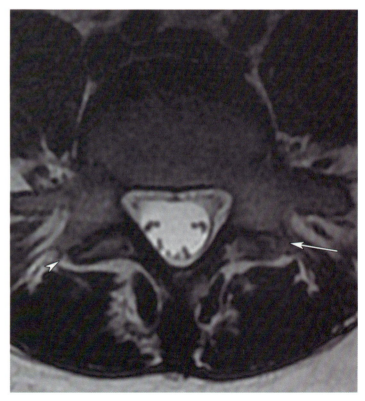

IMAGE 9 Axial T2-weighted image showing coronal orientation of the left L5-S1 zygapophyseal joint (arrow) and a more dorsolateral orientation on the right (arrowhead).

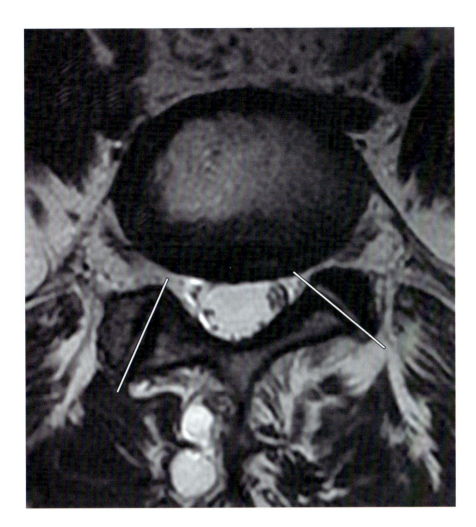

IMAGE 10   Axial T2-weighted image showing facet tropism. Note the differential orientation of the zygapophyseal joints (lines).

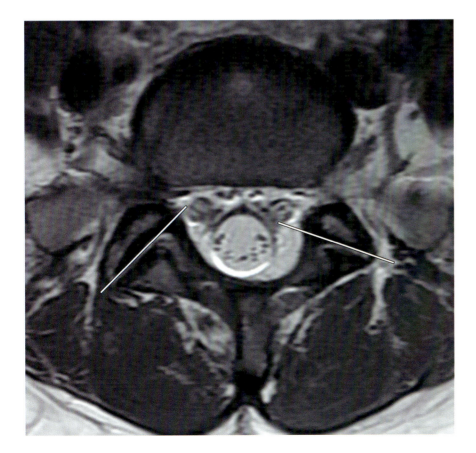

IMAGE 11   Axial T2-weighted image demonstrating facet tropism that is more pronounced than in Image 10.

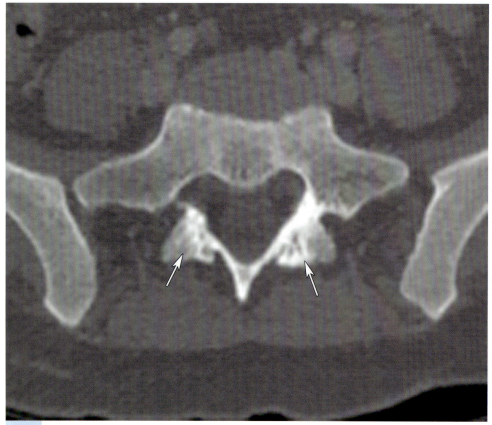

12a

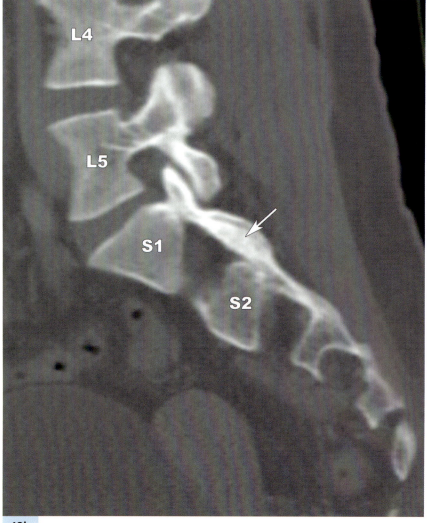

12b

IMAGES 12a,b (a) Axial and (b) sagittal CT images showing congenitally fused zygapophyseal joints at S1–S2 (arrows).

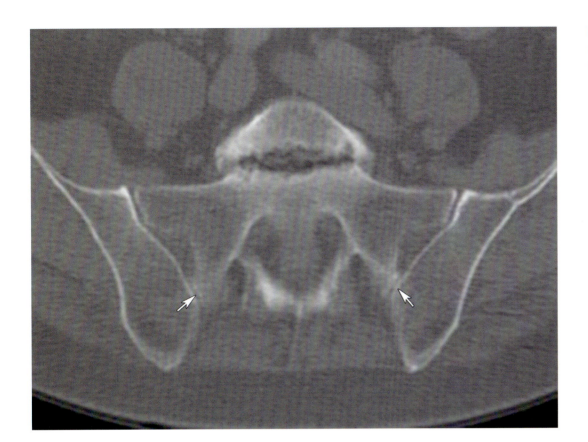

IMAGE 13   Axial CT image showing bilateral accessory sacroiliac joints (arrows).

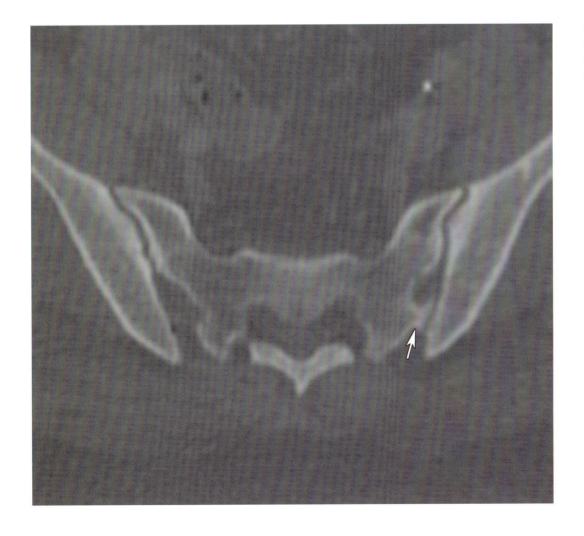

IMAGE 14   Axial CT image showing a unilateral accessory sacroiliac joint on the left (arrow).

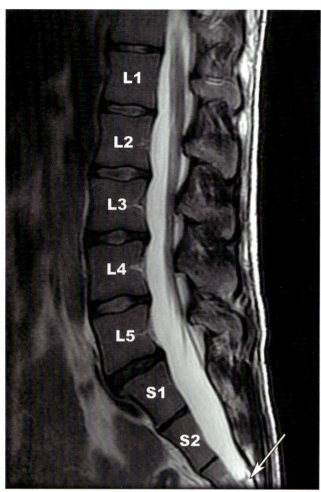

IMAGE 15 Sagittal T2-weighted TSE image demonstrating variant thecal sac anatomy. The fundus of the thecal sac is located at the caudal margin of S3 (arrow).

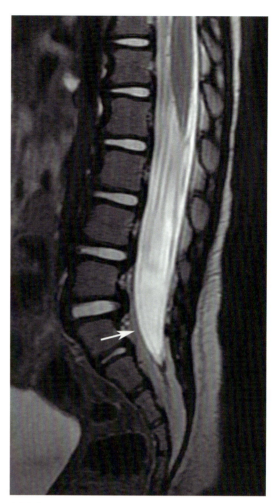

IMAGE 16 Sagittal T2-weighted TSE image showing a prominent ventral epidural fat pad that extends from L4 to the sacral canal (arrow).

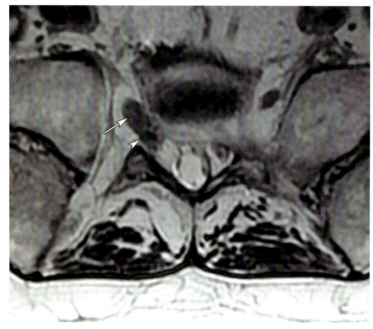

IMAGE 17 Axial T2-weighted TSE image displays conjoined right S1 (arrow) and S2 (arrowhead) nerve roots.

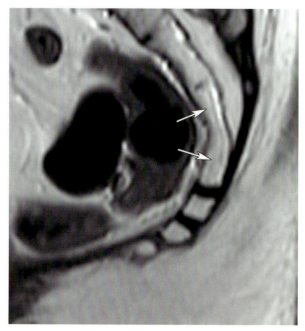

IMAGE 18 Sagittal T2-weighted TSE image demonstrating congenitally fused lower sacral segments (arrows).

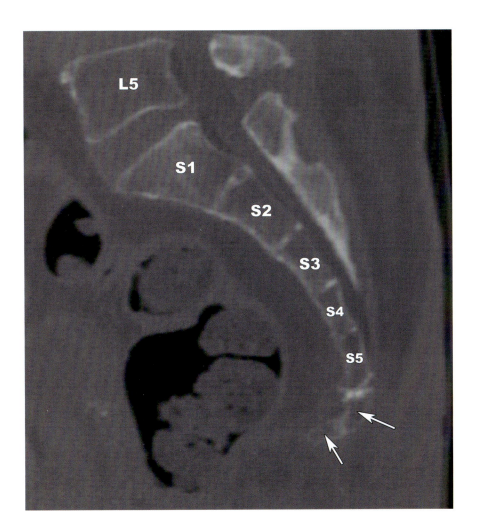

IMAGE 19 Sagittal reformatted CT image shows a two part coccyx (arrows).

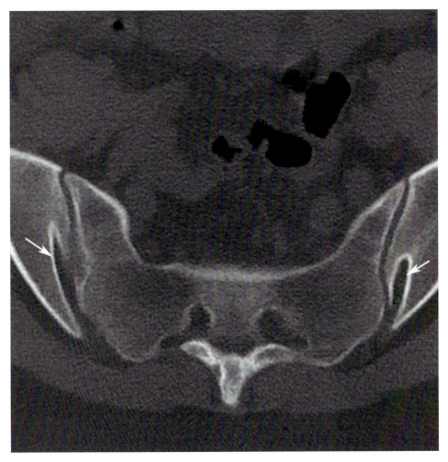

IMAGE 20 Axial CT image demonstrates bilateral bipartite iliac bone plates (arrows).

SUGGESTED READINGS

Abrams HL. The vertebral and azygous venous systems, and some variations in systemic venous return. *Radiology*. 1957;69:508–526.

Aihara T, Takahashi K, Ono Y, et al. Does the morphology of the iliolumbar ligament affect lumbosacral disc degeneration? *Spine*. 2002;27(14):1499–1503.

Alicioglu B, Sarac A, Tokuc B. Does abdominal obesity cause increase in the amount of epidural fat? *Eur Spine J*. 2008;17(10):1324–1328.

Bagnall KM, Harris PF, Jones PRM. A radiographic study of the human fetal spine 2. The sequence of development of ossification centres in the vertebral column. *J Anat*. 1977;124(3):791–802.

Bagnall KM, Harris PF, Jones PRM. A radiographic study of the human fetal spine 3. Longitudinal growth. *J Anat*. 1979;128(4):777–787.

Baque P, Karimdjee B, Iannelli A, et al. Anatomy of the presacral venous plexus: implications for rectal surgery. *Surg Radiol Anat*. 2004;26:355–358.

Bertram C, Prescher A, Furderer S, et al. Attachment points of the posterior longitudinal ligament and their importance for thoracic and lumbar spine fractures. *Orthopade*. 2003;32(10):848–851.

Bogduk N. The innervation of the vertebral column. *Aust J Physiol*. 1985;31(3):89–94.

Broome DR, Hayman LA, Herrick RC, et al. Postnatal maturation of the sacrum and coccyx: MR imaging, helical CT, and conventional radiography. *AJR*. 1998;170:1061–1066.

Cheng JS, Song JK. Anatomy of the sacrum. *Neurosurg Focus*. 2003;15(2):1–4.

Chotigavanich C, Sawangnatra S. Anomalies of the lumbosacral nerve roots. An anatomic investigation. *Clin Orthop Relat Res*. 1992;278:46–50.

Cohen MS, Wall EJ, Brown RA, et al. Cauda equina anatomy II: extrathecal nerve roots and dorsal root ganglia. *Spine*. 1990;15(12):1248–1251.

Cohen SP. Sacroiliac joint pain: a comprehensive review of anatomy, diagnosis, and treatment. *Anesth Analg*. 2005;101:1440–1453.

Cramer, GD, Darby SA. *Clinical Anatomy of the Spine, Spinal Cord, and Ans*. 3rd ed. St. Louis: Elsevier; 2014.

Crock HV, Yoshizawa H, Kame SK. Observations on the venous drainage of the human vertebral body. *J Bone Joint Surg*. 1973;55(3):528–533.

d'Avella D, Mingrino S. Microsurgical anatomy of lumbosacral spinal roots. *J Neurosurg*. 1979;51:819–823.

De Andres J, Reina MA, Maches F, et al. Epidural fat: considerations for minimally invasive spinal injection and surgical therapies. *J Neurosurg Rev*. 2011;1(S1):45–53.

Diel J, Ortiz O, Losada RA, et al. The sacrum: pathologic spectrum, multimodality imaging, and subspecialty approach. *Radiographics*. 2001;21(1):83–104.

Demondion X, Vidal C, Glaude E, et al. The posterior lumbar ramus: CT-anatomic correlation and propositions of new sites of infiltration. *Am J Neuroradiol*. 2005;26:706–710.

Djindjian M. The normal vascularization of the intradural filum terminale in man. *Surg Radiol Anat*. 1998;10:201–209.

Duncan G. Painful coccyx. *Arch Surg*. 1937;34:1088–1104.

Esses SI, Botsford DJ, Huler RJ, et al. Surgical anatomy of the sacrum: a guide for rational screw fixation. *Spine*. 1991;16(6):S283–S288.

Fortin JD, Washington WJ, Falco FJE. Three pathways between the sacroiliac joint and neural structures. *Am J Neuroradiol*. 1999;20:1429–1434.

Geers C, Lecouvet FE, Behets C, et al. Polygonal deformation of the dural sac in lumbar epidural lipomatosis: anatomic explanation by the presence of meningovertebral ligaments. *Am J Neuroradiol*. 2003;24:1276–1282.

Gilchrist RV, Slipman CW, Isaac Z, et al. Vascular supply to the lumbar spine: an intimate look at the lumbosacral nerve roots. *Pain Physician*. 2002;5(3):288–293.

Goswami P, Yadav Y, Chakradhar V. Sacral foramina: anatomical variations and clinical relevance in North Indians. *Europ J Acad Essays*. 2014;1(4):29–33.

Grenier N, Greselle JF, Vital JM, et al. Normal and disrupted longitudinal ligaments: correlative MR and anatomic study. *Radiology*. 1989;171(1):197–205.

Griessenauer CJ, Raborn J, Foreman P, et al. Venous drainage of the spine and spinal cord: a comprehensive review of its history, embryology, anatomy, physiology, and pathology. *Clin Anat*. 2014. doi:1002/ca.22354.

Haijiao W, Koti M, Smith FW, et al. Diagnosis of lumbosacral nerve root anomalies by magnetic resonance imaging. *J Spinal Disord*. 2001;14(2):143–149.

Hansasuta A, Tubbs RS, Oakes WJ. Filum terminale fusion and dural sac termination: study in 27 cadavers. *Pediatr Neurosurg*. 1999;30(4):176–179.

Hanson P, Sorensen H. The lumbosacral ligament. An autopsy study of young black and white people. *Cells Tissues Organs*. 2000;166(4):373–377.

Hauck EF, Wittkowski W, Bothe HW. Intradural microanatomy of the nerve roots S1-S5 at their origin from the conus medullaris. *J Neurosurg Spine*. 2008; 9:207–212.

Hasegawa T, Mikawa Y, Watanabe R, et al. Morphometric analysis of the lumbosacral nerve roots and dorsal root ganglia by magnetic resonance imaging. *Spine*. 1996;21(9):1005–1009.

Hellems HK, Keats TE. Measurement of the normal lumbosacral angle. *Am J Roentengol.* 1971;133(4):642–645.

Jackson H, Kam J, Harris JH Jr, et al. The sacral arcuate lines in upper sacral fractures. *Radiology.* 1982;145:35–39.

Jackson H, Burke JT. The sacral foramina. *Skel Radiol.* 1984;11:282–288.

Lazorthes G, Gouaze A, Zadeh JO. Arterial vascularization of the spinal cord. Recent studies of the anastomotic substitution pathways. *J Neurosurg.* 1971;35(3):253–262.

Lotan R, Al-Rashdi A, Finkelstein J. Clinical features of conjoined lumbosacral nerve roots versus lumbar intervertebral disc herniations. *Eur Spine.* 2010;19:1094–1098.

Mahato NK. Variable positions of the sacral auricular surface: classification and importance. *Neurosurg Focus.* 2010;28(3):1–7.

Mahato NK. Anatomy of lumbar interspinous ligaments: attachment, thickness, fibre orientation and biomechanical importance. *Int J Morphol.* 2013;31(1):351–355.

Oh CH, Park JS, Choi WS, et al. Radiological anatomical consideration of conjoined nerve root with a case review. *Anat Cell Biol.* 2013;46:291–295.

Ogoke BA. Caudal epidural steroid injections. *Pain Physician.* 2000;3(3):305–312.

Ohshima H, Hirano N, Osada R, et al. Morphological variation of lumbar posterior longitudinal ligament and the modality of disc herniation. *Spine.* 1993;18(16):2408–2411.

Panjabi MM, Oxland T, Takata K, et al. Articular facets of the human spine. *Spine.* 1993;18:1298–1310.

Phongkitkarun S, Jaovisidha S, Dhanachai M. Determination of the thecal sac ending using magnetic resonance imaging: clinical applications in craniospinal irradiation. *J Med Assoc Thai.* 2004;87(11):1368–1373.

Postacchini F, Massobrio M. Idiopathic coccygodynia. Analysis of fifty-one operative cases and a radiographic study of the normal coccyx. *J Bone Joint Surg Am.* 1983;65(8):1116–1124.

Puhakka KB, Melsen F, Jurik AG, et al. MR imaging of the normal sacroiliac joint with correlation to histology. *Skeletal Radiol.* 2004;33:15–28.

Rane A, Frazer M, Jain A, et al. The sacrospinous ligament: conveniently effective or effectively convenient? *J Obstet Gynaecol.* 2011;31(5):366–370.

Rongming X, Ebraheim NA, Gove N. Surgical anatomy of the sacrum. *Am J Orthop.* 2008;37(10): E177–E181.

Rydevik B, Holm S, Brown MD, et al. Diffusion from the cerebrospinal fluid as a nutritional pathway for spinal nerve roots. *Acta Physiol Scand.* 1990;138(2):247–248.

Scapinelli R, Stecco C, Pozzuoli A, et al. The lumbar interspinous ligaments in humans: anatomical study and review of the literature. *Cells Tissues Organs.* 2006;183(1):1–11.

Scheuer L, Black S. *The Juvenile Skeleton.* London: Academic Press; 2004.

Scuderi GJ, Vaccaro AR, Brusovanik GV, et al. Conjoined lumbar nerve roots: a frequently underappreciated congenital abnormality. *J Spinal Disord Tech.* 2004;17:86–93.

Sekiguchi M, Yabuki S, Satoh K, et al. An anatomic study of the sacral hiatus: a basis for successful caudal epidural block. *Clin J Pain.* 2004;20(1):51–54.

Senoglu N, Senoglu M, Oksuz H, et al. Landmarks of the sacral hiatus for caudal epidural block: an anatomical study. *Br J Anaesth.* 2005;95:692–695.

Song SJ, Lee JW, Choi JY, et al. Imaging features suggestive of a conjoined nerve root on routine axial MRI. *Skeletal Radiol.* 2008;37:133–138.

Tubbs RS, Murphy RL, Kelly DR, et al. The filum terminale externum. *J Neurosurg: Spine.* 2005;3: 149–152.

Vandenabeele F, Creemers J, Lambrichts I. Ultrastructure of the human spinal arachnoid mater and dura mater. *J Anat.* 1996;189:417–430.

Vleeming A, Schuenke MD, Masi AT, et al. The sacroiliac joint: an overview of its anatomy, function and potential clinical implications. *J Anat.* 2012;221:537–567.

Wall EJ, Cohen MS, Massie JB, et al. Cauda equina anatomy I: intrathecal nerve root organization. *Spine.* 1990;15(12):1244–1247.

Whelan MA, Gold RP. Computed tomography of the sacrum: 1. Normal anatomy. *AJR.* 1982;139: 1183–1190.

Wiltse LL, Fonseca AS, Amster J, et al. Relationship of the dura, Hofmann's ligaments, Batson's plexus, and a fibrovascular membrane lying on the posterior surface of the vertebral bodies and attaching to the deep layer of the posterior longitudinal ligament: an anatomic, radiologic, and clinical study. *Spine.* 1993;19(8):1030–1043.

Woodley SJ, Kennedy E, Mercer SR. Anatomy in practice: the sacrotuberous ligament. *NZ J Physiother.* 2005;33(3):91–94.

Woon JTK, Stringer MD. Clinical anatomy of the coccyx: a systematic review. *Clin Anat.* 2012;25: 158–167.

Woon JTK, Maigne JY, Perumal V, et al. Magnetic resonance imaging morphology and morphometry of the coccyx in coccydynia. *Spine.* 2013;38(23):E1437–E1445.

Woon JTK, Perumal V, Maigne JY, et al. CT morphology and morphometry of the normal adult coccyx. *Eur Spine.* 2013;22:863–870.

Yamamoto I, Panjabi MM, Oxland TR, et al. The role of the iliolumbar ligament in the lumbosacral junction. *Spine.* 1990;15(11):1138–1141.

The Paraspinal Musculature

*A*complete understanding of the anatomy of the spine must include knowledge of the paraspinal musculature. Functions attributed to the paraspinal muscles include protection of the spine, limiting excess motion, maintenance of spinal alignment, and motion. In this chapter, the anatomy of the paraspinal muscles of the cervical, thoracic, lumbar, and sacral spine is presented as a series of images in order from craniad to caudad with the use of two modalities, MR and CT.

CERVICAL PARASPINAL MUSCLES

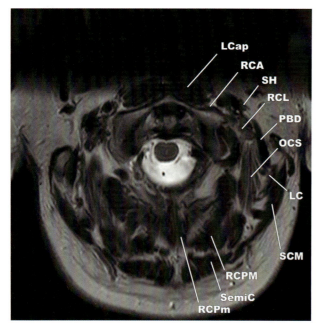

IMAGE 1 (MR)

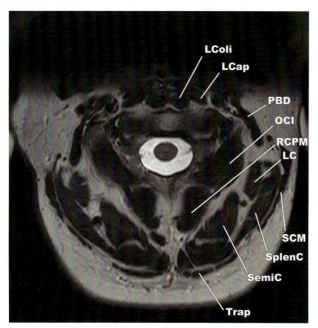

IMAGE 2 (MR)

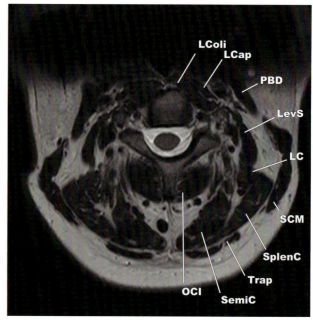

IMAGE 3 (MR)

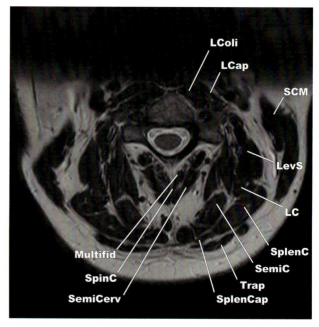

IMAGE 4 (MR)

KEY

LC	longissimus capitis muscle	RCPm	rectus capitis posterior minor muscle		
LCap	longus capitis muscle	RCPM	rectus capitis posterior major muscle		
LColi	longus coli muscle	SCM	sternocleidomastoid muscle		
LevS	levator scapulae muscle	SemiC	semispinalis capitis muscle		
Multifid	multifidis muscle	SemiCerv	semispinalis cervicis muscle		
OCI	obliquus capitis inferior muscle	SH	stylohyoid muscle		
OCS	obliquus capitis superior muscle	SpinC	spinalis cervicis muscle		
PBD	posterior belly of the digastric muscle	SplenC	splenius cervicis muscle		
RCA	rectus capitis anterior muscle	SplenCap	splenius capitis muscle		
RCL	rectus capitis lateralis muscle	Trap	trapezius		

*The iliocostalis, longissimus, and spinalis muscles are frequently referred to collectively as the erector spinae muscles.
**The semispinalis (capitis, cervicis, dorsi), multifidus, rotatores (cervicis, thoracis, lumborum), interspinales, and intertransversarii muscles may be referred to as the transversospinal muscles. These muscles function to extend and rotate the spine.

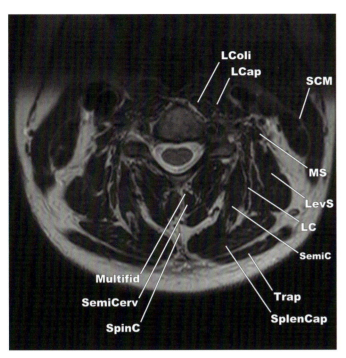

IMAGE 5 (MR)

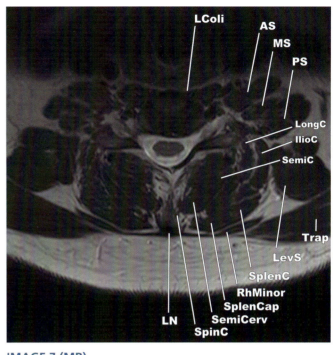

IMAGE 7 (MR)

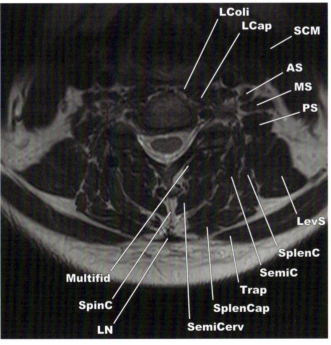

IMAGE 6 (MR)

KEY

AS	anterior scalene muscle	**SemiCerv**	semispinalis cervicis muscle
IlioC	iliocostalis cervicis muscle	**SpinC**	spinalis cervicis muscle
LC	longissimus capitis muscle	**SplenC**	splenius cervicis muscle
LCap	longus capitis muscle	**SplenCap**	splenius capitis muscle
LColi	longus coli muscle	**Trap**	trapezius
LevS	levator scapulae muscle		
LN	ligamentum nuchae		
LongC	longissimus cervicis muscle		
MS	middle scalene muscle		
Multifid	multifidis muscle		
PS	posterior scalene muscle		
RhMinor	rhomboid minor muscle		
SCM	sternocleidomastoid muscle		
SemiC	semispinalis capitis muscle		

*The iliocostalis, longissimus, and spinalis muscles are frequently referred to collectively as the erector spinae muscles.

**The semispinalis (capitis, cervicis, dorsi), multifidus, rotatores (cervicis, thoracis, lumborum), interspinales, and intertransversarii muscles may be referred to as the transversospinal muscles. These muscles function to extend and rotate the spine.

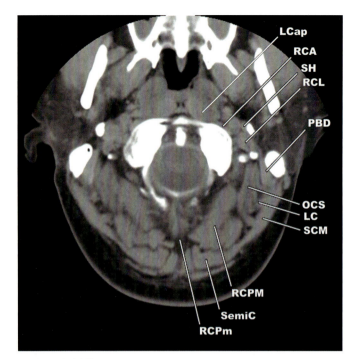

IMAGE 8 (CT)

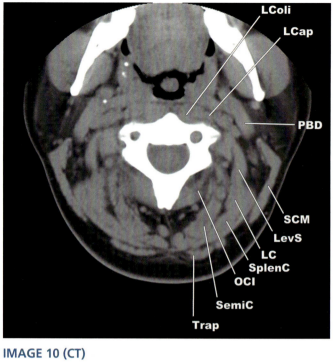

IMAGE 10 (CT)

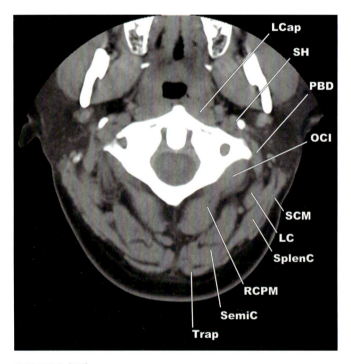

IMAGE 9 (CT)

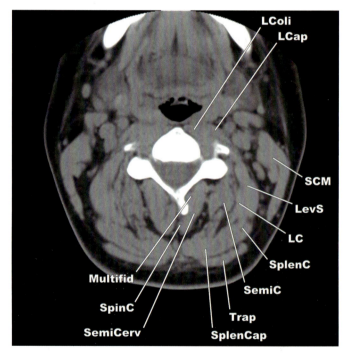

IMAGE 11 (CT)

KEY

LC	longissimus capitis muscle	RCPm	rectus capitis posterior minor muscle	*The iliocostalis, longissimus, and spinalis muscles are frequently referred to collectively as the erector spinae muscles.
LCap	longus capitis muscle	RCPM	rectus capitis posterior major muscle	
LColi	longus coli muscle	SCM	sternocleidomastoid muscle	
LevS	levator scapulae muscle	SemiC	semispinalis capitis muscle	**The semispinalis (capitis, cervicis, dorsi), multifidus, rotatores (cervicis, thoracis, lumborum), interspinales, and intertransversarii muscles may be referred to as the transversospinal muscles. These muscles function to extend and rotate the spine.
Multifid	multifidis muscle	SemiCerv	semispinalis cervicis muscle	
OCI	obliquus capitis inferior muscle	SH	stylohyoid muscle	
OCS	obliquus capitis superior muscle	SpinC	spinalis cervicis muscle	
PBD	posterior belly of the digastric muscle	SplenC	splenius cervicis muscle	
RCA	rectus capitis anterior muscle	SplenCap	splenius capitis muscle	
RCL	rectus capitis lateralis muscle	Trap	trapezius	

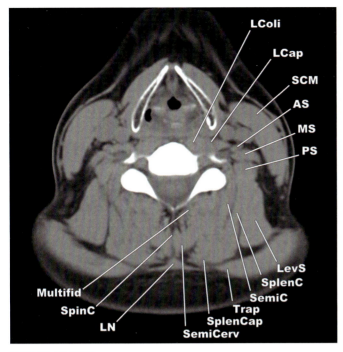

IMAGE 12 (CT)

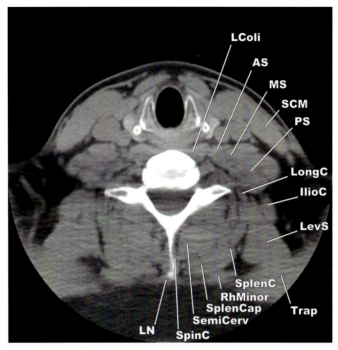

IMAGE 13 (CT)

KEY

AS	anterior scalene muscle	**PS**	posterior scalene muscle	
IlioC	iliocostalis cervicis muscle	**RhMinor**	rhomboid minor muscle	
LCap	longus capitis muscle	**SCM**	sternocleidomastoid muscle	
LColi	longus coli muscle	**SemiC**	semispinalis capitis muscle	
LevS	levator scapulae muscle	**SemiCerv**	semispinalis cervicis muscle	
LN	ligamentum nuchae	**SpinC**	spinalis cervicis muscle	
LongC	longissimus cervicis muscle	**SplenC**	splenius cervicis muscle	
MS	middle scalene muscle	**SplenCap**	splenius capitis muscle	
Multifid	multifidis muscle	**Trap**	trapezius	

*The iliocostalis, longissimus, and spinalis muscles are frequently referred to collectively as the erector spinae muscles.

**The semispinalis (capitis, cervicis, dorsi), multifidus, rotatores (cervicis, thoracis, lumborum), interspinales, and intertransversarii muscles may be referred to as the transversospinal muscles. These muscles function to extend and rotate the spine.

THORACIC PARASPINAL MUSCLES

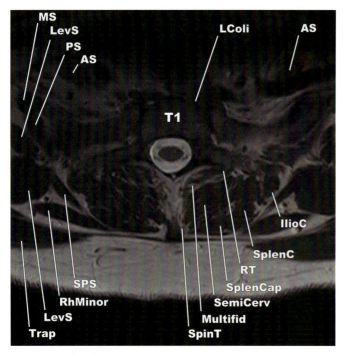

IMAGE 14 (MR)

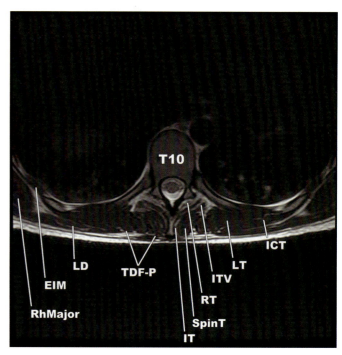

IMAGE 16 (MR)

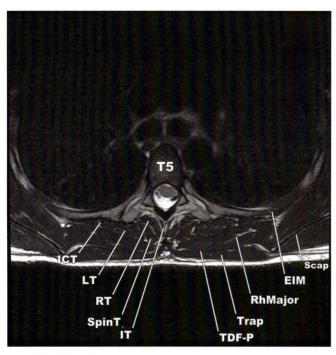

IMAGE 15 (MR)

KEY			
AS	anterior scalene muscle	**Scap**	scapula
EIM	external intercostal muscle	**SemiCerv**	semispinalis cervicis muscle
ICT	iliocostalis thoracis muscle	**SpinT**	spinalis thoracis muscle
IlioC	iliocostalis cervicis muscle	**SplenC**	splenius cervicis muscle
IT	interspinales thoracis muscle	**SplenCap**	splenius capitis muscle
ITV	intertransversarii muscle	**SPS**	serratus posterior superior muscle
LevS	levator scapulae muscle	**TDF**	thoracodorsal fascia (M—middle layer,
LColi	longus coli muscle		P—posterior layer)
LD	latissimus dorsi muscle	**Trap**	trapezius muscle
LT	longissimus thoracis muscle		
Multifid	multifidis muscle		
MS	middle scalene muscle		
PS	posterior scalene muscle		
RhMajor	rhomboid major muscle		
RhMinor	rhomboid minor muscle		
RT	rotatores thoracis muscle		

*The iliocostalis, longissimus, and spinalis muscles are frequently referred to collectively as the erector spinae muscles.

**The semispinalis (capitis, cervicis, dorsi), multifidus, rotatores (cervicis, thoracis, lumborum), interspinales, and intertransversarii muscles may be referred to as the transversospinal muscles. These muscles function to extend and rotate the spine.

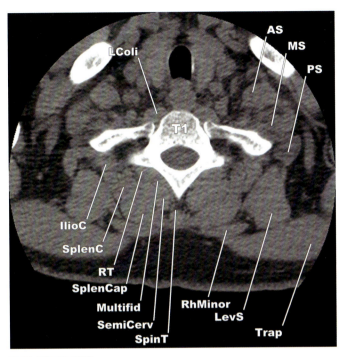

IMAGE 17 (CT)

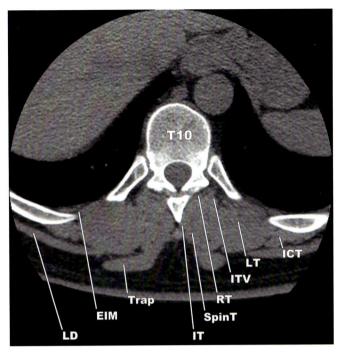

IMAGE 19 (CT)

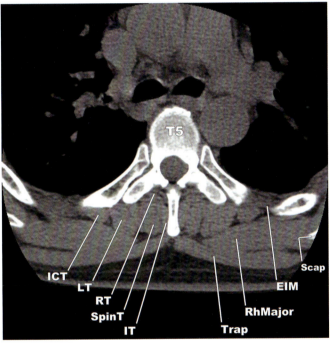

IMAGE 18 (CT)

KEY

AS	anterior scalene muscle	**RT**	rotatores thoracis muscle
EIM	external intercostal muscle	**Scap**	scapula
ICT	iliocostalis thoracis muscle	**SemiCerv**	semispinalis cervicis muscle
IlioC	iliocostalis cervicis muscle	**SpinT**	spinalis thoracis muscle
IT	interspinales thoracis muscle	**SplenC**	splenius cervicis muscle
ITV	intertransversarii muscle	**SplenCap**	splenius capitis muscle
LevS	levator scapulae muscle	**Trap**	trapezius muscle
LColi	longus coli muscle		
LD	latissimus dorsi muscle		
LT	longissimus thoracis muscle		
Multifid	multifidis muscle		
MS	middle scalene muscle		
PS	posterior scalene muscle		
RhMajor	rhomboid major muscle		
RhMinor	rhomboid minor muscle		

*The iliocostalis, longissimus, and spinalis muscles are frequently referred to collectively as the erector spinae muscles.
**The semispinalis (capitis, cervicis, dorsi), multifidus, rotatores (cervicis, thoracis, lumborum), interspinales, and intertransversarii muscles may be referred to as the transversospinal muscles. These muscles function to extend and rotate the spine.

LUMBOSACRAL PARASPINAL MUSCLES

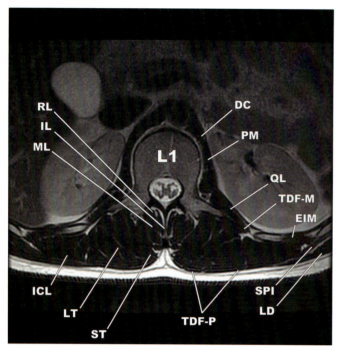

IMAGE 20 (MR)

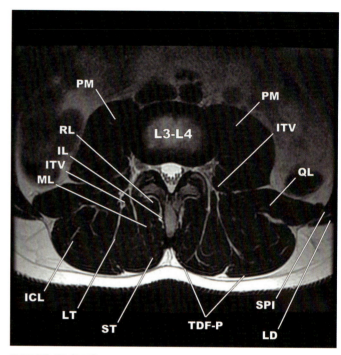

IMAGE 22 (MR)

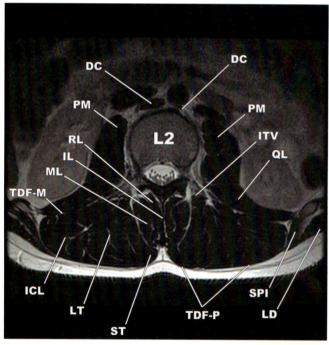

IMAGE 21 (MR)

KEY

DC	diaphragmatic crus	SPI	serratus posterior inferior muscle
EIM	external intercostal muscle	ST	spinalis thoracis muscle
ICL	iliocostalis lumborum muscle	TDF	thoracodorsal fascia (M—middle layer, P—posterior layer)
IL	interspinales lumborum muscle		
ITV	intertransversarii muscle		
LD	latissimus dorsi muscle		
LT	longissimus thoracis muscle		
ML	multifidus lumborum muscle		
PM	psoas major muscle		
QL	quadratus lumborum muscle		
RL	rotatores lumborum muscle		

*The iliocostalis, longissimus, and spinalis muscles are frequently referred to collectively as the erector spinae muscles.
**The semispinalis (capitis, cervicis, dorsi), multifidus, rotatores (cervicis, thoracis, lumborum), interspinales, and intertransversarii muscles may be referred to as the transversospinal muscles. These muscles function to extend and rotate the spine.

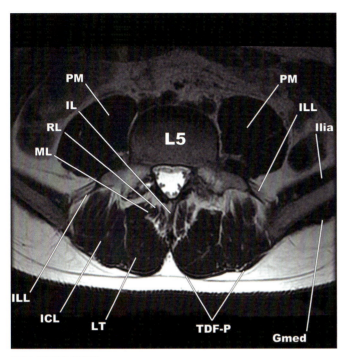

IMAGE 23 (MR)

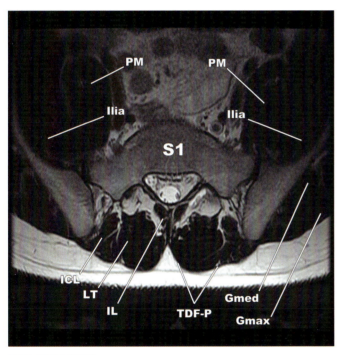

IMAGE 24 (MR)

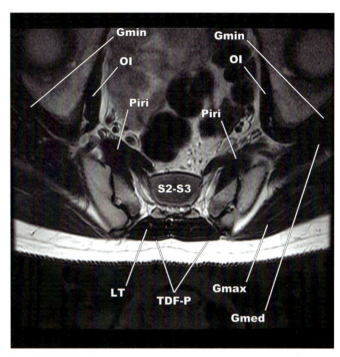

IMAGE 25 (MR)

KEY

Gmax	gluteus maximus muscle	**PM**	psoas major muscle
Gmed	gluteus medius muscle	**RL**	rotatores lumborum muscle
Gmin	gluteus minimus muscle	**TDF**	thoracodorsal fascia (M—middle layer, P—posterior layer)
ICL	iliocostalis lumborum muscle		
IL	interspinales lumborum muscle		
Ilia	iliacus muscle		
ILL	iliolumbar ligament		
LT	longissimus thoracis muscle		
ML	multifidus lumborum muscle		
OI	obturator internus muscle		
Piri	piriform muscle		

*The iliocostalis, longissimus, and spinalis muscles are frequently referred to collectively as the erector spinae muscles.

**The semispinalis (capitis, cervicis, dorsi), multifidus, rotatores (cervicis, thoracis, lumborum), interspinales, and intertransversarii muscles may be referred to as the transversospinal muscles. These muscles function to extend and rotate the spine.

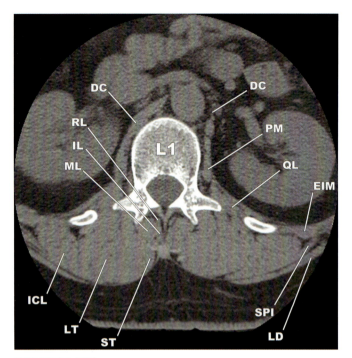

IMAGE 26 (CT)

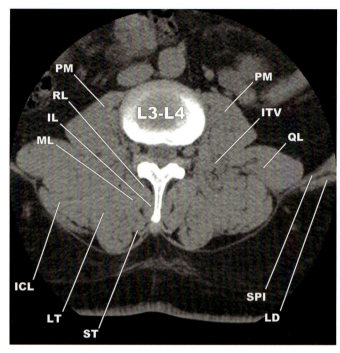

IMAGE 28 (CT)

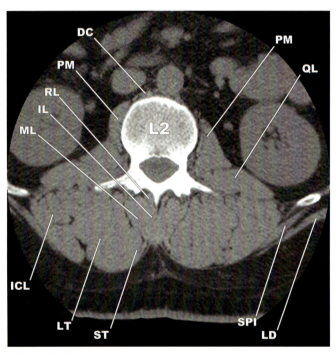

IMAGE 27 (CT)

KEY

DC	diaphragmatic crus	RL	rotatores lumborum muscle
EIM	external intercostal muscle	SPI	serratus posterior inferior muscle
ICL	iliocostalis lumborum muscle	ST	spinalis thoracis muscle
IL	interspinales lumborum muscle		
ITV	intertransversarii muscle		
LD	latissimus dorsi muscle		
LT	longissimus thoracis muscle		
ML	multifidus lumborum muscle		
PM	psoas major muscle		
QL	quadratus lumborum muscle		

*The iliocostalis, longissimus, and spinalis muscles are frequently referred to collectively as the erector spinae muscles.
**The semispinalis (capitis, cervicis, dorsi), multifidus, rotatores (cervicis, thoracis, lumborum), interspinales, and intertransversarii muscles may be referred to as the transversospinal muscles. These muscles function to extend and rotate the spine.

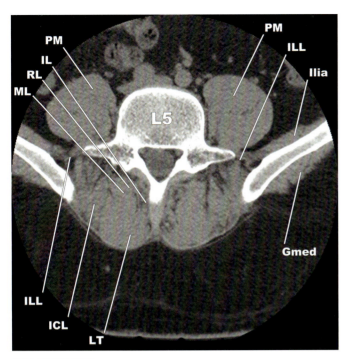

IMAGE 29 (CT)

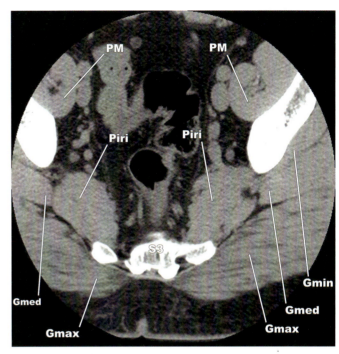

IMAGE 31 (CT)

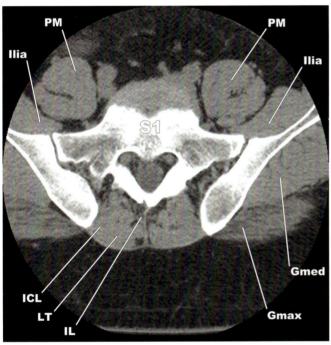

IMAGE 30 (CT)

KEY

Gmax	gluteus maximus muscle
Gmed	gluteus medius muscle
Gmin	gluteus minimus muscle
ICL	iliocostalis lumborum muscle
IL	interspinales lumborum muscle
Ilia	iliacus muscle
ILL	iliolumbar ligament
LT	longissimus thoracis muscle
ML	multifidus lumborum muscle
Piri	piriform muscle

PM	psoas major muscle
RL	rotatores lumborum muscle

*The iliocostalis, longissimus, and spinalis muscles are frequently referred to collectively as the erector spinae muscles.
**The semispinalis (capitis, cervicis, dorsi), multifidus, rotatores (cervicis, thoracis, lumborum), interspinales, and intertransversarii muscles may be referred to as the transversospinal muscles. These muscles function to extend and rotate the spine.

Master Legend Key

A

AA = anterior arch
AAA = anterior arch of atlas
AAOC = anterior arch ossification center
AB-CL = ascending band of cruciform ligament
AC = articular cartilage
ACA = anterior cerebral artery
ACC = anterior condylar confluence
ACS = acrocentral synchondrosis
ACST = anterior corticospinal tract
ACV = anterior condylar vein
ACV-HC = anterior condylar vein-hypoglossal canal
AD-IIA = anterior division internal iliac artery
ADS = apicodental synchondrosis
AEVP = anterior external vertebral venous plexus
AF = annulus fibrosis
AF = arcuate foramen
AF = articular facets
AFA = articular facet for the atlas
AICA = anterior inferior cerebellar artery
AIVP = anterior internal vertebral venous plexus
AL = alar ligament
ALA = alar ligament attachments
ala = sacral ala
ALAS = alar ligament attachment sites
ALL = anterior longitudinal ligament
ALV = ascending lumbar vein
AMAJ = anterior median atlantoaxial joint
AMSV = anterior median spinal vein
AMV = anterior medullary vein
AOAM = anterior occipitoatlantal membrane
AP = accessory process
AP = articular pillar
apex = (sacral) apex
AR = anterior rami
Arch = aortic arch
ARV = anterior radiculomedullary veins
AS = anterior scalene muscle
ASA = anterior spinal artery
AscCA = ascending cervical artery
ASCT = anterior spinocerebellar tract
ASTT = anterior spinothalamic tract
AT = anterior tubercle
AurS = auricular surface
AV = anastomosing vein
AV = azygous vein

B

B = basion
BA = basilar artery
Basi = basilar artery
b-FFE = balanced fast field echo
BP = basilar part of the occipital bone
bSP = bifid spinous process
BVV = basivertebral veins

C

C = centrum
C = clivus
C0–C1 = occipitoatlantal joints (C0–C1)
C1 = atlas
C1 = atlas vertebra
C1–C2 = atlantoaxial joint (C1–C2)
C2 = axis vertebra
CC = central canal
CCA = common carotid artery
CCAB = common carotid artery bifurcation
CCB = common carotid bifurcations
CCF = condylar canal/fossa
CCo = coccygeal cornua
CC-SC = central canal of the spinal cord
CE = cauda equine
CF = cuneate fasciculus
CIA = common iliac artery
CIV = common iliac vein
CL = cruciform ligament (transverse band or transverse ligament)
CM = conus medullaris
CMJ = cervicomedullary junction
Coc = coccygeal nerve
CP = costal process
CTA = computed tomography angiography
CTB = costotransverse bar
CTJ = costotransverse joint
CV = communicating veins
CVJ = costovertebral joint
CVP = coronal venous plexus

D

D = dens
DA-AL = dens attachment of the alar ligaments
DB-CL = descending band of cruciform ligament
DC = diaphragmatic crus
DF = dens facet
DF = dorsal funiculi

DH = dorsal horn
DLS = dorsolateral sulcus
DMS = dorsal median sulcus
DMS = dorsomedian septum
DOC = dens (basal) ossification centers
DR = dorsal root
DRG = dorsal root ganglion/ganglia
DS = dorsum sella
DS = dural sleeve
DSAS = dorsal subarachnoid space
DSF = dorsal sacral foramen/foramina
DSS = dorsal subarachnoid spaces

E
EC = echancrure
ECA = external carotid artery
EDS = extradural segment
EFP = epidural fat pads
EIA = external iliac artery
EIM = external intercostal muscle
EOC = external occipital crest
ETT = endotracheal tube

F
FEFP = foraminal epidural fat pad
FM = foramen magnum
FSE = fast spin echo
FT = filum terminale
FT = foramen transversarium
FT = foramina transversaria
FT = foramina transversarium
FV = foraminal vein

G
GC = gray commissure
GF = gracile fasciculus
Gmax = gluteus maximus muscle
Gmed = gluteus medius muscle
Gmin = gluteus minimus muscle
GRE = gradient-recalled echo
GSN = groove for spinal nerve
GTL = groove for the transverse ligament
GVA = groove for vertebral artery

H
HAV = hemiazygos vein
HC = hypoglossal canal
HP = hard palate
HPT = hairpin turn

I
I = ilium
IAF = inferior articular facet
IAP = inferior articular process
IC = iliac crest
ICA = internal carotid artery
ICL = iliocostalis lumborum muscle
ICT = iliocostalis thoracis muscle
IDF = inferior demifacet
IDS = intradural segment
IEA = inferior epigastric artery
IEP = inferior endplate
IIA = internal iliac artery
IJV = internal jugular vein

IL = interspinales lumborum muscle
ILA = inferolateral angle
ILEFP = interlaminar epidural fat pad
Ilia = iliacus muscle
IlioC = iliocostalis cervicis muscle
ILL = iliolumbar ligament
ILS = interlaminar space
IMA = inferior mesenteric artery
INL = inferior nuchal line
INMTA = innominate artery
INS = intraneural synchondrosis
IR = inferior recess
ISS = interspinous space
IT = interspinales thoracis muscle
ITV = intertransversarii muscle
IVC = inferior vena cava
IVD = intervertebral disc
IVDS = intervertebral disc space
IVF = intervertebral foramen
IVN = inferior vertebral notch
IVV = intervertebral vein

J
JB = jugular bulb
JF = jugular foramen
JP = jugular process

L
L = lamina
LA = levator ani
LA = lumbar artery
LC = longissimus capitis muscle
LC = lumbar cistern
LCV = lateral condylar vein
LCap = longus capitis muscle
LColi = longus coli muscle
LCST = lateral corticospinal tract
LD = latissimus dorsi muscle
LevS = levator scapulae muscle
LF = lateral funiculi
LF = ligamenta flava
LF = ligamentum flavum
LIV = left innominate vein
LM = lateral mass
LN = ligamentum nuchae
LongC = longissimus cervicis muscle
LSC = lateral sacral crest
LSTT = lateral spinothalamic tract
LSV = lateral sacral vein
LT = longissimus thoracis muscle
LV = limbus vertebra
LV = lumbar vein

M
MAL = mamillo-accessory ligament
MAN = mamillo-accessory notch
Mand = mandible
MB = muscular branch
MCA = middle cerebral artery
MDCT = multidetector computed
        tomography
MIP = maximum intensity projection
ML = multifidus lumborum muscle
MO = medulla oblongata
MP = mammillary processes
MPTB = mastoid portion temporal bone
MRA = magnetic resonance angiography

MReST = medial reticulospinal tract
MS = marginal sinus
MS = middle scalene muscle
MSA = median sacral artery
M-SSCM = multifidis-semispinalis cervicus
      muscle
MSC = median sacral crest
mSP = monofid spinous process
MSV = median sacral veins
MT = medial tubercles (transverse ligament
      attachments)
Multifid = multifidis muscle
MVL = meningovertebral ligament

N
N = nasion
NA = neural arch
NAOC = neural arch ossification center
NCS = neurocentral synchondrosis
NFNA = nonfused neural arch
NFTP = nonfused transverse process
NGT = nasogastric tube
NP = nucleus pulposis
NR = nerve root

O
O = opisthion
OA-AL = occipital attachments of the alar
      ligaments
O-ALL = ossification of the anterior longitudinal
      ligament
OB = occipital bone
OC = occipital condyle
OCCA = occipital artery
OCI = obliquus capitis inferior muscle
OCS = obliquus capitis superior muscle
OI = obturator internus muscle
OMS = occipitomastoid suture
O-PLL = ossification of the posterior longitudinal
      ligament
OST = olivospinal tract
OVB = omovertebral bones

P
P = pedicle
PBD = posterior belly of the digastric muscle
PCA = posterior cerebral artery
PCV = posterior condylar vein (in condylar canal)
PD-IIA = posterior division internal iliac artery
PEJV = posterior external jugular vein
PEVP = posterior external vertebral venous
      plexus
PI = pars interarticularis
PIA = posterior intercostal arteries
PIC = posterior iliac crest
PICA = posterior inferior cerebellar artery
Piri = piriform muscle
PIV = posterior intercostal vein
PIVP = posterior internal vertebral venous
      plexous
PLL = posterior longitudinal ligament
PM = psoas major muscle
PMSV = posterior median spinal vein
POAM = posterior occipitoatlantal membrane
PP = ponticulus posticus
PR = posterior rami

PRV = posterior radiculomedullary vein
PS = posterior scalene muscle
PSCT = posterior spinothalamic tract
PT = pharyngeal tubercle
PT = posterior tubercle

Q
QL = quadratus lumborum muscle

R
R = rib
RA = ring apophyses
RCA = rectus capitis anterior muscle
RCL = rectus capitis lateralis muscle
RCPm = rectus capitis posterior minor muscle
RCPM = rectus capitis posterior major muscle
RExZ = root exit zone
REZ = root entry zone
RH = rib head
RhMajor = rhomboid major muscle
RhMinor = rhomboid minor muscle
RL = rotatores lumborum muscle
RMA = radiculomedullary artery
RMV = radiculomedullary vein
RT = rib tubercle
RT = rotatores thoracis muscle
RuST/LReST = rubrospinal tract/lateral
      reticulospinal tract

S
S = sacrum
SA = segmental artery
SA/V = segmental arteries/veins
SacC = sacral canal
SAF = superior articular facet
SAP = superior articular process
SAS = subarachnoid space (V - ventral,
      D - dorsal)
SB = segmental branches
SB = spina bifida
SC = spinal cord
SCA = subcostal artery
SCA = superior cerebellar artery
SCan = spinal canal
Scap = scapula
SCM = sternocleidomastoid muscle
SCo = sacral cornua
SCS = suboccipital cavernous sinus
SDF = superior demifacet
SDS = subdental synchondrosis
SDSL = short dorsal sacroiliac ligament
SemiC = semispinalis capitis muscle
SemiCerv = semispinalis cervicis muscle
SEP = superior endplate
SF = sacral foramen/foramina
SH = sacral hiatus
SH = stylohyoid muscle
SIJ = sacroiliac joint
SLL = spinolaminar line
SMA = superior mesenteric artery
SN = spinal nerve
SOC = secondary ossification centers
SOVP = suboccipital venous plexus
SP = spinous process
SpCM = splenius capitis muscle
SPI = serratus posterior inferior muscle

SpinC = spinalis cervicis muscle
SpinT = spinalis thoracis muscle
SplenC = splenius cervicis muscle
SplenCap = splenius capitis muscle
SPM = superior pedicle margin
SPr = sacral promontory
SPS = serratus posterior superior muscle
SPSL = superficial posterior sacrococcygeal
      ligament
SR = superior recess
SS = sigmoid sinus
SSCpM = semispinalis capitis muscle
SSL = supraspinous ligament
ST = sacral tuberosity
ST = spinalis thoracis muscle
ST = spinous tubercle
STIR = short-TI inversion recovery
Subclav = subclavian artery
SV = segmental vein
SVC = superior vena cava
SVN = superior vertebral notch

T
T = trachea
TB-CL = transverse band of cruciform
      ligament
TCF = transverse costal facets
TCT = thyrocervical trunk
TDF = thoracodorsal fascia (M = middle layer,
      P = posterior layer)
TG = thyroid gland
TM = tectorial membrane
TM = trapezius muscle
TP = transverse process
TPC = transverse process of coccyx
TR = transverse ridges
Trap = trapezius
TS = thecal sac
TS = tuberculum sella
TSE = turbo spin echo

U
UP = uncinate process
UVJ = uncoverteberal joint

V
V1 = initial extraforaminal segment of vertebral
      artery
V2 = intraforaminal segment of the vertebral
      artery
V3/V4 = junction of V3 and V4 segments of
      vertebral artery
V3h = horizontal portion V3 segment of vertebral
      artery
V3v = vertical portion V3 segment of vertebral
      artery
V4 = intradural segment of the vertebral artery
VA = vertebral artery
VAVP = vertebral artery venous plexus
VB = vertebral body
VBJ = vertebrobasilar junction
VC = venous channels
VC = vertebral canal
VEFP = ventral epidural fat pad
VF = ventral funiculi
VFT = vein of the filum terminale
VG = vertebral gutter
VH = ventral horn
VLS = ventral lateral sulcus
VMF = ventral median fissure
VR = ventral ramus
VR = ventral root
VSAS = ventral subarachnoid space
VSF = ventral sacral foramen/foramina
VSS = ventral subarachnoid spaces
VST = vestibulospinal tract
VT = ventriculus terminalis

Z
ZJ = zygapophyseal joint

Index